Praise for Dianne Schwartz and *The Big Book of True Recovery from Food Addiction and Beyond*

The Big Book of True Recovery from Food Addiction and Beyond is a wonderful, well-written, easy-to-understand, comprehensive explanation of the relationship between food and addiction. It expands our understanding of addiction, laying bare the genesis of this disease. This book is bound to become a classic in addiction and recovery literature.

As the founder and CEO of Realization Center, I have witnessed the positive impact of Dianne's education series on our clients who come to treatment searching for an answer to their substance abuse dilemma. Her book is an in-depth, thorough presentation of the information she offers in her education series. The reader can't miss the message. This book makes it clear why and how the hijacking of the brain by eating issues leads to addiction. I believe this material should be taught in schools as a course in understanding the source of addiction.

The Big Book of True Recovery from Food Addiction and Beyond will help many people. The solution presented is a clear and simple guide for living in freedom from food addiction. It was Realization Center's pleasure to have the stage for the development of this understanding.

—Marilyn J. White, Founder and CEO of Realization Center

Dianne is widely known as one of the best in the clinical world for her expertise in food and substance addictions. *The Big Book of True Recovery from Food Addiction and Beyond: It's Not Broccoli* is a must-read and game-changer if you are truly tired of food robbing you of achieving your best life. Dianne's book lays out clear steps that you will want as your companion to accompany you as you cope with the ups and downs of your personal and work life journeys.

Food is socially sanctioned and supported until body size indicates the visible evidence of its overuse or underuse, which leads to shame and criticism about lack of willpower. We use food in building personal and work relationships, to cope with regrets, feed spirits, and to rejoice in triumphant celebrations. I believe that love and work are intimately tied and often managed by these relationships with food.

As a therapist and career/executive coach, my goal is to help clients to be their best personal and professional selves when it has been blocked by unhealthy relationships with food. This is why I look forward to sharing Dianne's secret of It's Not Broccoli with my clients!

—Mary Pender Greene, LCSW-R, CGP, Psychotherapist, Career/
Executive Coach, President & CEO of MPG Consulting

In her exciting new book, *The Big Book of True Recovery from Food Addiction and Beyond,* Dianne Schwartz describes her personal experience with multiple expressions of addiction and her blessed recovery which she shares as a recovering person and a professional in the field of addiction treatment. Her personal story describes the traps of addiction. By identifying for us the substances that kept her from achieving clean abstinence, she offers very valuable insights. I recommend this in-depth review of the facts of addictive disease and the processes of successful treatment and recovery. Thank you, Dianne for the many years you have been an effective front-line warrior against the disease of addiction.

—Kay Sheppard, MA, LMHC

I met Dianne Schwartz in 2013 as a principal at Realization Center, an outpatient substance use treatment clinic where I interviewed to be a moonlighting psychiatrist. The interview ended with Dianne extending a job offer followed by what I have come to refer to as "The Food Talk." Dianne took this opportunity to discuss addictive eating behavior and shared her belief that the fluctuating blood sugar levels resulting from consumption of refined carbohydrates were the culprit behind the recovering patients' challenges in staying sober, succumbing to the power of the cravings, and relapsing to alcohol/drug use.

Dianne went on to describe the use of food as a way to self-medicate and how addictive eating behavior activates the same dopamine mediated reward circuitry as all the other addictive substances. Through this same mechanism, the fluctuating blood sugar levels and resulting dopamine fluctuations lead to mood and energy problems characteristic of substance abuse and withdrawal syndromes. She highlighted her observation that when patients reported trouble with mood and energy, psychiatrists would frequently prescribe medications to treat a mood disorder not realizing these symptoms were the result of misusing food and not indicative of an underlying psychiatric illness. She ended her talk by relaying that these beliefs were embodied in an education series she developed and presented to most of the clients at the center.

Even though her ideas were derived from basic neurobiological concepts, it was new to relate poor eating behavior to maintenance of the brain circuitry behind cravings leading to relapse into substance use, and that mood and energy swings resulting from misusing food mimic brain chemistry imbalances that would normally require treatment with psychiatric medication. Needless to say, I was skeptical.

Over the years, I have had the opportunity to observe many patients at Realization Center who have changed their eating behavior after learning about the effects of their addictive eating practices through Dianne's education series; I have witnessed firsthand the dramatic improvement in their presenting problems of depression, anxiety, fatigue, brain fog, etc., with fewer relapses and more recovery. I have become a convert.

I've always been impressed with Dianne's passion about teaching and exposing the truth about the source issue underlying substance abuse, relapse, mood issues, energy issues, and life issues in general—the addictive eating of refined carbs. Her book, *The Big Book of True Recovery of Food Addiction and Beyond*, is highly readable, relatable, and remarkable in her development of the understanding of these ideas. She has succeeded in presenting a logical case for her beliefs and offers the solution to what has become a widespread struggle as logical, understandable, and doable.

—Dr. Maria Alikakos, DO, Board Certified in General Psychiatry, Child and Adolescent Psychiatry, and Addiction Medicine; Medical Director, Realization Center, NY

PERSONAL TESTIMONIALS

"With abstinence from binge foods and a program of sound nutrition, I discovered a freedom I never thought possible ...I am finally able to feel secure in my sobriety and my abstinence. Thank you, Dianne."

—Jim H.

"I feel so fortunate to be part of Realization Center...I am learning so much from you—about food, about being truly sober, [and] about how to polish some of my rougher edges."

—Kathy N.

"Drugs—Sugar—Caffeine. Today I don't have those issues. One day at a time. I love your class. You are an inspiration. Thanks."

—Jason K.

"I am so grateful to you and your Food Plan because it is the solution, and I am now...proof that True Recovery is attainable."

—Rachel P.

"My entire view of addiction and its relationship to food has been reworked. I truly believe that armed with [these] new facts, I will have a greater chance at maintaining sobriety."

—Dawn H.

"Realization Center...introduced me to the path to True Recovery [and] helped me to build a strong foundation through abstinence."

—Toni S.

"Realization Center has changed so many lives. I know it has changed mine!"

—Jaclyn E.

"Dianne, because of you, I am living my life again—happy, joyous, and free! I didn't think this would be possible without the Food Plan—which I pray I am on until the day I die."

—Chelsea R.

"I truly appreciate the invite to the food group presentation—it was an eye-opener. I hope to incorporate what I have learned into my daily life as well as in my counseling of others."

—Monty S.

"Dianne, you are one of my greatest teachers and guides. Thank you for all you have given me. You are so dear to me."

—Magdalaina C.

"I am so very grateful to you for all your wisdom and for your great kindness."

—Gloria P.

"Thank you for all your knowledge! You taught me a lot!"

—Yvette M.

"How can I ever thank you for your loving generosity and wisdom. The plan is working! You're an angel."

—Toni T.

"Thank you for giving me an understanding of my first true addiction, "food," but also helping me to realize the importance of a healthy diet."

—Joanne M.

"Thank you for teaching me life is not about food. Your love, commitment, and inspiration will always be a touchstone for me."

—Christine P.

"You are so precious to our group. Thank you for being such a great power of example."

—Jean N.

"You are such a gifted teacher and healer. Thank you for sharing your knowledge, working so hard, and giving so generously to us all. With gratitude, respect and affection."

—Jane S.

"Since I came to the U.S. ten years ago, I've been fighting and struggling with invisible days, also looking for the map that leads me [to] my real life. I was just sitting around waiting for my life to begin, while it was all just slipping away. I was tired of waiting for tomorrow to come, but this year was [an] extremely special year for me. So, I was able to find out firm hope of my future when I met you. You taught me we can make impossible possible. Also, you gave me braver[y], fortitude, to realize and to live. You are the person I admire. I really want to be like you. I really appreciate you, appreciate I was able to meet you in my life. I will make true recovery, then want to support with fighting people. Yes, I will do it!!"

—Michael N.

THE BIG BOOK OF TRUE RECOVERY FROM FOOD ADDICTION AND BEYOND

It's Not Broccoli

Dianne Schwartz, CASAC

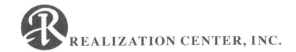

The publisher does not advocate the use of any particular healthcare protocol but believes the information in this book should be available to the public. The publisher and author are not responsible for any adverse effects or consequences resulting from the use of the suggestions, preparations, or procedures discussed in this book. Should the reader have any questions concerning the appropriateness of any procedures or preparation mentioned, the author and the publisher strongly suggest consulting a professional healthcare advisor.

Realization Center Inc.
19 Union Square West, 7th Floor
New York, NY 10003-3304
(212) 627-9600 • https://realizationcenternyc.com/

ISBN-13: 979-8-218-02354-6 (softcover)
    979-8-218-03484-9 (hardcover)

Copyright © 2022 by Dianne Schwartz

All rights reserved. No part of this publication may be reproduced, stored in a retrieval system, or transmitted, in any form or by any means, electronic, mechanical, photocopying, recording, or otherwise, without the prior written consent of the copyright owner.

Wherever necessary, permissions for copyrighted work have been graciously granted by the copyright holder(s). Appropriate notice appears with each work requiring permission for use.

Editor: Carol Killman Rosenberg • carolkillmanrosenberg.com
Cover & interior design: Gary A. Rosenberg • thebookcouple.com
Illustrations: Michael Allen • mikeallenart@gmail.com

Printed in the United States of America

Contents

Foreword: The Doctor's Opinion by Dr. Ronald Hoffman. xi

Introduction 1

Dianne's Story: My Addiction, My Recovery. 5

PART ONE: THE PROBLEM: FOOD ADDICTION 29

1. The Disease Concept of Addiction: The Biopsychosocial
Definition of Addiction 31

2. What Is Food Addiction?. 50

3. Little Food Addict in Training: An Illustration of How
Food Addiction Develops 91

4. Little Food Addict in the "War Zone":
Damaged Characteristics and Resulting Adaptation 118

5. Food Addiction: The Precursor/Gateway
to Chemical Dependency. 148

6. Understanding Metabolism and the Development
of the Disease of Food Addiction. 156

7. The Culprits and Triggers 175

8. Denial and Other Defense Mechanisms. 197

PART TWO: THE SOLUTION: ABSTINENCE. 217

9. What Is Abstinence? 219

10. The Basics of Nutrition 226

11. Realization Center Food Plan for True Recovery
from Food Addiction 237

PART THREE: DEALING WITH FOOD ADDICTION 257

12. Compliance versus Surrender 259

13. The Language of Feelings and Food Addiction 283

14. Self-Esteem and the Family System 309

15. Family and the Food Addict 357

PART FOUR: TREATMENT AND RECOVERY 383

16. 12 Step Food Recovery Fellowships and Relapse
    Prevention—Tools of Recovery 385

17. Sabotage and Relapse 412

18. Therapy and Treatment for Food Addiction 433

19. Recovery . . . Discovery 449

Conclusion: Last Words 463

Appendix: "Am I Addicted to Food?" Questionnaire 465

Acknowledgments 468

Resources 471

Endnotes 473

Index 483

About Realization Center 499

About the Author 501

*To all who knowingly or unknowingly suffer
from this life-draining disease . . .
and those who try to help.*

FOREWORD
The Doctor's Opinion

The sobering truth (forgive the pun!) is that recovery often fails or is incomplete. Alcohol relapse occurs in almost one-third of recovering alcoholics during their first year of sobriety. For drugs, the relapse rate may be even higher. For cigarettes, as any former smoker will attest, it takes many failed attempts, sometimes over years, to definitively quit.

That message was brought home to me when, as a medical student in the 1970s, I went on a "field trip" to observe an Alcoholics Anonymous meeting. Attendee after attendee stood to describe their tribulations in taking it "one day at a time." But what left a lasting impression on me was the pall of cigarette smoke that hung over the room, the ubiquitous overflowing ashtrays, the giant urns of coffee arrayed on a table next to sugar shakers at the back of the room, and the pyramids of doughnuts piled on big platters.

It was explained to me then that these addictive substances—nicotine, caffeine, and sugar—were part of the prevailing "risk mitigation" or "harm reduction" strategy. Surely, they weren't good for you, but asking alcoholics to go "cold turkey" on all forms of gratification at once was a gambit sure to fail.

It occurred to me then that, if these props remained in place, in addition to undermining the future health of the recovered alcoholics, they were an indication of an incomplete resolution of the root causes of addiction. To borrow the parlance of the 12 Steps, these individuals exemplified "dry drunk syndrome," which among other things has been defined as "replacing the addiction with a new vice (e.g., sex, food, and internet use)."

I've learned from my practice that there's a strong genetic basis for this. Many of my patients, like the author of this book, are children of alcoholic or drug-addicted parents. Some of their family members may have succumbed to suicide, indicating an inherited predisposition to depression. Others' forebears may have developed lung cancer or emphysema after a lifetime of smoking. Wary of their relatives' self-destructive habits, my patients studiously steered clear of classic addictive habits. They've applied a constructive correction. But, invariably, they retain one almost universal dependency: sugar. It continues to rule their lives.

The relationship of simple carbohydrates to mood problems and addiction has been recognized since the mid-twentieth century with the work of E. M. Abrahamson, who wrote the pioneering book *Body, Mind, and Sugar* (1951). He introduced the notion that carbohydrate dependency and dysregulated glucose metabolism are the keystones of many psychiatric disorders that ultimately lead to addictions.

In 1975, as a premed student, I came across William Dufty's *Sugar Blues* (1975), which amplified Abrahamson's work. It motivated my subsequent study of therapeutic nutrition as a way of alleviating psychiatric disorders.

Unfortunately, Americans' consumption of refined carbohydrates has only soared since then with the introduction of cheap high-fructose corn syrup and its infiltration into a myriad of processed foods and beverages. Our dependency on carbohydrates was further accelerated by misguided official recommendations to eschew saturated fat and cholesterol, to reduce consumption of animal protein, and to substitute low-fat alternatives—which invariably are laden with starch and sugar. On top of that, we've supersized our portions.

The result is a continuous stream of patients whose health is undermined by poor diet. Unfortunately, it's not merely a knowledge deficit that keeps them metabolically unfit and perpetuates the wrong food choices. If only it were so simple as to hand them a diet plan and urge them to summon self-discipline and adhere to it!

Unfortunately, their cravings are physiologically hardwired, not to mention psychologically reinforced. They are slaves to impulses that are near to impossible to control.

When it comes to reversing classic eating disorders, the statistics are dismal. For sufferers of anorexia nervosa, just 21 percent make a full recovery. Relapse rates for clients successfully treated for bulimia nervosa range from 31 to 44 percent during the first two years of recovery.

Nor do ordinary weight-loss subjects fare much better. *Scientific American* reports, "Research suggests that roughly 80% of people who shed a significant portion of their body fat will not maintain that degree of weight loss for 12 months; and, according to one meta-analysis of

The Doctor's Opinion

intervention studies, dieters regain, on average, more than half of what they lose within two years."[1]

Hence the urgent need for this book.

Having known Dianne Schwartz for twenty years, we've had many enjoyable conversations. I get her, and she gets me. I've been impressed with her passionate conviction, borne out of personal experience and long hours in the clinic, that our current models of addiction treatment are obsolete and need to be informed by understanding the key role that diet plays—a belief I share.

I've been an unflagging supporter of her book project, encouraging her to push past obstacles to complete it and get it published. It's remarkable to me that she had the tenacity to see it through, given her time-consuming professional commitments and the institutional barriers to publication of information that challenges the prevailing paradigm. The resulting work truly encapsulates her life's work, lent a particular immediacy by her personal experience transcending addiction. I'm so glad her labor of love has finally gained fruition after so much careful research and effort.

In this book, Dianne Schwartz updates the concepts of early nutrition pioneers with a thorough review of the latest scientific literature that now clearly delineates that poor eating habits change the brain and render people more susceptible to a vicious cycle of dependency.

Her central thesis can be found in the book: *"I believe that the high incidence of relapse with alcoholics and drug addicts is due to the fact that they never fully get clean. They continue to use by substituting any of the major triggering substances . . . for alcohol and/or drugs and therefore remain in craving."*

High on the aforementioned list: sugar, artificial sweeteners, flour products, refined carbohydrates like breakfast cereals, high-fat crunchy and/or salty snacks, caffeinated drinks, gums, mints, candies, energy bars—in short, foods or beverages that perpetuate a dopamine reward-craving cycle.

What's left? Wholesome, natural foods that are unadulterated and unrefined, delivering optimal satiety.

There's much more to it than that. Dianne Schwartz offers a nuanced discussion of the hallmarks of food dependency, including withdrawal symptoms that impede recovery. She tackles the issue of denial, which from a food standpoint is easily America's most ubiquitous evasion.

She broadens the scope of classic eating disorders to comprise ordinary societally condoned habits—we are, each and every one of us, situated somewhere on the spectrum of maladaptive food consumption patterns!

She also applies insights from developmental psychology on the origins of food dependency. This proceeds through stages until adulthood: *"By this stage, the disease is cemented; those with food addiction are well established in using food to cope with the challenges and conflicts present in developing committed relationships, discovering meaningful work, balancing play, negotiating differences, losses, and disappointments, and being comfortable with success and achievement."*

I wish I could make this book mandatory reading for the fleet of professionals who engage in the "diet industry," an enterprise that garnered 79 billion dollars in 2019. I'd also recommend it to not just addiction specialists but to *all* psychologists and counselors, because no matter what psychopathology they're tackling, diet is invariably a lynchpin, and unresolved dietary issues are an impediment to the resolution of long-standing conflicts. Finally, I'd make it required reading for doctors-in-training and my medical colleagues, who all too frequently are dismissive of patients' "lack of willpower" in implementing constructive lifestyle changes.

I've often thought to myself that we need to apply an addiction model if we're going to lick America's pandemic of avoidable degenerative diseases, three-quarters of which are driven by modifiable lifestyle choices: alcohol, tobacco, and drug use; sedentary habits; and dietary excess. Heart disease, stroke, diabetes, and hypertension; lung, kidney, and liver disease; certain cancers; and even Alzheimer's disease are largely preventable, and they saddle us with an enormous burden in medical costs and lost productivity. The Centers for Disease Control report that, as of 2020, 90 percent of the nation's 3.8 trillion dollars in annual healthcare expenditures are for people with chronic and mental health conditions—the majority of which are preventable.

Instead, we're saddled with bland exhortations to "kick the habit" without remotely addressing the true underpinnings of addiction—all the worse for our nation's health. *The Big Book of True Recovery* should spearhead a revolution in our thinking about how to tackle these enormous challenges. Our very survival is at stake.

—Dr. Ronald Hoffman

Introduction

For food addicts and non-addicts alike, food serves many purposes—as a distraction, to provide comfort, for social connections, as a quick way to self-medicate, and as a way to numb or even sedate ourselves. We turn to food for nurturing, to fill up our emptiness. Food also often serves as a substitute when someone is trying to stop an addiction such as smoking, drinking, or drugging. The real purpose of food, of course, is to fuel the body and keep it functioning. However, everyone, at one time or another, "uses" food. We're chewing or sucking or drinking or scarfing down something virtually all the time. If we're not doing any of that, we're thinking about chewing, sucking, drinking, or eating. Or we're thinking about what we will eat next or that we ate too much or too little at our last meal. We are generally obsessed with putting something in our mouths.

Whenever we use a substance to cope, be it alcohol, drugs, or food, we abandon ourselves; food is so easy to use to tamp down whatever it is we don't want to feel. No wonder we have abandonment issues and that we are so sensitive to rejection. When we grab something to deal with any difficulty, even gum, we are abandoning ourselves.

Many don't experience this "using" of food as a problem. Most of us don't stand back and look at how we are surrounded with things to chew, drink, or eat and see it as a problem. You can't buy a newspaper or magazine or even a bottle of water without being assaulted by a strategically placed array of gum, mints, cookies, cakes, muffins, ice cream cones, or pops. Not too long ago, we weren't presented with these little, "bite-sized" temptations of confections and sweets. Most of us might never think of buying an entire box of cookies or doughnuts, but we are lured in by those clever marketing ploys of "single-serving," snack sizes, handy packages, "mini" cookies, or "tiny" doughnuts. We don't buy these items and down them because we're hungry. It's all impulse eating; it feeds our food addiction. To make matters worse, manufacturers invest in producing foods that feed our society-wide food addiction. More and more processed foods, made with more and more sugar and flour, prompt us to crave, buy, and eat evermore. We give up good health for good taste. This results in dire health consequences that overburden our healthcare system at very high economical costs.

Sure, we all know that the purpose of eating is to sustain our wonderful machine, the body. However, eating represents so much more than just that. Many of us view eating as a time when we come together to be with one another. Sharing a meal with others can demonstrate our love. Food connects us to memories, tradition, emotions, togetherness, and belonging—being "a part of" rather than "a part from." In the preparation of food and cooking family recipes, the kitchen represents life. In *Food and Eating: An Anthropological Perspective*, Robin Fox expresses it this way:

> We have to eat; we like to eat; eating makes us feel good; it is more important than sex. To ensure genetic survival the sex urge need only be satisfied a few times in a lifetime; the hunger urge must be satisfied every day. It is also a profoundly social urge. Food is almost always shared; people eat together; mealtimes are events when the whole family or settlement or village comes together. Food is also an occasion for sharing, for distributing and giving, for the expression of altruism, whether from parents to children, children to in-laws, or anyone to visitors and strangers. Food is the most important thing a mother gives a child; it is the substance of her own body, and in most parts of the world mother's milk is still the only safe food for infants. Thus food becomes not just symbol of, but the reality of love and security.[2]

It is not uncommon for a food addict to admit that their "food problem" first presented itself at the family table and/or eating out of view of others. Eventually, eating food and/or not eating food became a painful and violent act instead of a loving and nurturing one. It was no longer a matter of togetherness, but of separateness and being alone, helpless and hopeless, with no solution in sight.

With all the literature that exists about eating disorders, no one has fully addressed or examined the issue that, at some point, almost everyone turns to food to do something that has nothing to do with nutrition. They use food for an unintended purpose, which sets us up for problem

Introduction

eating at an early age. Examining this, as we do throughout this book, is the first step toward true recovery for the food addict.

The Big Book of True Recovery from Food Addiction addresses all aspects of food addiction, which includes overeating, eating and purging, and undereating (that is, restricting food and/or starving). Keep in mind that not everyone fits the established criteria for having an eating disorder; however, many still experience daily life centered on food, eating, weight, and body image; they don't accept their bodies. Such people are not at peace and are uncomfortable with their eating behavior or weight. Maybe they were okay in these areas when they were younger, but now, as they've gotten older, they turn to more weight- and shape-control behaviors because they're not happy with the way they relate to food and it's showing on their bodies.

Be aware, too, that in our society, some women fly just under the radar because they don't meet the clinical definition of having an eating disorder. Society doesn't question them because they look functional and present well in so many other areas of life. But they are suffering nonetheless—with denial perpetuating the pattern. If we don't recognize that a problem exists, does that mean there's no problem? For example, one unaddressed concern is that, as women get older, they become more adept at concealing their eating problem, from both themselves and others. Their symptoms may be attributed to aging or mood or other causes. For some, dieting and the gym take over their lives. Age becomes an acceptable—if tacit—excuse for gaining weight, as well as for the "diseases of aging,"—e.g., diabetes, cardiovascular disease, joint pain, and memory problems. In truth, these are all diseases of poor lifestyle—food addiction and physical inactivity. Our bodies are made to move until the day we die, hopefully in the act of moving. Even if the eating doesn't increase, as a consequence of long-term food addiction, physical activity often decreases and food addiction creates a weight problem. Since we treat symptoms rather than causes, rounds of dieting continue.

This book addresses the problem of our seemingly unsolvable, challenging eating issues and, most important, *the* solution. It offers a perspective and understanding through the lens of addiction, then gives the sufferer hope that there *is* an answer, albeit one that takes work. The answer is **RECOVERY**, which offers so much more than being at peace with one's eating behaviors and one's body. This book provides information, education, support, and direction to find and live in the solution. It is an invaluable resource for the addict and those around them who are crucial to their recovery—family and loved ones, clinicians/therapists, and medical professionals who serve as a team to help the addict recover and live in their potential.

The basis of my personal recovery from food addiction, professional experience, and treatment philosophy is the understanding that biology plays a major role in the problem of and the solution to problematic eating. Today, there is science to explain how brain chemistry (in particular, our reward circuitry) is involved in what we regard as problematic eating behaviors. Looking at obsessive patterns as addiction allows us to understand how some have the problem because of genetic predisposition, a family "inheritance," along with an important component of how living in and surviving a dysfunctional family system affects us. This and so much is discussed throughout these pages. Let me begin by sharing my personal story of addiction and recovery, so that you can understand, beyond a shadow of a doubt, that true recovery from food addiction is possible.

A NOTE ABOUT GENDER

Numerous studies support the data that food addiction affects more women than men (even though more males are now being identified as co-sufferers); therefore, I use mostly feminine pronouns in this book.

Dianne's Story:
My Addiction, My Recovery

I came into the world in a palace.

My mother's alcoholism was a thief and robber—committing an act of more than grand larceny. Her disease robbed my "palace" of all its decorations. And I could not stop it. I was powerless—and frightened and angry that her disease could do that.

Her disease took my innocence, my spirit, my freedom, my trust, my voice. Her disease let me know that I didn't matter—that what I needed and wanted were unimportant—only <u>her</u> needs and wants mattered.

The Stage Is Set . . .

When I was just a toddler, I was sitting at the kitchen table in our house early in the day, probably waiting for breakfast, and I was sobbing. My mother asked why I was crying, and I told her, through my tears, that I had heard her and Daddy arguing the night before. "We were not arguing!" she yelled. "We were having a discussion. That's what married people do—have discussions." I got the message loud and clear at that early age: *Keep my mouth shut! Don't show my feelings! My reality is NOT my reality.*

My mother resembled a cross between Lucille Ball and Susan Hayward (the beautiful redhead in the forties with a turbulent Hollywood life and alcohol in the mix). My father, sixteen years my mother's senior, was a simple, kind man—successful in his trucking and warehousing businesses but clueless when it came to the complexities of his "Kewpie doll," emasculating wife. She was the alcoholic; he was the classic codependent enabler. My older brother, Peter, and I were always in competition with each other for our parents' attention and praise. We were a "looking good" family—our outsides appeared mainstream for a suburban, upper middle-class Jewish family. As such, my physical, financial, and educational needs were taken care of, but I learned from early on that it was safer to keep quiet, "defer" to everyone else's opinions or thoughts, and basically be on my own. I learned not to trust. Although I was very loved by my mother and father, it became clear that I was not understood and that my emotional needs were better ignored since it was evident they were not going to be met by people not equipped to handle them. I understand now that was about their limitations, their history.

Another memory that stands out took place a year or so later. I was with my mother in the Catskills at a bungalow colony. We were outside, and as some people approached us, I became frightened—they were strangers, and I hid behind my mother. As they came close to greet her, I heard her say in a sarcastic tone, "I don't know why she's like that." How painful those words were; they hurt me to my core. I felt alone, unprotected, uncared for, separate, and unattached to her, and criticized, belittled, shamed, and rejected by her. All I had at the time were the emotions; I did not have the words to describe those painful feelings. All my mother needed to do was pick me up and reassure me that these people were friends, not to be feared, and introduce me in a gentle and loving way. The stage—that is, my beliefs about myself—was being set.

My third significant memory—one that is still very fresh for me—was when I was about seven years old. My mother attempted suicide by taking pills, probably sleeping pills or tranquilizers. It was the middle of the night, and I was woken by a lot of commotion, noise, and lights from fire engines and police cars. I opened my bedroom door a crack and peered out (I had a direct view to the master bathroom), and I saw my mother's naked, limp body being propped up on a stool by my father and my father instructing my eleven-year-old brother to put his finger down Mother's throat, being careful not to scratch it.

I guess my father knew that my mother had taken a lot of pills. And I would guess that she had also been drinking. I saw huge firemen and policemen coming up the stairs, and then bringing my mother down the stairs on a stretcher. When they all left with my father, there was a welcome silence, and I was able to unfreeze, leave my bedroom, and go into my brother's room. He was trying to make a phone call, maybe to the hospital. I wasn't sure if my mother was dead or alive, so I asked Peter if Mother was all right, and he just told me to go back to bed.

Dianne's Story: My Addiction, My Recovery

The emotional messages that night and for the rest of my childhood were: *There's no one here for you, no one to protect you. No one cares. Your needs don't matter. You don't matter. Don't ask questions. Don't talk. Do what you're told. Don't bother anyone.* I was an afterthought.

My mother was gone for what seemed like a month. My father never spoke about what had happened—except to tell me that my mother would be back about a week before she actually returned. I remember worrying about her coming home. I don't think I wanted her to come back; her leaving had been so painful and traumatic that I didn't want to go through anything like that again. I had adjusted to her not being there, and I didn't want to readjust. Becoming "needless" was a position I took early in life. I was scared to see her again and didn't know what to say or do—afraid of how she might be. I had a jumble of feelings, and I was only seven years old!

As I write this, I'm seeing my reactions differently than I had before—I must have been very wary of my mother and her moods. It seems sad that, as a seven-year-old, I was already worried and treading carefully around her, fearful of being wrong or saying or doing something displeasing to her. I believe I knew from an even earlier age that something was wrong, and her alcoholism wasn't even in full force yet. The minefield I had to negotiate had already been well established.

There were more suicide attempts. During my childhood, my parents had horrendous arguments almost every night. My mother was always accusing my father of having a girlfriend and "getting laid." He would always deny the accusations. The arguments went on for hours and were both disgusting and terrifying to me. To get to sleep, I would eventually pound my pillow and scream into it, saying "die" over and over again. I wanted my mother to die to put me out of my shame and agony—and there was no one I could tell.

Around that time or perhaps a year later, another memorable exchange between my mother and me took place. She was picking out my clothes to pack for an annual weekend outing arranged by my father's lodge at a hotel in the Catskills. She pulled out a seersucker dress with a little white Eisenhower-type jacket that went with it. I said excitedly, "Oh, it's like a dinner jacket." She fired back, nasty and derisive, "Girls don't wear dinner jackets; only men do!" I instantly shriveled up. I tried to save some dignity by saying meekly, "I know."

That was a painful experience because it demonstrated that my mother didn't know me, didn't "get" me. I thought that men's jackets were so cool because they had pockets inside for stuff and didn't have to carry purses. I envied that. Of course I knew the difference between men's and women's clothing. She could have asked me *why* I thought the jacket was like a dinner jacket to show interest in my thinking and in me. But that's not how communication worked in my family. This was another nail in the coffin of my needing to reveal myself and be known by others.

An Unnecessary Childhood Prison Sentence

Two months before my ninth birthday, I was mistakenly diagnosed with rheumatic fever and "sentenced" to complete bed rest by Dr. Eugene Calvelli, the head of the St. Francis Home for Cardiac Children, in Port Washington, New York. I don't believe "second opinions" were even considered in those years, and besides, my parents had the authority of a "top doc" whom they didn't think to question. So, one moment, I was a tomboy out in the backyard helping one of my father's workers, Alley, build a brick barbeque, and the next moment, I was waving to Alley from my bedroom window. It felt unreal—like a bad dream. I was confused, and I didn't understand why I had been told to stay in bed. I felt fine. And no one could tell me how long I had to stay there. I think I was in shock.

I remained in my bed for the next three years. It was torture. I knew there was nothing wrong with me, but I also knew no one wanted my opinion—and I was made to doubt my sense of myself. Early on in my confinement, a playmate came to visit, but that soon stopped, probably because her parents thought I was contagious. Anyway, it was no fun to visit me. We couldn't do anything interesting—just talk. During that time, I gained a substantial amount of weight and was put on my first diet by my mother. I felt very deprived because my meals were all I had to look forward to. A teacher from the school system came to give me my lessons, but food remained the highlight of my day.

One morning my mother came into my bedroom to make my bed and get me organized for the day, the usual morning routine. This particular morning, she didn't talk to me. I felt her anger and was frightened, so I kept quiet (something I became very good at). This silent treatment went on for days. It was gut-wrenching. I didn't know what it was about, and I felt isolated and abandoned. Finally, one morning when I couldn't

Dianne's Story: My Addiction, My Recovery

stand to keep my pain inside anymore, I started to cry when she came in, and she angrily asked me why I was crying. I was terrified to talk, but I couldn't keep the words in. I sobbed, "You're mad at me, but what did I do?" She walked out without saying anything. The next morning, she left a stuffed monkey (I never liked dolls) on the hospital-like countertop table that went across my bed. I knew it was her way of telling me it was okay, that she was no longer angry, and that she cared about me.

I know now that the silent treatment wasn't about me. She must have been overwhelmed by the situation of my "illness" as well as issues with my brother, the responsibility of running a big home, grieving the recent loss of her mother, and not having the kind of emotional support from my father that she needed. During the time of my "illness," she started to see a psychoanalyst, Cornelia Wilbur, M.D., for help. Dr. Wilbur was the psychiatrist who treated Sybil, known for her multiple-personalities disorder, and whose story was later made into a film.

Real communication in my immediate family was still nonexistent. It would have meant so much to me to have a discussion about this awful circumstance, my "illness." I believe my mother at that time had been talking with my uncle, her brother-in-law, a psychiatrist. They must have been concerned about the psychological effects of my confinement. One day, when I was about ten years old, my mother asked if I would like see a doctor. When I asked what kind of doctor, she said, "A talking doctor." It sounded scary, but I said yes—anything to get out of the house. She brought me to see Dr. Podolnick, the psychologist for the Great Neck school system. What a dear man he was—he saved my sanity. The first time I met him, he asked me a lot of questions in a kind and caring way. It felt like he really understood what I was feeling—feelings I was not even aware of. He touched my pain, and I cried a lot during that first visit. When it was over and I went out to get into my mother's car, I was still crying. She asked if I wanted to go back to see him and, through tears, I said, "Yes!"

I don't remember how long I continued to see Dr. Podolnick, but he was my guardian angel. He got me to talk—no small feat—which, in retrospect, was very healing. In the beginning, he held my sessions in a small kitchen in the garden apartment that was his office, and it had a child-size table. As we talked, I worked on building a model airplane. After a number of sessions, he asked me if I would like to come into his office instead of the kitchen. I knew that he thought I was comfortable or mature enough to talk to him without the distraction (or security) of the airplane. I was always insightful and could often figure out people's motives—but rarely spoke about what I saw (my survival rule of "don't talk" was well entrenched by then).

During one of our sessions, Dr. Podolnick asked me to describe how the cardiologist examined me during my bimonthly visits. He informed me that the procedure used by the cardiologist was antiquated, and, I learned later, dangerous, because I was being exposed to significant amounts of radiation (the cardiologist used a fluoroscope, a form of X-ray, to see my heart while trying to sketch the outline of my heart and compare the new sketch to his sketch of my previous exam to see if my heart had gotten larger or smaller). Dr. Podolnick explained that the current techniques for heart exams were very different from what the cardiologist had been doing. I'm sure he discussed that with my parents, which prompted a visit to a prominent cardiologist in New York City. I still have the 1954 letter from the New York cardiologist to Dr. Podolnick, which he gave to me, with his conclusions about his more contemporary exam: "She is a well developed young girl . . . I find no present evidence of organic heart disease in Dianne. I believe that she may lead an unrestricted life." So, after three years of fruitless isolation, my imprisonment was over. But I was left with a sense of being overweight—feeling fat, ugly, and awkward with poor social skills and really low self-esteem. I felt very ashamed of myself. My yardstick was my attractive, personable mother, and I just did not measure up.

Adolescence and the Start of Addiction

A few months before my sixteenth birthday, I had a nose job, believing that if I fixed my outsides, I would feel more acceptable and normal. Earlier on, at age fifteen, I asked my mother to take me to a doctor to help me lose weight. She took me to Dr. Milton Kemp, who, without hesitation, wrote a prescription for Dexedrine, an amphetamine. Those pills more than did the job. They not only reduced my appetite—they launched me into a twenty-year addiction to amphetamines. I loved them! Not only did my appetite diminish and allow me to be in control of it, but I felt powerful. I could move furniture and, best of all, I didn't need anybody. The pills helped me concentrate and be focused and motivated me to do things and get things done—especially schoolwork—and *not feel anything.*

The pills also helped me numb feelings about my mother's active alcoholism, which had gotten worse during my teenage years. Being home with her was a horror, until she found AA and got sober for about a year. I attended an AA meeting with my father where my mother celebrated a year of sobriety and expressed her gratitude for being sober and gratitude for her family. She even referenced the hard time she had given us. What a revelation that was—that she had the awareness and was able to speak quite comfortably in front of an audience. Obviously, the members of my family knew little about each other's insides. Actually, there was one evening when my mother spoke with me about her drinking and that she was sorry she had hurt me. I know now that she was making amends to me, the AA "ninth step." I found that so uncomfortable and painful that I tried not to hear her and think I tried to stop her by saying, "I know, I know."

Sadly, her sobriety didn't last long. Looking back today, I know she would have greatly benefited from antidepressants, antianxiety medication, and solid treatment/therapy, but it wasn't meant to be.

One afternoon, I was walking home from high school, and I saw a local taxi pull up to our house. My thoughts started to race. What was a taxi doing at our house? Mother was supposed to be in Manhattan per her weekly routine—on Wednesdays, take the LIRR into the city, meet my father and go out for the evening, and then drive back to Great Neck. This time, however, she obviously did not make it past one of the bars near the Great Neck train station. The taxi driver got out and went around to open the rear passenger door, scooped up my mother in his arms, and was carrying her limp body toward the house.

I panicked, thinking, *"Oh my God, she's dead,"* then realizing if she were dead he wouldn't be bringing her to the house, then thinking she's drunk, maybe dying. I instinctively raced to the house, getting there as the driver was putting her on the bed in the master bedroom. The housekeeper had let them in and was standing over her, trying to figure out what to do. I went into action, taking off her shoes, and, as she started to revive and began to be sick, I got pots for her to throw up in.

That went on for a while, and then she wanted to hold me—so I got onto the bed with her so she could hug me, cry, scream, and carry on about how awful life was and yelling that she didn't want to live. This went on for hours. I was repulsed and terrified; I felt trapped, powerless, and helpless, afraid to pull away, afraid she would do something crazy or dangerous. I don't remember if I became hysterical or was so shut down that I stayed cool. She finally passed out, and I was able to get up and leave. I didn't know she was experiencing a blackout and that she would not remember the next day that I didn't stay with her for the whole episode. I had been afraid that she would be angry with me, and that was intolerable.

There were many similar episodes. During her blackouts, she would writhe on her bed screaming, "All right!" over and over again for hours. I never knew what that was about for her, but now I think it had something to do with her being sexually molested by her father. All I wanted was for her to stop; it was so painful and crazy-making. Often, my father or brother would call our family doctor, Dr. Kemp, who would come over to the house and give my mother an injection of a sedative to, I used to think, put us out of our misery. Then, the following morning, she would get up around 8 am, smoke a cigarette, drink a cup of strong coffee, and start her day, which included preparing for dinner for that evening. She always managed to make sure there was dinner for the family—trying, I guess, to create some semblance of normalcy. She tried to not let her alcoholism interfere with her responsibilities, which she took very seriously. There would never be any word of what took place the night before. We lived with an elephant in our living room. Everyone knew and was affected by her drinking, but no one dared talk about it.

In some respects, the diet pills saved my sanity—at the very least, I was not eating my brains out in an effort to deal with the pain of living in my family. My father, however, clearly used food to cope with his feelings. He seemed to be always in the kitchen eating something. He didn't know what to do. None of us did.

Unfortunately, the pills deceived me into believing that I could not function without them. I believed I needed them to be successful in any effort to do anything. I believed they got me through high school, college, the CPA exam, the requirements of my jobs, and the requirements of living in general. I thought I was highly functional. In retrospect, my functioning was limited, although I couldn't acknowledge it at the time. The pills were my big secret. Because I attributed my functioning, including

Dianne's Story: My Addiction, My Recovery

any success I achieved, to the pills, I felt like a fraud—I believed that without the amphetamines, I'd be nothing. Actually, if I weren't taking the amphetamines, I knew I would have been eating out of control.

The amphetamines did, however, interfere with going to sleep, so I eventually added alcohol to help me "come down" in the evening. Although I swore I would never be like my mother—meaning, in part, that I would never drink—I started to drink, and I liked the way it made me feel . . . or not feel. I could go to sleep, but then I couldn't get up in the morning—without a pill, coffee, and a cigarette. I was fully caught in the cycle of addiction.

If only I had known that a simple food plan and a plan of recovery were the answer to my difficulty with functioning and controlling my appetite, that is, being thin. But it wasn't meant to be—not then.

College Years—The Addiction Continues

I spent my freshman year of college at the University of Miami. It was not really a match for me, but I was the first member of my family to attend college, and there was no one to give me direction. I wanted to go to college. It seemed to be my next step in life after high school, but the choice of school was more by default; a number of my peers from Great Neck were applying to the University of Miami, so I followed suit. I also did not have a wide choice, since my grades and SAT scores were average, and my extracurricular activities were nil; those three years in bed, my mother's active alcoholism, and our family dysfunction in general took its toll on my academic performance.

One of my general goals was just to get out of my house. Years later, in a rare intimate conversation with my brother, Peter, I learned that his method of escape was marriage. My mother had wanted me to live at home and go to secretarial school, as she had done. I don't think my father cared what my decision was—he would have been supportive of anything that would make me happy. I also think he must have been proud that I was going to attend college. (He had immigrated to the United States from Russia when he was eleven years old and only had an eighth-grade education because he had to work instead of finishing his primary education.)

I initially enrolled in the School of Liberal Arts, which required that I take a foreign language. Although I had studied Spanish in high school,

I did so poorly on the entrance exam that they placed me in elementary Spanish. Because it was like a review course, I did well, but the second semester brought with it the next level of Spanish. This challenge scared me so much that I switched to the business school, which did not require a language. I was always scared of academic challenges and avoided them, believing I was not very smart. I missed so much because of my negative, erroneous beliefs about myself. The first time I set foot on Spanish soil in 1963, I fell in love with Spain—and I regretted my decision not to learn Spanish. Today, my Spanish proficiency is almost intermediate, and I would like to have the time to improve it. I love the language and enjoy speaking it. How ironic!

There was a benefit, however, to being in the School of Business: I took my first accounting course and loved it. It quenched my thirst for ideas and education. Growing up with my mother's alcoholism, and the unpredictability and inconsistencies that came with it, I longed for predictability and consistency. Accounting has that, along with enough complexity to be interesting, the kind of challenge I could deal with. I also started to envision myself going into my father's business—but since I couldn't major in trucking and warehousing, I knew I could not go wrong majoring in the language of business, that is, accounting. Over the years, one of the things I've learned about myself is that I'm pretty left-brained. I think logically and analytically, and I am very good at figuring out the details.

As time passed, I felt too geographically distant from my family while in Miami. The school really didn't work for me. I didn't make many friends and the opportunity to "play" didn't appeal to me. I became the serious one I my family—it was one of my survival mechanisms; someone had to be the serious one, and I've carried that throughout my life. The social scene at the university didn't suit my personality at the time. I felt too inadequate to venture out. I hung out mostly with my roommate and a few classmates. Truth be told, I'm not a very social person. One of my roles growing up in my alcoholic family is that of "Lost Child" (discussed in Chapter 15: Family and the Food Addict). I'm attached to things and pets, and I have become too comfortable being alone. Even so, I'm rarely lonely.

I wanted to transfer to a college closer to New York when the year ended. So I transferred to American University for my sophomore year. That first semester I did not take any diet pills (I had no dealer, aka doctor), and my focus, concentration, and motivation were poor. I know

Dianne's Story: My Addiction, My Recovery

my eating behavior was also poor, and, of course, I gained weight, which depressed me. My academic performance was correspondingly poor, and I was put on academic probation. I did, however, get my "A" in Accounting II. I received a letter from the college administration telling me that my grades had to improve. They recommended the school's tutoring program to get help. I was ashamed, embarrassed, and scared. I also reacted to their invitation in a very addict-like, ACOA (adult child of an alcoholic), defiant way—*Help? Me go for help? I'll show them!*

I went to a doctor in Washington, D.C., and I went back on the diet pills. That next semester I made the dean's list. And I lost the weight I had gained. I don't think anyone in the history of the university had ever gone from probation to dean's list. I can't image what they thought, but I had my secret. Through the grace of the amphetamines, I studied like a maniac, and with the help of my roommate, who clued me in to likely test questions on the philosophy final, I rose out of the ashes.

There Is No Escape

There was another major force working against me and my functioning at the time. During my time at American University, my mother was in the throes of her alcoholism. I would call her weekly on Saturdays to check in. She was usually drunk or on the way to getting drunk—and threatening to commit suicide. I would be on the phone with her for hours on end, trying to convince her not to kill herself, to keep living. It tore my insides out. I felt it was my responsibility to keep her alive. Yet it was such a trap. I felt obligated to call and stay on the phone to save her. I was so frightened she would kill herself. I was caught up in her depression and despair.

I realize now that I had allowed myself to be tormented. There was no one around to tell me I was talking to a bottle and to hang up—that I had no power or control to keep her from killing herself. My dear friend, my roommate, in a way tried to tell me, but I couldn't hear it. The irony is that my mother eventually stopped drinking and lived to three days short of her eighty-eighth birthday—and *I* had nothing to do with it. I should have been going to Al-Anon meetings, but who knew back then? I go now. Because all that codependency runs so deep, I need the support and guidance of a program of recovery from all the effects of growing up with a parent's alcoholism.

I made the calls to my mother with trepidation. I never knew if she would be drunk or not. If she wasn't drinking, the conversation would be very pleasant, a "normal" conversation between a mother and her daughter away at college, sharing details of their lives. But this unpredictability was very stressful. When Mother wasn't drinking, she was warm, caring, understanding, generous, really funny, and even somewhat supportive, and those times created a false idea for me in believing they would last.

In some respects, the trusty amphetamines again saved my sanity. They allowed me to put away my feelings of guilt and inadequacy, and some of my negative thoughts, and focus on studying. And once more, I wish I could have had a do-over—as a sober, abstinent young adult without the burden of my mother's depression and alcoholism.

When graduation approached, I worried about my mother's behavior at the ceremonies and festivities. That year, 1963, graduation was especially a big deal because the university had succeeded in getting President John F. Kennedy as the commencement speaker. I was overwhelmed with feelings of loss—I had successfully reached my goal of graduating from college, but I felt enormous fear of what was coming next in my life: the great, scary unknown. I had little confidence in myself. At the same time, I was beside myself worrying about my mother making a spectacle of herself (and me)!

I was able to screw up my courage and asked her not to drink while at the graduation ceremonies. She didn't drink, but she was moody, angry, and sullen. I'm assuming it had to do with her complying with my request, but maybe not. Maybe she'd had an argument with my father on the drive down to Washington, or maybe she was angry with my brother, who had made a condescending grand gesture of sacrifice to fly to Washington to celebrate my accomplishment. Peter was quite obnoxious at the event, jealous because he never attended college and I was getting so much attention and kudos from my parents, making critical remarks wherever he could. My mother and I suspected that my father or Peter locked the camera in the car trunk, so there are few pictures of the graduation. Mother tried to be pleasant but was stiff and cold.

During a Memorial Day weekend soon after, mother added too much Librium to whatever she was drinking (often vodka) and ended up in the emergency room at North Shore Hospital to have her stomach pumped. Because she refused to go to a private rehab program that we (mainly,

Dianne's Story: My Addiction, My Recovery

me) were trying to convince her to go to, that led to a six-week confinement in a state psychiatric facility. Just another terrifying episode with her that tore up my insides and made me want to withdraw from her, my feelings, and myself! Again, thank God for the amphetamines—to some degree they allowed me to numb out from these traumas.

Adulthood Begins

In 1963, I moved into Manhattan with my college roommate and two other friends. Working at a full-time job and studying for the CPA exam, I found a diet doctor, a "feel-good doctor" on Central Park South who had a "pill" practice. I could get the diet pills I wanted to keep me going. One day, I walked into his office for my monthly appointment and replenishment of my supply of amphetamines. He took one look at me and said, "I can't give you any medication." I was quite thin at the time, and he couldn't justify handing me his normal array of amphetamines for the morning, afternoon, and night—I didn't weigh enough. He was caught up in the congressional investigation of the rampant "feel-good doctors" of that time, and he had become cautious about whom he treated with his diet formulations.

So I was caught without a NY "dealer." At that time, however, I had been taking business trips to Spain and discovered that I could buy diet pills over the counter in their *farmacias*. After I lost Dr. Feel-good as my supplier, I would periodically go to Spain and stock up. I knew every drugstore in Madrid where I would make the rounds to get a six-month stash to last me until I returned. What an addict I had become.

I loved Spain and figured out how I could move there, partly because of my attachment to the country and partly because of my addiction and the ease of getting my amphetamines there. Just prior to moving to Spain, I called my mother to tell her my plans and to say goodbye. I believed I was not coming back except for visits. At this point, I actually hadn't been in contact with her for about five years. It had been too painful. She was now pretty stable, and it was the beginning of our reconnection—on a healthier level.

To Spain and Back

So I did it. I moved to Spain, believing I would be able to get all the diet pills I needed, stay thin, open a business, and have an interesting life. It lasted two years. The amphetamines stopped working as well as they had. I would get up in the night and compulsively eat various concoctions, trying to stay away from caloric foods, but my night eating always ended up in binge foods. Then, to avoid the consequences of my growing loss of control—weight gain—I started using laxatives. At the same time, I was drinking more coffee to boost the effect of the amphetamines, to no avail. I was in trouble. My ravenous appetite was overriding the amphetamines. I was gaining weight. I was really scared. And I was running out of money. I was a mess—emotionally, socially, and financially.

I did not understand it at the time, but I was morally and emotionally bankrupt, dreading the recognition that I had no control over my self-destructive eating no matter what I tried. I was powerless. It became clear that I couldn't stay in Spain. I made arrangements to move back to the United States. My father financed my return to New York and supported me for the next two years.

At the time, I was sharing my life with a significant other, so I didn't feel totally alone. I was also dependent on this person for support, companionship, and convenience. We moved back to New York City the week of the bicentennial—July 4, 1976. I had just turned thirty-five. I had enough amphetamines to last until the middle of August. We found an apartment on the East Side, moved in, and waited for the days to pass. When I took the last amphetamine, I knew my life would change, but I didn't know how. I was not thinking clearly. I think I was scared and even angry. For all the years I had used the drug, I believed I could not function without it. I thought my life was over. I slept for two weeks straight—but every time I woke up, I would go to the refrigerator and eat whatever was in there because I was starving. My body was reacting to twenty years of being starved and drugged sleep. I didn't know it, but I was in withdrawal.

Within what seemed like a flash, a few weeks, a month, I gained twenty pounds. I was miserable. I felt like a blob. My brain must have been mush. I would try not to eat during the day, but my appetite always took charge during the evening and night. This went on until December 1976.

Beginning Recovery

I was with my friend in a supermarket. I overheard a conversation between my friend and another shopper on the caloric value of yellow

Dianne's Story: My Addiction, My Recovery

onions versus white. My ears perked up as I heard this woman say that she had just lost twenty pounds. I watched her disappear in the aisles of the supermarket. Part of my head was yelling, "Go find her and ask her how she did it!" and the other—shy, ashamed, fearful—was holding back.

The voice inside finally won, and I took a deep breath and started to search the aisles for her. I found her and asked her how she had lost the weight. She was very nice and said (as she opened her coat and proudly flashed her slim body), "It was OA." I asked what OA was, and she said, "Overeaters Anonymous."

At that point, I lost the nerve to ask anything else. But when I got back to the apartment, I looked it up and called the number listed. There was a recording announcing the time and place of meetings. I went to my first meeting at the Lenox Hill Neighborhood Association on East 76th Street. That was the beginning of my new life. I had entered the world of recovery. Actually, I had only put one foot into the world of recovery. The beginner's kit had the basic literature, including a pamphlet describing four food plans. Of course I chose the most restrictive, believing it would give me the maximum weight loss. This meal plan eliminated starchy veggies and grains, and was printed on gray paper (which eventually became a separate fellowship "GreySheeters Anonymous"). I understood the "three meals a day with nothing in between" concept but focused on "EXCEPT non-sugar gum, diet soda, coffee and tea."

Because their plan allowed the use of addictive substances, i.e., sugar substitutes and caffeine, I never went through the detox process necessary to be free of cravings. I continuously used gum and diet soda to feed my cravings. I was chewing unbelievable amounts of Trident and drinking bottles and bottles of diet soda daily. My stomach was bloated, and of course, I had a lot of gas. I did lose those twenty pounds I had packed on.

I believed that OA was the answer to my eating issues. Right away I began to attend meetings religiously. But though I went to OA meetings, followed this plan of eating, and chewed sugar-free gum and mints and drank diet soda to keep my cravings under control, I remained isolated and fearful. I was too scared to speak at meetings or talk to the members. I knew, though, that was my great challenge—to become known and connected. I saw others sharing confidently and socializing with each other at the meetings, and I wanted to be able to do the same. I especially liked certain weekend meetings that were called the "Home Group." They were meetings held at the West Side apartment of an amazing, generous, kind, strong, warm, colorful Hungarian woman, Margit.

About a year after I started going to OA meetings and losing all the weight I wanted, it all started to unravel. I started, to my dismay, to eat again. I don't exactly remember the process, but I began to binge again—at night, as was always my pattern. I was beside myself. I was frightened and depressed. I knew what the missing piece was: putting both feet in the program, participating in the fellowship of OA—sharing freely, connecting with other program members at meetings and on the phone. But I was in a trap, knowing what I had to do but feeling too frightened to make myself do it.

I did see an answer, however. After one OA meeting at Margit's, I mustered up all my courage and went up to her and said words I had never said in my entire life: I tearfully said to her, "Please help me." Through tears, I told her I was eating again and couldn't stop. She put her arms around me and comforted me and invited me to join a small writing group of women that she had organized and ran. She told me to sit in her living room and disappeared into another part of her apartment. She came back with a young woman whom she introduced to me as my new food sponsor. Her name was Susan, and she was blind. We made arrangements to speak every morning about my food plan for the day, and I would read passages to her from the literature of various recovery organizations, including *Alcoholics Anonymous Big Book*, OA literature, and *Twelve Steps and Twelve Traditions*.

Going to Margit's OA writing group was invaluable and life-saving. It was the beginning of me becoming me, finding out who I am. I learned that I could write and, more important, that I could talk. At the start of each session, Margit would pose some questions relevant to compulsive eating and recovery. We would all write responses to her questions and then talk about what we had written. It was a small group, so I felt safe enough to open up and talk. Margit was so supportive and loving that she created just the right atmosphere for me to venture out and expose my thoughts and feelings. I'm sure others felt as I did. Because of her kindness and compassion, she was very beloved by many in those rooms.

In time I found more comfortable food plans and became "abstinent" from bingeing. I eventually let go of the gum. For a long time, I held on to Equal (aspartame), but I was developing a tolerance to it, so I was using more and more—even putting it into Diet Coke, because it didn't taste sweet enough without it. I became so addicted to it that I poured the packet into my palm and put it into my mouth with my hand. One day I could no longer stand my behavior with Equal. I knew I was totally out of control, and it couldn't go on. I called my program friend Liz and told her that I had to stop. She said, "OK, stop right now." I said I couldn't stop in the middle of the day, but starting tomorrow morning, it was over, which it was—thank God! And the diet soda went with it! Double thank God.

Slow Change

Attending OA meetings became part of my life. Over time, I was changing, albeit slowly, growing up and feeling, little by little, more self-confident. I was leading meetings from time to time. I had a year or two of abstinence from bingeing—but then I would relapse and go back to being lost in food, again.

As I mentioned earlier, I was an inveterate smoker—starting from the age of fifteen, I had become very addicted to nicotine; I loved to smoke. As with other addictive substances, I developed tolerance and had to have more. I was eventually smoking four packs a day. Clearly, I knew I was out of control with smoking and in trouble. I was even getting up in the middle of the night to take a few drags—because after a few hours of sleep, I went into withdrawal and had to get nicotine back into my system. One day in 1979, I woke up in the morning and found it hard to take a deep breath—I was actually gasping. I said to myself, "I have to stop smoking." At that point, I made a decision to stop and take my brother's suggestion to sign up for SMOKENDERS. So in June 1979, I committed myself to their program, and on June 9 I had my last cigarette—that was my "cutoff day." That was one of the hardest things I had ever had to do. The withdrawal process was torture, but I was determined to stop.

In retrospect, my life has been a process of letting go of those self-destructive addictive substances and behaviors that I grabbed onto to help me survive—emotionally.

During that summer, I met someone I was romantically interested in, and in August, I went to Oklahoma City to explore the potential of having a relationship. When I got there, I was totally rejected and was told there was no chance of a relationship. I was devastated—in shock. I called a friend in New York who told me to come back to where I was loved and cared about and not try to make something out of nothing.

In September 1979, my father died. He had split from my mother years before and was living with a woman who was taking good care of him in Florida. He had health issues. He was eighty-three years old. I was very sad. I'm so sorry he never got to see me as a success—becoming the real me—productive and functional. He would have been happy and very proud.

In December 1979, I started to eat non-stop. The combination of giving up cigarettes, losing my father, and being rejected was too much for me and any thought I might have had that I could handle these events on my own. I didn't use my support system, and I wasn't honest enough with myself about my feelings. Because I grew up with alcoholism, I developed an ability to override feelings and just move on to the next thing on my "to do" list. Beyond that, I think my food wasn't "clean enough" for me to hold on to my "abstinence."

I binged for four months up to a size 14 or 16. For reference, I have a small frame, and I am five-foot-one. I was never so heavy in my entire life. I didn't recognize myself. I continued to go to meetings, despite the disgust and despair I felt—I believed I had nowhere else to go.

I joined a few OA friends who were also having trouble with their abstinence and became part of a relapse group. We would meet weekly in each other's homes, using a relapse group format to structure our meeting and weekly assignments. It was very helpful. I felt a lot of support—I didn't feel so alone in my struggle.

Recovery Continues

In March 1980 I stopped bingeing. I don't remember the precise circumstances, but, with the groups, I became willing to stop. It has always been difficult for me to ask for and receive help, which I think was one of the obstacles that allowed my disease so much power and control over my

Dianne's Story: My Addiction, My Recovery

life. Over the ensuing years, I had periods of abstinence and long periods of relapse, but never so severe as when I binged for four months straight. I always knew, though, that each time I relapsed, I was holding on to some food substance that was always my undoing.

Although I didn't understand it at the time, the abstinence I thought I had was undone by one of the following substances, which kept me in trouble with cravings:

- Nicotine—four packs a day, as described earlier.

- Gum—addicted to having something in my mouth; I was basically holding on to the sweet flavor from the aspartame. It was too uncomfortable to just be with me without a "mouthy" distraction.

- Diet soda—I needed to feel full (addiction) and get that sweet taste.

- Caffeine—I eventually stopped drinking regular coffee and started on decaf.

- Decaf coffee—I finally became honest with myself and owned up to the fact that I was drinking so much decaf that I was still consuming a lot of caffeine. When I finally stopped the decaf, I experienced real caffeine withdrawal. A few days into the caffeine detox period, I joked about killing for a cup of decaf. I was finally being honest and upfront about my coffee dependency.

- Vegit and Butter Buds—I used these seasonings (which contained maltodextrin, a form of sugar) on everything. I was so addicted to them that I carried them with me. I was buying Butter Buds by the case.

- Equal (aspartame)—as described earlier.

- BranCrisp Bread—I carried these bran crackers to every meal.

- Rice cakes/puffed cereals—These are processed carbs. Once grains are "blown up," they are no longer complex. They become refined/processed carbs, which spike glucose levels and then trigger excessive insulin production, leading to a "crash," that creates, among other symptoms, cravings that no one (let alone food addicts) can manage successfully.

A WORD ABOUT SUGAR

I'd started listening to Carlton Fredericks, Ph.D. (1910–1987) on the radio station WOR in the late 1950s. He was a health educator and a pioneer in the health food nutrition field. He talked a lot about sugar and how harmful it was, and how it wreaked havoc with blood sugar levels. He wrote *Low Blood Sugar and You* in 1976, which I embraced, believing I suffered from episodes of low blood sugar. I think that's when I eliminated refined sugar from my life. But I still held on to wanting the taste of sweetness, so I used sugar substitutes (Saccharin, Sugar Twin, and eventually Equal), thinking that that was okay. (See the discussion about Equal on page 177.)

Realization . . .

My work life evolved to where I had my own accounting practice, and I eventually developed a specialization in litigation support services to lawyers in the area of valuations and financial investigations. I was growing professionally but always working on my recovery.

In 1988, I met Marilyn White, an amazing, energetic, and entrepreneurial addiction-counseling expert, passionate about addiction recovery, who was in the early stages of establishing an outpatient addictions treatment center, Realization Center. Because so much of my life dealt with recovery, I was attracted to the idea of a business devoted to helping alcoholics and drug addicts find recovery. I started giving her some professional business advice, and the next thing I knew, there was a fork in the road of my professional life—and I took it. I joined with her, took on her dream of creating a large recovery center, and we have more than accomplished our goal. She told me that my food issues were addiction—although I really didn't quite understand the implications of that at the time.

It became clear to me and others that I had the ability to engage clients and that I enjoyed being part of their treatment process. In the beginning, I acted as intake coordinator and explained aspects of treatment to clients, including their financial arrangements. My therapist at the time encouraged me to obtain my CASAC (Credentialed Alcoholism and Substance Abuse Counselor; CAC at that time—Credentialed Alcoholism Counselor). I attended the New School for alcoholism treatment courses

Dianne's Story: My Addiction, My Recovery

and attended courses at our Center: At that time, we had an education and training division. After I had completed the required courses, I took the long test and, lo and behold, I passed! It was the first time in my adult life that I had studied and prepared for an important test without the "help" of amphetamines. It was a very special experience that I was very mindful of. I learned that my brain could absorb, retain, and interpret information, and then use it in a test environment. I was proud of myself.

Because of my passion for recovery from eating issues, we invited an eating disorders counselor I knew to bring her knowledge and expertise to the program at Realization Center. I learned much from her. And, in 1995, I attended a conference, Food Addiction 2000, at the Robert Woods Johnson campus in New Jersey. It modified and expanded my understanding of my and other people's problems with eating. Even though my colleague Marilyn had early on identified my issues with food as addiction, it had still been unclear as to how it fit.

Evolution

Over time, my food recovery was evolving. I was letting go of more and more of the "culprits"/triggers to eating problems as addiction. Up until that time, I referred to my problem as "compulsive overeating," and I called myself a "compulsive overeater." That's what I had learned in the rooms and from the OA literature. Of course, what I know now is that compulsive overeating is just a manifestation or symptom of the disease of food addiction—it's not the problem itself. Just like "overdrinking" is a manifestation/symptom of the disease of alcoholism.

When I was first introduced to the OA program, embarking on my journey of recovery, I knew at the outset that my answer lay in the OA program. What I did not hear over the years of attending meetings was that the illness was biochemically based. I regret that that's not talked about in either the literature or meetings. Food Addicts Anonymous (FAA) is the 12-step program that addresses eating problems as being biochemically based. If it had been discussed, it would have shortened my quest to find peace with my cravings, my need to be thin, my body, my being. I started to understand that those culprits (alcohol, sugar, sugar substitutes, flour, wheat, caffeine, high fat) kept me enslaved. As my path narrowed, as I let go of those culprits, I came to find the peace

I so wanted. I internalized this basic knowledge of my disease, and my biology—and my struggle ended. I found true abstinence.

The Promises of Recovery

I have been sober since October 1979, and abstinent for almost twenty-five years. I continue to be in awe of and very grateful for my body size, my energy level, my brain function, and my health in general. As a result of my abstinence and sobriety, my body has stayed thin (and I do not starve, diet, or count calories), I have amazing energy, and I love my brain. It works better than ever. My health is wonderful (*pooh, pooh, pooh*[3]). I love recovery. It has given me back everything I lost except for the years lost to being caught in the disease. I always believed that God would give me the good stuff in my later years because I had lost so much in the early ones.

I have been blessed to receive the promises of recovery (as listed in the book *Alcoholics Anonymous*), especially "We will not regret the past nor wish to shut the door on it." My past was the path to my future and my experiences in it are mine to offer others so they might see themselves and trust enough to let go. I recommend without hesitation this journey of awareness, trust, and hope. Being abstinent is an amazing way to live.

How This Book Came About

Using my growing knowledge of eating problems and my deepening understanding of addiction in general, I put the pieces together and started to develop the Food Addiction Treatment Program at Realization Center. (See "About Realization Center" on page 483.) What evolved is an eighteen-week lecture series that presents the "how's and why's" of food addiction, and what the solution is. Over time, I became better and better at presenting the information, and many clients started to respond positively by changing their eating behavior—i.e., consuming less sugar, eliminating the other addictive/triggering food substances, starting their day with "the breakfast," and being amazed by how much better they felt by simply eating a simple breakfast meal, as we define it. Many became "abstinent" during the series. The idea of writing a book embodying the series eventually became my mission. I am both amazed at and proud of the result.

I believe that all addicts start with food as their first addictive substance and that addressing the food issue is key to an addict's process of recovery, and that food recovery is the basis of all recovery. Becoming abstinent by following the Realization Center food plan is the ideal. This book provides all the information in the eighteen-week lecture series and beyond.

PART ONE

The Problem: Food Addiction

CHAPTER 1

The Disease Concept of Addiction
The Biopsychosocial Definition of Addiction

No amount of willpower will change the biological factors at the root of addictive illness.

Due to current advanced brain-imaging technology, there is much new knowledge about the brain's reward system. Understanding the biological basis of food addiction—that brain reward is "driving the bus" (along with family messages/culture about eating and body image)—can help the food addict experience a reduction in the crippling shame that comes with out-of-control eating behavior by recognizing that their "flawed solution" is not just impaired judgment, but faulty circuitry. Clients have commented something to the effect of, "Now I understand why I get so depressed and anxious before I binge and feel such a pleasant 'afterglow' when I'm done. I love it, until the guilt and remorse come back."

Understanding that brain circuitry works on a dopamine-mediated reward system—and that eating, restricting, and purging are flawed attempts to experience that reward—helps motivate food addicts to seek healthier rewards, which is a large component of recovery. Hopefully, the food addict learns that switching substances (substituting or masking one substance with another) is not the answer to one's food addiction, nor is it recovery. Alcohol, drugs, gambling, work, exercise, smoking, sex, shopping, and the like are not the solution, and they all have their own addictive potential. The expression that describes the attempt to "escape" from an addictive behavior by using another addictive behavior is like "changing deck chairs on the Titanic."

In a speech to the American Clinical & Climatology Association in 2008, Dr. Robert L. DuPont stated:

"Addiction is unique in the way it corrodes the character and the relationships of the sufferer. The addict not only has the disease but over time, the addict *becomes* the disease. Addiction often remains hidden, even from those it is killing. This stealthy disease has been called by people who live close to it 'cunning, baffling and powerful.' It is that."[4]

He further noted:

"The disease concept of addiction means that the addict is not simply addicted to a specific drug but that he or she is addicted to brain-rewarding chemicals in general. Addictive behavior is sustained not by fear of withdrawal, but by the longing for the brain-reward resulting from drug use."[5]

As they say in the rooms of 12 Step Recovery Fellowships, "A drug is a drug is a drug." Any substance that triggers brain reward can be classified as a drug.

The purpose of my lectures and of this book is twofold: 1) to explain why most people's out-of-control eating behavior is addiction, and 2) to present the solution. Many individuals who suffer from out-of-control eating behaviors have gone to great lengths to find an answer, including various weight-loss programs, visits to doctors and nutritionists, going on umpteen diets, taking diet pills (both prescription and over-the-counter), stomach surgery (gastric bypass or sleeve, and now, the "safer" alternative, lap band), various forms of induced purging (vomiting, laxatives, exercise), and the hope of all hope, psychotherapy.

The reason these approaches fail is that the problem is *not* the weight! It's addiction—*food addiction,* a biochemical illness. Addiction does not resolve with therapy. I have never met any addict among the thousands of addicts I have encountered who was "therapized" out of addiction. I describe this as follows:

Traditional therapy says, "If we deal with your FEELINGS, that will help you change your THOUGHTS, which then will change your BEHAVIOR."

The Addiction Model of Treatment says, "If you change your BEHAVIOR, your THINKING will then change, and then your FEELINGS will change."

The Addiction Model of Treatment is based on the understanding that addiction is a biochemical problem—and that needs to be dealt with first.

HISTORY OF THE "DISEASE CONCEPT"

Prior to the founding of Alcoholics Anonymous in 1935, and for a long time thereafter, the world viewed "drunks" as crazy, weak-willed, spineless, immoral, shameless, self-indulgent, shiftless, and lazy. And if you had one in your family, everyone tried to keep it a secret because it was so shameful. The belief at that time was that drinking was a choice.

Alcoholics Anonymous (AA) had its start because Bill Wilson, a stockbroker and a seemingly hopeless drunk, joined with Bob Smith, a physician and also a seemingly hopeless drunk, to find a solution to their drinking problem. They discovered, each with the support of the other, that if they did not pick up the FIRST drink and they helped another alcoholic, they could stay sober, one day at a time. What an amazingly simple idea. A wonderful doctor at that time, Dr. William D. Silkworth, did what he could to help support people like Bill Wilson and Bob Smith, and, in doing so, became a specialist in alcoholism. In "The Doctor's Opinion," he explained alcoholism as an allergy, as follows:

> "We believe, and so suggested a few years ago, that the action of alcohol on these chronic alcoholics is a manifestation of an allergy; that the phenomenon of craving is limited to this class, and never occurs in the average temperate drinker[...] All these, and many others, have one symptom in common: they cannot start drinking without developing the phenomenon of craving. This phenomenon, as we have suggested, may be the manifestation of an allergy which differentiates these people, and sets them apart as a distinct entity. It has never been, by any treatment with which we are familiar, permanently eradicated. The only relief we have to suggest is entire abstinence."[6]

This explanation makes sense to anyone who suffers from the inability to control their drinking and, by extension, drug use. Of course, today, thanks to brain-imaging technology, we understand more about the brain's involvement in alcoholism/addiction; however, that doesn't change the understanding that it is a physiological problem.

This was the beginning of our society's changing its view of alcoholics.

Nonetheless, it did take a long time for us to finally understand that alcoholism/addiction is an illness. We call this understanding the "disease concept." And, with that, we have also come to understand that it is a biopsychosocial disease, meaning that there are three parts to this illness: 1) biological, 2) psychological, and 3) social.

Applying the Disease Concept to Eating Problems

The idea that a person's eating problems could be an addiction is *beginning* to be seriously considered. However, it will take a long time for society as a whole—including the traditional medical establishment—to embrace the disease concept as it relates to food addiction. This is because collective denial is a major obstacle to looking at the facts and acknowledging that food addiction is a disease. (See Chapter 8: Denial and Other Defense Mechanisms for a discussion of how denial is used to refute or negate the idea that a sufferer has no control over their behavior because admitting that would suggest there is no hope of change.)

I believe that mainstream thinking with regard to food addiction is at the same place alcoholism was in 1930s when the idea of its being a disease was introduced. The term had been used much earlier in medical literature, but narrowly so. Society, including the medical establishment, had much resistance to, and denial of, the disease concept. That seems to be the case today. Like the early thinking about alcoholism, many people, including doctors, believe that food addicts whose illness is evidenced by overweight lack willpower, moral aptitude, discipline, and intellect, and are shameless, self-indulgent, lazy, spineless, and so on.

SATISFACTION VERSUS CONSEQUENCES

Behavior in general is controlled much more by short-term positive effects than by long-term negative ones. The immediate satisfaction of eating outweighs the thought of long-term consequences (i.e., weight gain and/or compromised health). Euphoric recall is an emotional memory with a high value in implicit memory (memories that are things we know but aren't always aware of how we learned them), and it takes the place of healthy pleasures and coping mechanisms. Implicit memory is more authentic, difficult to forget, and can be said to be a deeper part of memory. It's no wonder that recovery takes a lot of work and some authentic, fundamental changing. New

The Disease Concept of Addiction

35

> habits have to form to overcome implicit memories—a good reason for 90 meetings in 90 days. Sobriety/abstinence is learning a new way to live and involves reprogramming memory. It takes a lot of doing, but the good news is that it is entirely possible. The work of recovery does work.

RESEARCH AND STUDIES THAT SUPPORT THE CONCEPT OF "FOOD ADDICTION"

We are not at a loss for substantiation of the brain-behavior connection in food addiction. In a Summer 2009 article in *Paradigm*, Michael Prager wrote: "The medical establishment has yet to acknowledge the links among foods, food behaviors, and addiction, and they ought to know better. More than 2,400 peer-reviewed studies establish the causes and conditions for food addiction."[7]

Scientific research using both animal models and human brain-imaging studies strongly supports the concept of food addiction. Here are a few of them, along with other notable studies:

- Brain-imaging work conducted by Dr. Mark Gold and researchers at the McKnight Brain Center at the University of Florida suggests "[t]here are important similarities between overeating highly palatable and hedonic foods and the classic addictions." Gold explains that in the past, addiction was defined by tolerance and withdrawal: "After our work and that of others on cocaine, it was clear that addiction was more like a pathological, often fatal attraction. The definition of addiction was changed [. . .] overeating and obesity are candidates for Addictive Disease." Gold states that food, especially highly palatable food, can produce the same effects as drugs of abuse. He says, "It is common for people to eat more than they intend [to] despite dire consequences. Failed diets and attempts to control overeating, preoccupation with food and eating, shame, anger, and guilt look like traditional addictions."[8]

- An even earlier study, published by Dr. Ernest Noble and researchers at UCLA in 1994, found that the brain's D2 dopamine receptor, already implicated in alcoholism, was also involved with obesity and with cocaine and tobacco dependence.[9] The D2 dopamine gene marker for alcoholism and drug addiction was found in overeating obese adults who are not alcohol- or drug-addicted.

- In December 2009, Princeton psychology professor Bart Hoebel presented research to the American College of Neuropsychopharmacology that found that all the characteristics of alcoholism and drug addiction appear in addiction to sugar.[10] Hoebel and his team have been studying signs of sugar addiction in rats for years. His current research studies the craving and relapse aspects of addiction. Previously the rats under study showed a behavioral pattern of increased intake, then showed signs of withdrawal—two of the three elements of addiction. His lab animals, trained to become dependent on high doses of sugar, were denied sugar for a prolonged period after learning to binge, worked harder to get it when it was reintroduced to them. They consumed more sugar than they ever had, suggesting craving and relapse behavior. Their motivation for sugar had grown. Hoebel has shown that rats consuming large amounts of sugar when hungry, describing it as "sugar-bingeing," undergo neurochemical changes in the brain that appear to mimic those produced by substances of abuse, including cocaine, morphine, and nicotine. "In certain models, sugar-bingeing causes long-lasting effects in the brain, and increases the inclination to take other drugs of abuse, such as alcohol."

  The Hoebel team found that dopamine is released in the nucleus accumbens region of the brain (the brain's "pleasure circuit") when hungry rats drink a sugar solution. This chemical signal is thought to trigger motivation and, eventually, with repetition, addiction. Hungry rats that binge on sugar provoke a surge of dopamine in their brains. After a month, the structure of the rat brains adapts to increased dopamine levels, showing fewer of a certain type of dopamine receptor than they used to have and more opioid receptors. These dopamine and opioid systems are involved with motivation and reward, systems that control wanting and liking something. Similar changes are also seen in the brains of rats given cocaine and heroin.

- S.H. Ahmed's research in France (2007) showed that intense sweetness—not just that of refined sugar, but also artificial sweeteners—surpasses cocaine as a reward in laboratory animals.[11]

The Disease Concept of Addiction

- Eric Stice, Ph.D., a neuroscientist at the Oregon Research Institute, has conducted ten prospective studies investigating risk factors for future increases in eating pathology, body mass, and depression, including three that involve brain imaging, genotypes, and their interactions. He has also conducted eleven randomized efficacy and effectiveness prevention trials and two treatment trials targeting eating disorders, obesity, and depression. Dr. Stice has stated that sugar is much more addictive than originally recognized. His work had evidenced that sugar activates our brains in a special way—that is reminiscent of drugs like cocaine. In the *60 Minutes* CBS episode, "Sugar," Dr. Sanjay Gupta climbed into an MRI scanner with a straw rigged to deliver a tiny sip of soda into his mouth. Just as the soda hit Dr. Gupta's tongue, Dr. Stice noted that the scanner detected increased blood rushing to certain regions of Dr. Gupta's brain. He stated that in the images, the yellow areas showed that Dr. Gupta's reward region was responding to the sweet taste. Dopamine—the chemical that controls the brain's pleasure circuit—was being released, just as it would in response to drugs or alcohol. Dr. Gupta commented that he had experienced some pleasure from the Coke, a euphoric effect. Dr. Stice said that by scanning hundreds of volunteers, he's learned that people who frequently drink sodas or eat ice cream or other sweet foods may be building up a tolerance, much like drug users do. As strange as it sounds, that means the more you eat, the less you feel the "reward." The result: You eat more than ever. If you overeat these on a regular basis, it causes changes in the brain that basically blunt the reward region's response to food, so you eat more and more to achieve the same satisfaction you felt originally.

- According to articles published in *Physical Behavior and Obesity Research,* research indicates there is scientific consensus that some humans who binge on food, restrict, and then continue this binge/restrict pattern, produce endogenous opioids.[12,13] Endogenous opioids (endorphins—a morphine-like substance originating from within the body, the brain) are produced when the body experiences pain or stress. Endorphins are called the natural opiates of the body. When endorphins are produced, the body feels good, high, or euphoric, and feels relief from pain (analgesia). It is understandable then, that endorphin levels go up when a person exercises, goes into labor, or is stressed out. Bingeing or purging are stressful activities to the body—generating the production of endorphins, thereby making those behaviors feel pleasurable—even euphoric and resulting in the desire to continue the behavior.

- Research shows evidence that markers on the ob (obesity) gene and deficiency in the biochemical leptin are related to disorders in satiation and to problems self-assessed food addicts call addiction to volume eating of all foods.[14]

- Scientists from Boston Children's Hospital and Harvard Medical School found that consuming a meal high in refined carbohydrates stimulates the nucleus accumbens (the brain's "pleasure circuit"), acting in much the same way as cocaine and heroin. In subjects who had consumed high-carb meals, the researchers also observed increased hunger [craving], decreased glucose levels, and heightened regions of the brain stimulated for hours after eating [desire for more refined carbs]. They observed that this was a critical period that affects eating behavior at the next meal. This study demonstrates that refined carbohydrates cause symptoms consistent with addiction.[15]

- Consumption of food (other than eating from hunger), and some drug use, are initially driven by their [brain] rewarding properties, which in both instances involves activation of mesolimbic dopamine pathways.[16]

- There are case studies of obese patients who for years could not diet, but after treating themselves as food addicts and eliminating all binge foods completely from their food plan, they were successful in losing and keeping off the weight.[17]

- There is outcome research showing that some members of a food-related 12 Step fellowship are successful when treating themselves as food addicted.[18]

- There are case studies of obese patients who could not stay on traditional diets and were not being treated successfully by doctors using an addiction model.[19]

The Disease Concept of Addiction

- One study investigates how food intake is regulated by dopamine-containing pleasure circuit of the brain.[20]

- Animal research used to test for alcoholism and drug addiction has shown that some animals can be addicted to sugar, other forms of sweeteners, and excess fat.[21]

Some of the other important research linking brain reward chemistry to eating behavior is cited here:

Avena, Nicole M., Pedro Rada, and Bartley G. Hoebel. "Evidence for Sugar Addiction: Behavioral and Neurochemical Effects of Intermittent, Excessive Sugar Intake." *Neurosci Biobehav Rev* 32, no. 1 (2008):20–39. doi:10.1016/j.neubiorev.2007.04.019.

Blumenthal, Daniel M., and Mark S. Gold, "Neurobiology of Food Addiction." *Current Opinion in Clinical Nutrition and Metabolic Care* 13, no. 4 (July 2010):359–365. doi: 10.1097/MCO.0b013e32833ad4d4.

Gerhardt, A. N., S. Yokum, P. T. Orr, E. Stice, W. R. Corbin, and K. D. Brownell. "Neural Correlates of Food Addiction." *Archives of General Psychiatry* 68, no. 8 (April 2011:808-16. doi: 10.1001/archgen psychiatry.2011.32.

Hellikere, Kevin. "Food May be Addicting for Some." *The Wall Street Journal.* Updated April 5, 2011. Accessed May 31, 2018. www.wsj.com/articles/SB100014 24052748703712504576243192495912186.

Himpens, MD, Jacques; Guy-Bernard Cadiere, MD, PhD; Michel Bazi, MD; Michael Vouche, MD; Benjamin Cadiere, MD; and Giovanni Dapri, MD. "Long-term Outcomes of Laparoscopic Adjustable Gastric Banding" *Archives of Surgery* 146, no. 7 (July 2011):802-7. doi: 10.1001/archsurg.2011.45.

Ifland, Joan, H. G. Preuss, M. T. Marcus, K. M. Rourke, W. C. Taylor, K. Burau, W. S. Jacobs, W. Kadish, and G. Manso. "Refined Food Addiction: A Classic Substance Use Disorder." *Medical Hypothesis* 72, no. 5 (May 2009):518-26. doi:10.1016/j.mehy.2008.11.035. (Research showing that some overeaters have all the characteristics of food as a Substance-Use Disorder.)

Leibowitz, Sarah. "Over-Consumption of Fats: A Vicious Cycle from the Start." Paper presented at Seattle Summit on Food Addiction: The Obesity Epidemic Connection, 2009.

Park, Madison. "Why isn't there a safe weight-loss pill?" CNN.com. April 15, 2011. Accessed May 31, 2018. www.cnn.com/2011/HEALTH/04/15/diet.drugs.fail/index.html.

Sheppard, MA, LMHC, CEDS, Kay. "The Science of Refined Food Addiction." *Counselor Magazine.* September 28, 2009. Accessed May 32, 2019. kaysheppard.com/articles/refined-food-addiction/.

ADDICTION AS A COMPLEX BIOPSYCHOSOCIAL DISEASE

As the term suggests, the *biopsychosocial model* suggests that addiction has biological, psychological, and social aspects. Biological factors have been found to include genetics, in utero damage, and temperament. As described by Alan Leshner, Ph.D., psychologist, neuroscientist, and former director of National Institute on Drug Abuse (NIDA), addiction is fundamentally a brain disease and is itself a result of a combination of environmental factors, historical factors, and the physiological state of individuals, including their genetic background.[22] They all coalesce through the brain to produce addiction.

The area in the brain that has been identified thanks to our sophisticated technology (including MRIs and PET and CAT scans) in the addiction process is called the "reward circuit." When triggered, the reward circuit produces a number of chemicals, called neurotransmitters, one of which is dopamine, which allows us to experience pleasure, joy, and euphoria. The basic tenet of the reward center of the brain is:

What feels good will be repeated and pursued.

What doesn't feel good will be avoided or eliminated.

The new definition of addiction, developed in 2011 by the American Society of Addiction Medicine (ASAM), is as follows:

> "A **primary, chronic** disease of **brain reward**, motivation, memory, and related circuitry. Dysfunction in these circuits leads to characteristic biological, psychological, social, and even spiritual manifestations. This is reflected in an individual pathologically pursuing reward and/or relief by substance abuse and other behaviors.
>
> Addiction is characterized by inability to consistently abstain, impairment in behavioral control, craving, diminished recognition of significant problems with one's behaviors and interpersonal relationships, and a dysfunctional emotional response. Like other chronic diseases, addiction often involves cycles of relapse and remission. Without treatment or engagement in recovery activities, addiction is progressive, and can result in disability or premature death."[23]

Food addiction falls right into this new definition of addiction. This definition is so important and comprehensive that you will see it again later. Meanwhile, the ASAM clarified this new definition in a set

The Disease Concept of Addiction

41

of frequently asked questions. The ones pertinent to food addiction are included here:

Question: What's different about this new definition?

Answer: This new definition makes clear that addiction is not about drugs ("substances" such as alcohol, heroin, marijuana, speed, or cocaine)—it's about brains. It is not the substance a person uses that makes them an addict; it is not even the quantity or frequency of use. Addiction is about what happens in a person's brain when they are exposed to rewarding substances or behaviors, and it is more about reward circuitry in the brain and related brain structures than it is about the external chemicals or behavior that "turns on" the reward circuitry. We have recognized the role of memory, motivation, and related circuitry in the manifestation and progression of this disease.

Question: This new definition of addiction refers to addiction involving gambling, food, and sexual behaviors. Does ASAM really believe that food and sex are addicting?

Answer: The new ASAM definition departs from equating addiction with just substance dependence by describing how addiction is also related to behaviors that are rewarding. This is the first time that ASAM has taken an official position that addiction is not solely "substance dependence." This definition says that addiction is about functioning and brain circuitry and how the structure and function of the brains of persons with addiction differ from the structure and function of the brains of persons who don't. It talks about reward circuitry in the brain and related circuitry, but the emphasis is not on the external rewards that act on the hard-wired reward system. Food, sexual behaviors, and gambling behaviors can all be associated with the "pathological pursuit of rewards" described in this new definition of addiction.

Question: Who has food or sex addiction? How many people is this? How do you know?

Answer: We all have the brain reward circuitry that makes food rewarding. In fact, this is a survival mechanism. In a healthy brain, this reward has feedback mechanisms for satiety or the "enough" trigger. In someone with addiction, this circuitry becomes dysfunctional, such that the message to the individual becomes "more," which leads to the pathological pursuit of rewards and/or relief through the use of substances and behaviors. So anyone with addiction is also vulnerable to food addiction.

Actually, there are some forces at work to now categorize eating disorders as addiction, so that insurance companies will have to reimburse treatment providers using the "substance abuse" benefit, which is a much better benefit than the "mental health" benefit currently being used. Addiction is *not* a mental health problem, and it's *not* a mental illness, though mental illness can be a factor in food addiction and drug use and can coexist alongside addiction. They are two separate and distinct diseases.

The best explanation of food addiction as addiction comes from Kay Sheppard, a licensed mental health counselor. She is a pioneer in the recognition and treatment of food addiction. She wrote:

"The biochemistry of food addiction follows a path which is initiated when ingestion of refined carbohydrates [sugar, flour] [also wheat, volume, hard cheeses] flood the brain with dopamine, serotonin, and norepinephrine. As the brain becomes flooded with these neurotransmitters, a feeling of well-being [pleasure] results, and craving is stimulated.

"This reaction simultaneously creates a deficiency in the brain, because the carbohydrates block the recycling of neurotransmitters. Thus the brain becomes depleted of its needed neurotransmitters.

"This feast, followed by famine, of brain chemicals upsets the hypothalamus. Since the hypothalamus is the brain's center for emotions and survival, mood and cravings go out of control.

"The result is that one is walking around drunk on refined carbohydrates. During this process, an insufficiency of neurotransmitters leaves receptor sites unfilled. This puts the brain in a condition of imbalance, resulting in distress and depression as well as cravings. It takes increasingly larger and more frequent amounts of carbohydrates to bring the brain back into balance. Over long periods of time, the food addict is unable to get back to baseline. To feel better, she continues to eat that which makes her feel worse."[24]

Although it fails to mention the involvement of brain chemistry as a driving force, a good description of food addiction by Ann Crumpler, LCSW, appeared in *Paradigm*, Summer 2006, in an article titled "Understanding Addictions":

The Disease Concept of Addiction

"Food addiction is a disorder characterized by preoccupation with food. Food addiction involves the repetitive consumption of food against the individual's better judgment, resulting in loss of control or the restriction of food, and preoccupation with body weight and image. Types of food addiction include compulsive overeating, bulimia, and anorexia. Food is used to cope with life stressors. Cravings lead to eating followed by a period of stimulation with increased energy, activity and satisfaction. The gratification is short-lived and followed by decreased energy, irritability, and renewed cravings. *Bulimia Nervosa* is described as binge eating and compensatory behavior to prevent weight gain [and eliminate the feelings of fullness]. Like overeaters, individuals become ashamed of their eating behavior and attempt to conceal symptoms through secret rapid consumption [and purging] of food. Other behaviors include: misuse of laxatives, fasting, and excessive exercise. Anorexia is characterized by intense fear of gaining weight. Self-esteem is dependent upon body shape and weight. Weight loss is seen as an achievement and an example of extraordinary self-discipline."[25]

The question, however, arises, "WHY?" Many of us who treat food addicts believe the answer is "the body, the brain." How does it happen that with these three different forms of food addiction, once started, they seem to take on a life of their own?

The main idea for food addiction is based on the principle that quickly metabolized carbohydrates trigger a craving for more carbohydrates, establishing an addictive cycle. Specific substances include sugar, all sugar substitutes, flour, caffeine, or anything eaten in volume. Sugar takes zero time to metabolize. The body uses it quickly and immediately calls for more. Flour takes a little longer to metabolize, but it also is quickly turned into sugar (glucose). Caffeine increases adrenaline, causing an overproduction of insulin, which also sets up a craving mechanism. Anything eaten in volume is stored as fat. When the body uses this material, it's turned first into glycogen (main storage form of glucose in the body), then into glucose, setting up the craving mechanism cycle again.

After a detoxification period, physiological cravings gradually disappear if these substances are removed through use of a specific food plan (not the quirky "diets" promoted by Weight Watchers, Jenny Craig, Nutrisystem, and the like) designed to eliminate triggering foods/substances. The food plan in Chapter 11 is especially designed to exclude/eliminate those triggering substances and create stabilized blood-sugar levels.

CRAVING VERSUS URGES

There is a distinction between "cravings" and "urges." It's useful to make this distinction because there is a difference between the drive to use food when the food addict is active in the disease and the drive when they are abstinent, or in recovery.

Cravings

Cravings are a physiological phenomenon. They come from the brain reward pathways discussed earlier. Once the addict is triggered and they're in craving, they will do virtually anything to get it satisfied. "The horse has left the barn," "the train has left the station"—nothing can stop the compelling power of the craving. Those are the times the addict has broken their commitments ("I'll never use again"), broken their promises, hurt those they love, manipulated, lied, cheated, or stolen to get their fix. And, certainly, willpower is impotent in the face of this biological force. (As established earlier, willpower comes from a different part of the brain and doesn't have the power to override the triggered reward pathways.)

The concept "euphoric recall" helps us understand cravings from another perspective. Euphoric recall is the intensely pleasurable memory of the "high" one achieved through taking a drink/drug or trigger food, the "high" that the chemically/food-addicted person continues to seek. The positive memory tends to outweigh all of the negative memories or side effects and repercussions that always accompany any substance abuse. Our brains tend to forget or minimize the memory of pain.

Urges

Urges, on the other hand, as I make this distinction, come from the heart and feelings. They can never be experienced until the addict is no longer in craving, which happens when they are abstinent, abstaining from those chemicals that trigger the addictive response and the cravings. Urges can appear when, for example, you feel let down, disappointed, hurt, criticized, shamed, misunderstood, or misrepresented by those you most want to trust. Or you feel lonely, frightened, anxious, stressed out, depressed, or enraged, and your historical solution to deal with your feelings is to bury your face in an Entenmann's cake or go to bed with "Ben & Jerry." But this time, since the drive is NOT from your brain, *and* you're

The Disease Concept of Addiction

45

working a program of recovery (FAA, OA, GreySheeters, CEA-HOW), you can think the urge through and do something other than eat, such as call a program fellow, go to a 12-step meeting, read program literature, write about your feelings, and otherwise do something program related. Until they are abstinent, I believe the food addict and anyone else who is chemically addicted, has never experienced an URGE, as I define it, since from the beginning of their lives, they have been ingesting those triggers that disturb brain chemistry, creating cravings on some level.

Causes of Cravings

Dopamine (the "feel-good" neurotransmitter) is released when major triggering substances are ingested, allowing us to experience pleasure. If one is genetically predisposed to addiction, having faulty feedback circuitry, and is therefore prevented from experiencing satiety (enough!), once the pleasure (dopamine) begins to subside, she will be left with an overwhelming need for more of the same or another triggering substance—which is the phenomenon of craving. (See the discussion on "brain-switch analogy" on page 47 later in this chapter.) We will discuss the culprits and triggers in depth in Chapter 7: The Culprits and Triggers. At Realization Center, we post the following for a quick glance (see chart on next page).

I believe that the high incidence of relapse with alcoholics and drug addicts is due to the fact that they never fully get clean. They continue to use by substituting any of the major triggering substances (listed above) for alcohol and/or drugs and therefore remain in craving. Then, there are times during their recovery when life goes to a scary place, when a candy bar just won't do it. But they know what will do it (euphoric recall; see page 47)—a drink or a drug! (For more on this, see Chapter 5: Food Addiction: The Precursor/Gateway to Chemical Dependency.)

Through their sponsors and fellow recovery members, AA actually encourages alcoholics and drug addicts to eat sugar and drink coffee because doing so satisfies their cravings. It's true that the refined carbs will satisfy their cravings, but the cravings will return, again and again, demanding to be satisfied. That's why many recovering addicts gain weight when they stop using; they're managing their cravings with the triggering substances mentioned earlier. They don't think of them as triggers, but we know otherwise!

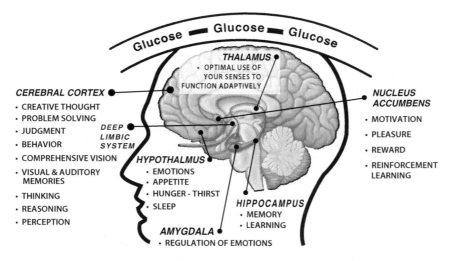

The Culprits/Triggers

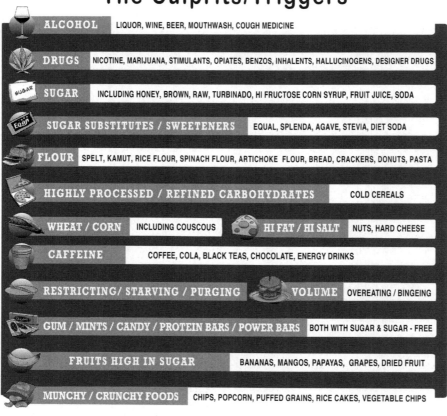

WHY SOME PEOPLE GET ADDICTED AND OTHERS DO NOT

There is a mechanism in the brain of the addict that differs from that of the non-addict. A genetic predisposition combines with environmental stressors to create susceptibility to addictive illnesses. As is said in scientific circles, "The genetics load the gun, and the family [environment] pulls the trigger!" The "brain switch" is my way of explaining the brain reward mechanism. We all come into the world with a brain switch. When we take in one of the substances listed on page 46, our brain switch goes to the "on" position and we experience pleasure (the *ahhhhh* effect). Then the switch goes into the "off" position and we say, "That was wonderful! I enjoyed that; that was ENOUGH."

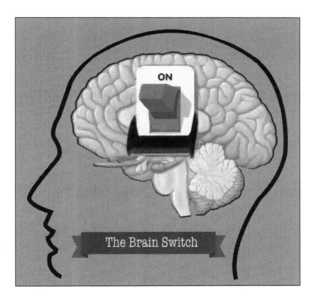

Some of us, however, have a defect or deficiency in this mechanism. When we take in any of the trigger substances, our switch goes to the "on" position and we experience that pleasure, joy, euphoria, and we say, "That was wonderful, good, I enjoyed that, I WANT MORE!" Our switch does not go into an "off" position because it doesn't have an "off" position. That's craving—"I want more!"

The addict, food and otherwise, has to go the distance, keep using, until some force interferes with it—e.g., no more food (usually the sugars, refined carbs) or other drugs, feeling sick, passing out (food addicts prefer to call that "going to sleep"), overdosing, and death. This is the phenomenon that causes addicts to go past their bodily limits, because the craving, the disease, is in charge. Examples of addicts exceeding their body limits include Michael Jackson, Philip Seymour Hoffman, Whitney Houston, Janis Joplin, Amy Winehouse, Heath Ledger, Elvis Presley and, sadly, many more.

That "more" phenomenon exists either because we have a genetic predisposition to this phenomenon or, because of our consistent overuse of these substances, something has changed in our brain. Ultimately, this is the true meaning of powerlessness. Once this craving phenomenon has been triggered, the addict is no longer in charge—the brain chemistry is, the disease is, the addiction is. The addict cannot predict how much will be consumed, when the urgency will stop, what the end of the "binge" will look like, be it alcohol, drugs, or food. This is why addicts unintentionally overdose, and why food addicts can die—purging and bingeing, bingeing and purging, blowing out their esophagus, choking on their vomit, rupturing the esophageal wall, etc. And those who binge and don't purge will often want to die, being so stuffed with food. That's the biology of addiction.

A SUMMARY OF THE SCIENCE

For some insight into how prominent world researchers in the field summarize the science for health professionals and the general public, watch the video clips from the 2009 Obesity and Food Addiction Summit by visiting www.foodaddictionsummit.org/agenda.htm.[26]

THE PSYCHOSOCIAL ASPECTS OF ADDICTION

Psychosocial factors of addiction include the family, the community or the school, and peers. Family and its influence on the psychological condition of the young addict will be discussed at length later in the book. Problems in social areas of life are magnified by the disease, but they are *not* the cause of addiction. A good explanation of the psychosocial characteristics of addiction can be found within the "Long Definition of Addiction" from the American Society of Addiction Medicine (ASAM):

The Disease Concept of Addiction

Other factors that can contribute to the appearance of addiction, leading to its characteristic psycho-social-spiritual manifestations, include:

a. The presence of an underlying biological deficit in the function of reward circuits, such that drugs and behaviors which enhance reward function are preferred and sought as reinforcers;

b. The repeated engagement in drug use or other addictive behaviors, causing neuroadaptation in motivational circuitry leading to impaired control over further drug use or engagement in addictive behaviors;

c. Cognitive and affective distortions, which impair perceptions and compromise the ability to deal with feelings, resulting in significant self-deception;

d. Disruption of healthy social supports and problems in interpersonal relationships which impact the development or impact of resiliencies;

e. Exposure to trauma or stressors that overwhelm an individual's coping abilities;

f. Distortion in meaning, purpose and values that guide attitudes, thinking and behavior;

g. Distortions in a person's connection with self, with others and with the transcendent (referred to as God by many, the Higher Power by 12-steps groups, or higher consciousness by others); and

h. The presence of co-occurring psychiatric disorders in persons who engage in substance use or other addictive behaviors.

Thoughts and beliefs about self and the world evolving from early childhood "War Zone" experiences and messages and continued use of substances leads to impairment in psychosocial functioning. (The "War Zone" will be discussed in detail later.) There is nothing in our lives that escapes the impact of addiction—not internally (brain and body) nor externally (our place in the world).

CHAPTER 2

What Is Food Addiction?

*Food addiction destroys. It robs us of our dreams.
It isolates and alienates us from friends and family.
It can even kill. But our food addiction doesn't have
to keep us from having a long, fulfilling life. Finding
the solution begins with identifying the problem.*

We all have to eat; it's the way we survive. Food is the fuel for our bodies. Eating is a fundamental activity of life. So how can it be an addiction? Let's discuss what happens when a person can no longer control how much or what they are eating or not eating—which is addiction.

Some "eating disorder" professionals and institutions reject the very idea that food could be an addiction. They see it as an emotional/mental disorder and strive to help their patients or clients eat in moderation. They believe that they can help a person eat, for example, *one* cookie, then stop and want no more, or *one* brownie and stop. I don't believe this is possible for someone who has lost control. As you are aware, I believe that eating problems are addiction, and are first and foremost based in the brain chemistry of the suffering individual.

Addiction is a pathological relationship to any mood-altering experience (substance, person, behavior, or process) that has life-damaging consequences.

Historically, aberrant eating behaviors were thought to be caused by lack of willpower. Our beliefs are being altered by our deeper understanding of the genesis of these behaviors. As Ann Crumpler, licensed clinical social worker/therapist experienced in treating addictions, states in her Summer 2006 article for *Paradigm* titled "Understanding Addictions":

"The idea that addicts lack willpower has long ago been debunked.

What Is Food Addiction?
51

Blaming attitudes keep individuals from seeking treatment, which fosters shame and fear around their illness. Addicts and those who love them are often the last to accept the disease concept, since they are engrossed in shame, denial, and the need to prove they are in control. Shaming addicts for their behavior is counterproductive; it creates barriers to recovery and complicates the recovery process. Addicts use substances/behaviors to medicate shame, fear, anger, and pain. Adding to the shame spurs increased addictive behaviors."[27]

Common characteristics are shared by all addictions; they follow a sequence of experiences that leads to loss of control and inability to manage daily living. Addiction causes changes in the brain, which include physiological, chemical, and even anatomical changes, with accompanying thought and behavioral changes. Initially, the substance/activity causes feelings of pleasure and concomitant changes in emotion. This initial euphoria creates an obsession to reconnect with that experience. In other words, addiction is both a physical and psychological dependence, independent of the need to avoid the pain of withdrawal. The body develops a physical tolerance to the substance/activity so that addicts must take/engage in increasingly larger doses to get the same effect. Removal of the drug/activity, inevitably, causes painful withdrawal symptoms.

According to Dr. Sam Sugar of the Pritikin Longevity Center & Spa in Florida, food addiction is a very real, everyday dilemma. He says:

"If you want to take a look at what's the most addictive, other than heroin and narcotics, go to a fast food place and see what they have been selling for the past 40 years. High salt, high sugar, meat, fat, cheese and chocolate—all of which are the most addictive foods known to man. Deep in our brains we know that those over-processed breads, decadent desserts, and soft drinks aren't the healthiest things we could be eating, but another deeper, darker part of our brain is prompting us to eat more of them. The brain works on a simple 'make me happy or suffer' level."[28]

Dr. Sugar goes on to say that these foods cause a significant elevation in the brain's dopamine levels, and the attendant feelings of pleasure and reward are thought to be similar to what addicts experience when using drugs, as touched upon in the previous chapter. The more you eat, the more you want. This is why supersizing is so popular.

As with all addictions, the body/brain builds up a tolerance to these foods and the pleasure circuit gets blunted. The food addict needs more and more to get the needed reward.

With the easy availability of foods of all kinds, it's no wonder that so many people are dealing with addiction and epidemic obesity. What we are seeing for the first time in 3.5 million years is that people are more likely to die of obesity than starvation. Though starvation is a stranger to most people in the United States, our brains are still programmed to store calories.

A major benefit of food addiction recovery (abstinence) is that by removing the "trigger/culprit" foods (e.g., sugar, artificial sweeteners, flour, wheat, high fat, high salt, hard cheese, caffeine, and alcohol) from the diet and creating a structured plan of eating, we give the brain a chance to rewire itself and become less dependent on the harmful "treats" for those good feelings. Let's examine the nature of this.

More Definitions of Addiction

Disease: any condition of a human being that makes a part of their body or themselves unable to function in a healthy way.

Stop for a moment and think about this definition. Which part of it jumps out and/or has the most meaning for you? Is it "any condition," or "their body or themselves," or "unable to function [...] in a healthy way"? (For me, it's the "functioning" part; to me, being able to function well is everything! One wants to be highly functional to the end.)

The word "addiction" comes from the Latin root *addictus*, which means "to be enslaved" (interesting that the Romans had a word for this terrible affliction). Using this meaning to develop a definition of addiction yields:

Slavish physical and/or emotional dependence on a mood-altering substance and/or behavior.

Again, think about this in relation to your behavior with food. What in this definition stands out for you? *Slavish? Physical/emotional dependence? Mood-altering?*

- Slavish—Does eating/not eating dictate your behavior?

What Is Food Addiction?

53

- Physical/emotional dependence—Do you make life decisions based on your access to specific foods?

- Mood-altering—Because of your eating/not eating behavior, do you experience mood swings? Do you look to eating to alter your mood?

The treatment field now officially recognizes alcoholism and addiction as a disease. As we discussed earlier, Alcoholics Anonymous (AA) has done this since the 1930s. In 1950, the medical establishment (AMA) officially recognized addiction as a disease, listing it in the Diagnostic and Statistical Manual of Mental Disorders, or DSM (the diagnostic "bible" used to define mental/behavioral conditions and illnesses) with the relevant diagnostic codes for alcoholism, cocaine addiction, opiate addiction, and so on. Sixty-one years later, the establishment took a critical next step. Sadly, the wheels of understanding and acceptance turn very slowly.

As presented earlier, in 2011, the American Society of Addiction Medicine published a long-awaited definition that finally officially recognized the biological basis of addiction. It's not simply a behavioral or social or moral problem. This definition finally opened the door to eating issues being included as an addiction. Although I included this definition earlier, I am including it here again to emphasize it:

Addiction is a **primary, chronic** disease of **brain reward**, motivation, memory, and related circuitry. Dysfunction in these circuits leads to characteristic biological, psychological, social, and spiritual manifestations. This is reflected in an individual **pathologically pursuing reward** and/or relief by substance abuse and other behaviors.

Addiction is characterized by the inability to consistently abstain from the problem behavior, impairment in behavioral control, craving, diminished recognition of significant dissonance with one's behaviors and interpersonal relationships, and a dysfunctional emotional response. Like other chronic conditions and diseases, addiction often involves cycles of relapse and remission. Without treatment or engagement in recovery activities, addiction is progressive, and can result in advancing disability or premature death.[29]

Consider the first word—*primary*—which means "first or main." So, how many primaries can one have? Just one. Now think about who, or what, is *your* primary relationship. Is it yourself, your spouse, your girlfriend or boyfriend, your parent, your child, or maybe your higher power? Really think; take your time. . . . Whatever you just said or thought—it's wrong!

As long as you are addictively *using any* substance, *that* is your primary relationship—for example, are you smoking or vaping? Do you *have to have* sugar or other sweetener every day? Would your life not be worth living if you had to "give up" Entenmann's cake, soda, coffee, or something else? To what lengths have you gone to make sure you have your "stuff"? Are you always careful to make sure you have enough cigarettes? Ice cream? Cookies? Cake? Candy? Sweet cereal? NutraSweet or other sweetener? How much space in your brain does the concern about maintaining your stash take up? Does it take up more space than you assign to what or who you designated as your primary relationship?

The word "primary" in this definition actually means "coming first"—that nothing precedes it. It isn't a secondary symptom of something else. So addiction is an illness *in and of itself*; **it isn't a symptom of another underlying disease.**

Food addiction is a primary disease. It stands alone, with its own causes and history. It is not an outgrowth of other disease processes such as emotional or psychiatric problems but an illness in its own right. It's not caused by, or a response to, a difficult life situation such as stress, external abuse, childhood trauma, or a bad marriage; it's not a substitute for something psychologically lacking, such as love, self-esteem, or confidence; and it's not the result of a moral deficiency, like weak will. The common belief that these conditions cause a person's overeating allows for the misunderstanding that "fixing" them will stop the problematic eating. How many food addicts sought psychotherapy to solve their eating issues—trying to get insight, understanding of their psyche, motivations, and pain, in hopes it would solve their eating problems? I have never met anyone, personally or professionally, who was "therapized" out of any addiction, including food addiction.

One of the secondary symptoms of being a food addict is weight gain. Most people have had the experience of losing weight. Most often, the weight comes back, plus. Gaining weight is not the problem, nor is losing weight the solution. The primary problem is food addiction. That's why diets don't work—they don't address the addiction, only the symptom!

What Is Food Addiction?

In her wonderful 1988 book *Lick the Sugar Habit*, Nancy Appleton, Ph.D., discusses cases of people with major secondary health problems that resolved when sugar was removed from their diets. Her work highlights how the medical field and those with health problems wrongly believe they have primary illnesses and focus all their attention on the symptoms. (Not to say that there aren't individuals who suffer from illnesses/diseases that are primary.) The point is that until the food addict sees the secondary issues of weight gain, depression, gas, constipation, etc., as stemming from food addiction, these conditions cannot be cleared up.

"Pathological" means changed by the course of a disease, something that is diseased, or arising from disease. We know this word from the phrase "pathological liar"—someone who lies and can't help it. The body/brain of the food addict reacts differently to trigger foods (see page 46) than that of a non-food addict and experiences the phenomenon of craving—resulting in compulsive behavior with food—i.e., overeating, purging, and restricting—with the menu of adverse effects.

A comprehensive definition of *addiction* is found in the literature of the 12-Step Program Sex and Love Addicts Anonymous:

> The use of a substance or activity for the purpose of lessening pain or augmenting pleasure, by a person who has lost control over the rate, frequency, or duration of its use and whose life has become progressively more unmanageable as a result.

Let's narrow this down to a specific definition.

Food Addiction: Pathologically pursuing pleasure/reward by engaging in unmanageable episodes of overeating, undereating, and/or eating/ purging despite the adverse consequences, injuring health, and/or interfering with social, economic, or emotional functioning on a continual basis, by a person who has lost control over the rate, frequency and duration of their behavior.

The substance most often abused is sugar as well as foods that are quickly converted to sugar (glucose) in the body. These foods, or binge foods, include the obvious sugary foods such as candy and ice cream, but also include refined carbohydrates such as flour products (breads, cookies, and pasta).[30]

EXAMINING THESE "ADVERSE CONSEQUENCES"

Food addiction has far-reaching physical, emotional, and social consequences, as discussed in this section.

Injuries to Health/Medical Issues

Possible medical complications vary according to the specific food addiction. The following is a brief discussion of each. Also see the further discussions in Chapter 4: Little Food Addict in the "War Zone" and Chapter 12: Compliance versus Surrender.

- *In anorexics*—Anorexics are often thin to the point of emaciation but are deathly afraid of gaining weight. Medical complications of anorexia can include liver and kidney problems, metabolic and bone changes, and damage to the endocrine system. Symptoms related to severe weight loss include dry skin and hair, cold hands and feet, general weakness, constipation and other digestive problems, insomnia, and amenorrhea (a cessation of menstruation). In addition, the body begins to grow hair (called lanugo) in an effort to keep itself warm. As weight loss progresses, more severe problems may develop, such as increased susceptibility to infections, stress fractures, ketosis (severe chemical imbalance), and progressive weakness of the heart muscle, which can lead to death.

- *In bulimics*—Bulimics may be of average weight or, more usually, slightly above average weight. They do most of their bingeing and purging secretly and experience rapid weight gains and losses. They purge through self-induced vomiting, abusing laxatives and diuretics, and/or fasting or overexercising. They are subject to medical problems occasioned by their purging methods as well as their eating habits.

  Vomiting causes the body to release endorphins, natural chemicals that make us feel good. Eventually the bulimic may make herself vomit even if she has not overeaten, so she can feel good. Soon the bulimic loses control over the binge-purge cycle. Repeated vomiting, fasting, exercising too much, or misuse of laxatives, diuretics, ipecac syrup, or enemas will eventually cause serious, long-term health problems in a variety of organ systems. Bulimia can result in dehydration, constipation and other digestive disorders, esophageal tearing, severe dental damage, and muscle weakness.

What Is Food Addiction?

As bulimia progresses, ulcers and life-threatening cardiac irregularities (from electrolyte imbalance) and heart failure may develop. Excessive laxative use can destroy natural bowel function and tonicity and can lead to ongoing diarrhea and rectal bleeding. As with repeated induced vomiting, abuse of laxatives can, in extreme instances, lead to death. Overuse of medications such as ipecac syrup to induced vomiting can lead to diarrhea, weakness, low blood pressure, chest pain, and trouble breathing. Prolonged overuse of these medications can lead to death.

- *In compulsive overeaters*—Compulsive overeaters are often overweight and may develop obesity. Overweight and obesity can lead to hypertension, stroke, varicose veins, and heart attack. Issues with overweight and obesity may also lead to metabolic syndrome, heart and related problems (high blood pressure, fluid retention, and so on), diabetes, digestive problems (reflux, indigestion, GERD, gas, bloating, constipation, diarrhea, colon polyps, diverticulitis, diverticulosis), some cancers, sleep issues (apnea), joint problems (e.g., arthritic conditions), fogginess (decline of brain function), cravings, and loss of libido.

Interference with Social Functioning

People with food addiction often isolate themselves, preferring to stay home, eat, and watch TV or read. They may feel uncomfortable in social settings because of their weight, so they avoid these gatherings. When they do socialize, it is often with "eating buddies" where the focus is on eating. They may feel so tired that the idea of being with other people is too much and avoid going out with friends. They look to food for nurturing, not realizing that true nurturing comes only from people; see Chapter 3: Little Food Addict in Training. Studies have shown that dieters and/or restrictors who maintain their weight at lower-than-normal levels (starvation mode) may experience loss of the sense of caring about others, love, and compassion. Breakdown of family ties is also seen where a person can become a loner, mistrustful, malicious, and even cruel to family members. A person in starvation mode shuts down physically, mentally, emotionally, and spiritually, and heightens his or her attention to food.

Interference with Economic Functioning

People with food addiction often spend more than they intended to on their binge foods, including fast food, even though it is relatively inexpensive. They may miss days at work as a result of their eating, eating/purging, and/or restricting behavior, and lose income due to their absence as a result. In some cases, they may work at a job that pays less than they are capable of earning because their motivation and energy level are compromised.

Interference with Emotional Functioning

This is *the* big one. When emotional functioning is unstable or dysfunctional, nothing else in the food addict's life can work right; health, social, and economic functioning are all affected. The eating behavior causes the addict's blood sugar level to "roller-coaster," causing a host of symptoms such as irritability, crankiness, depression, nervousness, anxiety, panic attacks, sweaty palms, lightheadedness, headache, occasional migraine, brain dysfunction (fogginess, poor focus and concentration, memory and thought-processing issues, poor decision-making, poor perception, poor judgment, low motivation), and/or craving (when the food addict is in craving mode, obsession takes over and nothing else matters). Executive functioning is exponentially affected, leading to poor judgment, poor decision-making, and avoidable errors. The components of executive functioning are discussed in the inset on page 59.

With regard to emotional functioning, in *Facts On: Food Addiction* by Nancy Fiorentino and Katie Regan, the authors write:

> "Food addiction also has emotional and spiritual dimensions. Emotional dimensions may include loss of self-esteem, anxiety, and an emotional 'roller-coaster' ranging from hysteria to depression, and often including suicidal thoughts. Spiritual dimensions may include hopelessness, the perception of a 'void' in one's life, and an absence of faith and trust in oneself or others. Addiction suppresses the ability to ask for, give, or receive help, and isolation is the result."[31]

WHAT IS EXECUTIVE FUNCTIONING?

The executive functioning of the brain is impaired in the food addict. Executive functions of the brain include the ability to monitor one's own performance in social situations (e.g., getting along with people); ability to properly and simultaneously attend to, and track more than one task (e.g., time management); ability to shift set; abstract thinking/creativity; appropriate and adaptive responses to novel stimuli; attentional processes; categorization; conceptualization (e.g., learning and synthesizing information); goal-directed behavior; inhibition of unwanted behavior: insight and judgment (e.g., from what to wear to whom to marry); memory; mental flexibility; planning and decision-making; rule application; special processing (e.g., musical, artistic skills); and the ability to appropriately and appreciate consequences (instant gratification versus long-term satisfaction/impulse control/criminal behavior).

All of these features are subsumed under the neuropsychological rubric of "executive function" or, when impaired, "executive dysfunction." Fortunately, this impairment is not permanent and is repaired by "The Solution" (discussed in Part Two: The Solution: Abstinence).

FURTHERING OUR UNDERSTANDING OF FOOD ADDICTION

Illustrating the impact of the consequences of food addiction and how we have adapted to and normalized them, an anonymous letter published in the "Letters to the Editor" in the October 2005 edition of *The Sun* magazine encapsulates the syndrome:

> What kind of day I'm having depends on what I've eaten. Some fruit and a plain waffle? Good day. Just coffee? Great day! Chocolate and cookies? Bad day.
>
> I've never been overweight. When I was fifteen, I was anorexic and weighed just a hundred pounds. *Look at all those other people eating*, I would think. *They have no self-control.* I was often light-headed, cranky, and reclusive, but I was thin.
>
> Sometimes I still long to feel that empty and light, to believe again that I have control.[32]

Do you identify with this? Does this sound like someone you know?

To increase our understanding of food addiction, we must closely examine its characteristics, which are similar to those of chemical dependency and other addictions. These characteristics include denial, primary, chronic, fatal, tolerance and progression, craving, obsession/preoccupation, compulsion, time wasted, loss of control, physical dependency, *treatable*, and more. Let's take a look at each characteristic in turn in the following sections.

Denial

There is an extensive discussion of denial in Chapter 8, but let's touch upon it here, too. Addiction is a disease that says, "You don't have a disease." Addiction is so powerful that it convinces you that it's not a problem, and according to Marilyn J. White, "It's the only disease that allows you to enjoy your own death!"[33] Think about how much of one's health and functioning is compromised and diminished by a pathological and addictive relationship with food.

For overeaters who do not purge, weight is usually the symptom that gets the attention. Most people with weight issues have attempted many diets. If they are successful, we don't hear about them again. But if they aren't, what we hear is that they have to go on another diet. Their denial was a failure to admit that what wasn't working *really* wasn't working. They would diet, lose weight, and regain it, and while their denial was operative, they would say, "I have to try again." They think they didn't work hard enough. "I have to do better, more, put more effort into it." However, it was the *diet* that failed, not the dieter.

It's important to understand that when it comes to addiction, denial works against, or covers up, the physiological/biochemical issue: there is a craving for a substance that leads to obsession. The reason for this is that the addict's body finds it more critical to get food than to act rationally. To put it into "food language," the body mistakes hunger for starvation. The overeater/food addict felt hungry but acted as if she were starving. She isn't eating to just satisfy hunger; she's eating to avoid dying. Hungry people eat until they're satisfied and then stop. They can do that because their biochemistry, genetics, and brain chemistry are not dysfunctional in the way a food addict's are.

It is understood clinically what happens when a person is starving: they start obsessing about food and can think of nothing else. That's not

What Is Food Addiction?

hunger; it is a chemical-medical state. In a food addict, however, hunger perceived as starvation is a biochemical reaction; there's nothing the addict can do about. Think about this: If your body is having a reaction to hunger, it is making an erroneous connection and then thinking it is starving and then the brain starts figuring out how to get food. The addict gets a brain-biochemical message that she is starving and will eat regardless of what she'd been thinking before that happened. Then, it is like a patient trying to stay alert when they have been given an anesthetic prior to an operation. All of a sudden, they enter into a euphoric state, start thinking about other things, and then they are gone. That's the power biochemistry has over our bodies as addiction progresses.

The problem is that same faulty biochemistry produces all sorts of lies. In addition to telling us we're starving when we're just hungry, it also tells us that it's okay to eat even though we committed not to. It tells us to think, *I'll start my diet tomorrow, even though I said this is the most important thing in my life.* The biochemistry says it's okay to starve myself as a way of not letting this happen; it says it's okay to purge every day so I can continue to eat as much as I want and not gain weight. All of this seems crazy—that is, unless you're in the mind of the food addict: *Well, that makes sense; I can eat all I want and just have to throw it up—perfect solution! I can eat as much as I want and get to weigh just what I want, not realizing, or forgetting, what's happening to my body— hydrochloric acid coming back up and starting to gnaw at the enamel on my teeth, burning my throat, starting to change the electrolyte balance in my body. As I'm beginning to purge more and more, I'm having to hide it as I'm starting to purge on my good clothes, as I'm lying to my friends about why I'm purging.*

Denial is a hallmark of addiction, and food addicts need to fail more than one test of various "Do you have food addiction?" questions before they begin to believe that their relationship to food is addictive. (See Appendix: "Am I Addicted to Food?" Questionnaire.)

In the 1990s publication *Facts On: Food Addiction,* Nancy Fiorentino and Katie Regan discuss this destructive, dangerous characteristic this way:

> "Denial of food addiction is especially pervasive, since overeating is as socially acceptable in American culture as motherhood and apple pie. It is extremely difficult for even the most committed 12-step member

in stable, long-term recovery from alcohol and other drug addiction to believe that obesity is a result of addiction to food. Many simply believe that their addictive behavior is under control and that eating a bag of chocolate-covered raisins can hardly be considered a lack of spiritual centeredness. This polarization of mind and body is another form of denial, and another way of maintaining an addiction."[34]

Denial on an individual level is about saying, "It's okay, it's just cookies, it's not like I'm using [drugs and alcohol]." Societal denial is also a factor as it does not attach the same level of seriousness to the "use" of food as it attributes to drug and alcohol use and abuse.

Primary

As stated previously, addiction is *the disease*, not a symptom of some other disease. And it's not an outgrowth of another condition.

Chronic

This characteristic means that the condition is ongoing and will not go away on its own. The dictionary definition of *chronic* is constant, continuing, constantly recurring, of long duration. In *Disease Concept of Food Addiction,* Charles and Peggy Starks clarify this characteristic:

"Food addiction, like alcoholism, is not a temporary misalignment, nor is it a product of faulty learning or psychological trauma. It is not something that is outgrown. Like the alcoholic, the food addict who remains abstinent for a long period can return to full-blown addiction in a heartbeat if the addictive chemical is taken into the body. This is true regardless of the reason that the addictive chemical is used. The body does not know the difference between the drink of Champagne that celebrates a daughter's wedding and the shot of whiskey gulped from a hidden flask. Similarly, the body cannot discriminate between the piece of cake eaten at a parent's fiftieth wedding anniversary and the candy bar scarfed down in the grocery store parking lot. When the addict's body experiences some, it craves more. This is true today, tomorrow, and for the next 40 years."[35]

The disease of addiction, any addiction, is a permanent condition, and not curable and, therefore, must be managed on a daily basis. The disease progresses even when we are doing the work of recovery. When

What Is Food Addiction?

63

relapse occurs, the addictive eating behavior is worse than any previous addictive eating behavior. And when the food addict has achieved abstinence, they have to do the emotional and spiritual work of recovery or return to the active disease state.

Treatable

Food addiction can be arrested, but it can't be cured. That's because it is a chronic condition. However, like other chronic conditions, it is entirely treatable. Treatment can take various routes, as discussed in Chapter 18. If you are a food addict, this is probably not the first book in which you have looked for an answer. Eating behaviors cannot be solved with a self-help book, but this book can serve as a launching pad for embarking on a journey of recovery. Understanding the nature of the addiction is the beginning of living in the solution.

Fatal

People who are overweight, who purge, and/or who are anorexic tend to have a shorter life span. The truth is, we can still know that and still engage in the behavior due to denial, another characteristic of food addiction discussed earlier. I believe that the "cause of death" listed on most death certificates in the United States is inaccurate and should actually be listed as "[consequences of] food addiction." Instead, we see diseases of the heart (i.e., cardiovascular diseases, stroke, heart attack [cardiorespiratory failure]) and some cancers (i.e., pancreatic cancer, colorectal cancer), diabetes, infection, or autoimmune illness. The overuse of sugar prevents the body from protecting itself from the vectors of disease.[36]

The line between good health and poor health is invisible. The price the food addict pays is usually over a long period of time because the diseases created by food addiction are those with a long incubatory period. The clinical symptoms are usually not seen until substantial damage has been done. This long period adds to the addict's denial. The addict thinks, *See, I'm getting away with it (eating the way I do, eating the junk I eat, starving all day and bingeing at night, etc.), my health is okay, my energy is okay, my brain function is fine, maybe my weight is okay.* That's another lie of the disease.

Food addiction *is* a terminal illness. If a person with food addiction does not become abstinent, they will die of a complication, because they are not clear about what they suffer from. They keep trying, unsuccessfully, to work on their weight and never encounter an effective treatment for food addiction.

What's even more alarming with regard to this "fatal" characteristic of food addiction is that it can progress to helplessness and hopelessness, which can lead to suicide. There is an increased rate of suicide among teens,[37] which can be connected to this demographic's increased use of drugs, but as a society, we don't really consider the role that failed attempts at controlling eating problems play in teen suicide—i.e., overeating, bulimia, and anorexia, which leads them to depression and worse. Likewise, some fatal car accidents can be attributed to drugs or alcohol in the driver's system, but the driver's sugar levels are never taken into consideration. Also, how many accidents or near accidents were caused by someone who was eating while driving? We'll never know, but I suspect the number is larger than anyone would think.

Active food addiction is a living death—the living death of being obsessed with food and being unable to manage life's challenges and problems.

DID YOU KNOW?

Do you remember Terri Schiavo? Terri was the young woman who went into an irreversible vegetative state in 1990. The legal case between her husband who wanted to remove her feeding tube and her parents who wanted life-support measures to continue brought much media attention. However, little or no attention was given to the reason Terri was in that state in the first place. She had out-of-control bulimia. It became so severe that the purging eventually deprived her heart of the necessary levels of potassium and her heart stopped beating. Although the paramedics were able to get her heart beating again, it was too late; she had suffered irreversible brain damage. Her death certificate did not indicate the cause of her death as a consequence of purging.

Two more sample cases of the fatal quality of food addiction include Anna Nicole Smith and Karen Carpenter. Anna Nicole Smith was a model and television personality who was known, in part, for her fluctuations in weight. Her addiction to drugs, which eventually killed her, had at its roots in weight control. She was using drugs to curb her appetite and keep her weight down. Karen Carpenter, the wonderful lead singer of The Carpenters, suffered from anorexia. At age thirty-two, her heart finally gave out after years of starving herself, and she died.

What Is Food Addiction?

65

> Overweight in her teenage years, the singer found that she could "control" her weight by starving herself, which eventually led to her being "out of control." So what at first seemed like a solution quickly became a problem—a terminal illness.
>
> And while these next examples don't fall into the same category as the three women mentioned above, they still illustrate the disastrous effects of eating sugar.
>
> Remember the chimpanzee, Travis, who brutally attacked his owner's neighbor and tore her face and hands off? That chimp had eaten a meal of fish and chips and then Carvel ice cream prior to the attack. Could such a crazy, unhealthy human diet creating ups (blood sugar spikes) and crashes (low blood sugar episodes) have caused his aggressive and out-of-control behavior? What about the shooting of Harvey Milk, a gay councilman in San Francisco, by a man who invoked the "Twinkie" defense and got his sentence reduced because he claimed that he was addicted to Twinkies and was suffering, at the time of the shooting, from a resultant hypoglycemic episode (like the chimp) and was acting out aggressively from his "old/primitive brain" because the thinking/decision-making/moral part of his brain was shut down because of the hypoglycemia? And the court bought his claim as being legitimate—because it was!

Tolerance and Progression

Building a *tolerance* is brain adaptation through the presence of high concentrations of mood-altering substances. When we ingest toxins and trigger substances and take large quantities of food into our bodies, our bodies go on "tilt"! In other words, our body penalizes us somehow. If we continue to put in these substances often enough, the body has no other choice but to metabolically adapt. Eventually, the body becomes dependent on them, because it has been forced to adjust to their intake. Then without them, a host of uncomfortable symptoms (withdrawal) are experienced. These symptoms are then relieved when these substances are again taken in. For the food addict, these substances are mostly refined carbohydrates and excess quantities of food.

The Big Book of Alcoholics Anonymous explains this well: We become "restless, irritable and discontent" until we get the substance. In the book *Food Addiction: The Body Knows,* Kay Sheppard writes:

> "For the food addict, as food intake increases, the physiological level of tolerance to binge foods increases. The body depends on the presence of refined carbohydrates and develops the need for greater quantities.

As time goes on, it takes more to get the job done. Early in the progression small amounts provide the desired effect. As time passes it begins to take much more to give the food addict relief. Increased tolerance demands increased intake of binge foods. There is not enough binge food in the world to satisfy the body's demands. *One bite is too many, a thousand is not enough*, for the food addict caught in the pain of addiction."[38]

Do keep in mind that, as you read this discussion, I am talking about physiology. This is a developing biological dependence, and although the psychological/emotional dependence grows with it, it is not the operative force.

The progression of food addiction is also similar to other addictions. It may begin with occasional eating or fasting for relief and then proceed to preoccupation with food, weight, and image; constant dieting or bingeing; deception; loss of interest, loss of control; and physical, spiritual and emotional deterioration. Like with the example of Karen Carpenter on page 64, what was once the solution is now the problem.

Addiction, like other major illnesses, progresses unless it is treated. At some point, the addict experiences total loss of control. This is where almost all of their life is reduced to and centers on "feeding" their addiction, or dieting, constantly involved in "fat madness." It takes over. They are now totally controlled by the addictive process and their addictive personality. This stage occurs because addiction works so well at producing pain, fear, shame, loneliness, and anger. It becomes too much for the person to handle, and they start to break down.

As the addict continues to seek relief from these feelings through eating, purging or starving, they continue to get worse to the point where they do not know how to function anymore and work just to survive. By the next stage, acting out no longer produces much pleasure, but there is a heavy burden of pain from which to escape. Now the addict has to use larger amounts or act out in more dangerous ways in an attempt just to get numb. For bulimics, the magic (purging) that seduced them into the addictive process does not work anymore.

As you've probably realized, to gain clarity around food addiction, we often relate this disease to our understanding of alcoholism. In alcoholism, we identify three stages: early, middle, and late stage. In the early and middle stages, we see a growing tolerance to alcohol. As tolerance develops, the alcoholic needs more and more to get the same desired effect. (That's what accounts for the progression of the illness.) In the late stage, however, there is *reverse tolerance.* It doesn't take much alcohol to get the alcoholic drunk. This is where the food addict departs from the alcoholic. In food addiction, there isn't any reverse tolerance. The food addict keeps going. Tolerance keeps building. The disease keeps progressing. That's why we sadly see bigger and bigger people. They can't stop eating. The purger (bulimic) needs more and more food and more and more purging to get rid of the excess food. The anorexic needs more and more starving.

One food addict describes the evidence of the progression of his food addiction in terms of how much time it was taking in his life. He says that when he was a young kid, it took very little, just the energy to sneak his food. Then he started dieting, and it took some time. Then he started dieting and failing, and his weight was increasing so he had to put a lot more energy into it. Eventually, it consumed his day.

Craving

We spent some time discussing this characteristic in Chapter 1, and we'll do so again throughout the book. What's important to note here is that once the craving has been triggered, obsession takes over. Craving is not a conscious or controllable choice; it is a biological process that takes place in the brain. When an addict has taken a triggering substance into their body, the obsession for "more" of the same or something related assumes control, as discussed next.

Obsession/Preoccupation

A great deal of time is spent thinking about food. Many of my clients have best described this as: "I can't think of anything else!" The mind can contain just so many thoughts. Even though it has a huge capacity, it isn't infinite. Once the thought about a binge food or bingeing begins, it fills every nook and cranny in the brain like butter on the proverbial English muffin. (Apologies for the food analogy.) There's no room for anything else because the brain is totally preoccupied.

Studies have shown that people with disturbed eating devote a great deal of time to thinking about food—often to the exclusion of friends, family, and other interests. Obsession with food becomes a way of life and the force of desire for food is irresistible. The addict becomes preoccupied with getting, preparing, and eating food. Food controls their thoughts and soon controls their actions.

In *Food Addiction*, Kay Sheppard explains her view of obsession in this manner: preoccupation with food is an early symptom of food addiction. Most kids spend some time peering into the refrigerator. The food-addicted child will spend an inordinate amount of time seeking, talking about, and involving herself with food. Movies mean popcorn, trips to the store include ice cream cones, Easter offers baskets of marshmallow chicks and chocolate bunnies, and Christmas and Thanksgiving entail huge amounts of traditional food. For food addicts, the holidays revolve around those special treats. Those in the throes of the disease are unable to assign any meaning other than eating to the activities of life.

The food addict sees life in relationship to the next opportunity to eat. Coffee is the "reward" for getting out of bed. Getting through the morning brings the reward of lunch. The afternoon is bearable because the afternoon snack and dinner await. Then there is evening, blessed evening, when serious eating takes place. Evenings are free time for lots of bingeing without interruption. A 1999 publication from the American College Health Association titled *Eating Disorders: What Everyone Should Know* states:

> "People with food addiction spend a lot of time thinking about eating, food, weight, and body image—they may count and recount the calories in their meals, weigh themselves many times a day, and place themselves on severely restrictive diets, regardless of their weight. They often "feel fat" when their weight is normal or abnormally low, or feel uncomfortable after consuming a normal-size or small meal. Generally, they categorize foods as "good" or "bad", and make judgments about themselves based on how well they control what they eat. Believing that others are judging them based on their control of food, they frequently feel anxious eating when people are around."[39]

Note how the addiction has taken over everyday life and normal functioning—unmanageable and chaotic.

Compulsion

Like obsession/preoccupation, the best description of *compulsion* comes from clients who have experienced it: *I can't do anything else!* The dictionary defines *compulsion* as a strong, usually irresistible impulse to perform an act, especially one that is irrational or contrary to one's will. That's why "willpower" doesn't and can't work to control compulsion. Someone who is experiencing compulsion is up against a biochemical process.

Compulsions can be thought of as behaviors that serve to relieve the anxiety caused by the obsessive thoughts. The cycle begins with *craving* (as a physiological phenomenon), which sets in motion the preoccupation, or obsession, with eating and then the irresistible impulse to act out with the food and ends with the act of eating/bingeing (which may require purging if that's what the food addict does), which then reduces the preoccupation and satisfies the cravings.

Time Wasted

A great deal of time is spent engaging in the addictive behavior: Acting out the compulsion—i.e., eating, eating and purging, or restricting. The food addict is consumed with planning the binge, spending time in supermarkets, cooking, lying in wait (weight) to be alone, hiding their addictive behaviors and the consequences, lying to themselves and others, surreptitious visits to doctors and dentists, perhaps the gym—not to mention the time spent attending various diet programs and nutritionists and scoping out the bathrooms in every venue.

Loss of Control

Once the food addict starts eating, there is no way to predict how much will be eaten, how long it will take, or how it will end—either with passing out (some think of it as just going to sleep, but it is technically passing out), calling 911, or purging. Once an episode of eating starts, the food addict is no longer in control (the addiction is), and the eating will run its course. That's why most food addicts find it easier to *not* start eating. Trying to avoid out-of-control eating, they often successfully restrict during the day (which is easier because of the day's distractions), but then lose the battle with dinner and going on into the middle of night and ending in one of the ways mentioned above. With regard to loss of control, Anne Katherine, in *Anatomy of a Food Addiction: The Brain Chemistry of Overeating,* says the following:

> "Loss of control can mean difficulty stopping eating once it's started. Or it can mean that strong urges [cravings] to eat are difficult to resist. We get a picture in our heads of a certain food and feel driven to obtain it and eat it. The drive is so powerful and yet so nearly unconscious that we may in some ways not even be aware of it, even though it propels us to figure out how to get the food and get it in our mouths."[40]

Loss of control is evidenced by unsuccessful efforts to cut down or stop the behavior. Further evidencing the loss of control are more diligent attempts at control, including purchasing over-the-counter diet pills, fat blockers, shakes to curb the appetite by filling up, and/or liquid meals; getting a doctor to prescribe medications to diminish appetite (dangerous ones at that); using antidepressants and amphetamines, which diminish appetite as a side effect; purging either by vomiting, using laxatives, enemas, or excessive exercising (either in a gym or running); and of course, now the latest (desperate and drastic) approach/ fad, gastric bypass surgery or lap band surgery. Some people (women more often than men) start drinking alcohol or using drugs (i.e., cocaine or methamphetamines) to kill their appetite but then end up with a serious alcohol or drug addiction. Clearly, the lengths to which the food addict will go to achieve some semblance of control are far-reaching and often dangerous.

Additionally, loss of control can be evidenced by choosing to eat only particular types of foods. Most often chosen are sugary foods and drinks such as candy, cake, ice cream, sodas, and juices; refined carbs, including breads, pastas, sugary cereals, doughnuts, bagels, and rolls; or fatty foods/ salty foods (crunchy snack foods and fast foods), or by eating excessive quantities of food (or, as we say, *volumizing*). Some food addicts who try to eat "healthy" evidence a loss of control by overeating healthy foods. Some who claim to be in recovery because they are following a plan do not adhere to the portions designated and are in powerful denial as a result; the truth is they are *not* abstinent.

Another example of loss of control is eating at inappropriate times or places. *Grazing* is a fairly new word in our vocabulary; it describes the act of eating all the time. (In our society, more and more people eat in this out-of-control manner, which is why we need a word to describe

What Is Food Addiction?

it.) Grazing behaviors can include having a snack or another meal after a meal, having meals in between meals, and, when at home, continuously going back and forth to the kitchen. Other examples include eating at places where it's not permitted (e.g., at work); sneaking food in situations or settings where eating is not the norm; keeping food in a desk drawer at work where eating is not acceptable; or keeping food in your bedroom or bathroom and waiting for the "coast to be clear" (e.g., waiting for family members to fall asleep); or going against one's values or standards to get a "fix."

With regard to going against one's values, Anne Katherine states in her book *Anatomy of a Food Addiction*:

> "The drive [compulsion] may be so strong that we lie or manipulate others in order to satisfy it. We may lie, even though we are deeply religious or spiritual and fastidiously honest in all other areas of our lives. It's the crossing of our own moral boundaries that is a hallmark of addiction. The urge [craving] to eat is so strong we'll defy our own moral standards."[41]

Eating while shopping at the supermarket is good example of not being in control enough to wait, at least until after checkout. The addiction is driving the behavior, and it can be downright dangerous in many cases. Anne Katherine points out:

> "Yet another instance of loss of control is taking extreme measures to obtain a particular food, even possible risking injury to get it. To risk an accident by veering across three lanes of traffic because the urge (craving) for a sweet is so strong you can't waste time driving another half-block and turning at the light, or dipping into your lap for a potato chip while driving 55 miles an hour on the interstate, or getting dressed at 10 p.m. to drive through rainy, slick streets to get a sweet—these are all signs that food is in control, not you."

On some level, the food addict knows that these out-of-control eating behaviors are strange, harmful, or dangerous—yet they can't stop. This is loss of control. Like all aspects of food addiction, it is a thief because a great deal of time is spent engaging in the behavior (see "Time Wasted" on page 69).

Physical Dependency/Withdrawal Symptoms

When the body has become physically dependent on mood-altering substances (including certain foods as I've been discussing), withholding the food or eating behavior results in withdrawal symptoms. The common ones experienced or that might come to mind in no particular order, include the following:

- Headaches

- Dizziness/light-headedness

- Nausea

- Mood swings/moodiness (wide fluctuations of mood in very brief periods of time)

- Irritability

- Depression

- Restlessness/agitation/ nervousness/anxiety/ jumpiness/panic attack(s)/ heart palpitations/ hyperactivity

- Tiredness/drowsiness

- Thirst

- Salt craving

- Blurred vision

- Itching

- Tinnitus

- Sweating

- Tingling sensations

- Sleep disturbances (both insomnia and early waking)

- Digestive problems

- Appetite disturbances

- Short attention span

What Is Food Addiction?

- Cravings—for sweets and/or refined carbs (cravings may be so intense that the food addict wants to eat anything not nailed down; don't give in; they will pass in four and a half days)

- Paranoid ideation

- Brain dysfunction—memory/loss, lapses, impaired abstract cognitive functioning, fogginess, cloudiness, fuzzy brain, confusion spaciness, thinking not clear (temporary)

- Hunger/starving

A person in withdrawal may experience some or all of these symptoms at varying levels of intensity. It's important to understand that if withdrawal symptoms are occurring, you are in the presence of addiction. If the food plan in Chapter 11 were to identify broccoli as a trigger to craving and you therefore eliminated broccoli, you would *not* experience broccoli withdrawal. There is nothing in broccoli that taps into the brain's reward circuit to create physical dependency—ergo, no withdrawal symptoms. See the additional discussion of withdrawal symptoms in Part Two: The Solution: Abstinence.

WITHDRAWING FROM TRIGGER FOODS

When certain foods are eliminated from our bodies, we experience withdrawal symptoms. These symptoms will disappear quickly if we consume the trigger foods during the withdrawal stage. However, they will recur when those foods are eliminated again. The symptoms of withdrawal will only truly stop when the withdrawal process is complete, which is typically in four to five days. Think of it this way: Have you ever had a hangover? A hangover is, in fact, a symptom of withdrawal from alcohol. A known "remedy" for a hangover is to take drink ("hair of the dog"). It stops the withdrawal symptom by reintroducing the drug to the body so that the body is no longer in withdrawal. That's what happens when a trigger food is consumed during withdrawal.

Behavioral Changes

Behavioral changes include withdrawing from social, occupational, and/ or recreational activities. The more the food addiction progresses, the more the food addict withdraws. The eating/not eating/purging behavior becomes the primary relationship of the food addict to the exclusion of other people and sacrifices all that is good in life. Values, attitudes, and beliefs are eroded.

Distorted Body Image/Poor Body Image

Having a distorted or poor body images means that the food addict finds some part(s) of their body unacceptable. Generally speaking, it is usually dissatisfaction with one's body's size or shape. In particular, it's the belief is that they are not thin enough. To determine that a part of one's body is "too" anything, it has to be compared to the standard we've been taught to believe is acceptable. Of course, the media, films, celebrities, models, and society in general are rife with the message that thin is success, smart, and the only acceptable standard. Young, impressionable girls (mostly), unsure of their persona, buy in to the message, and families (often parents) can support the unhealthy message and launch their beloved child into looking for "magic." They also have peers who are experiencing the same messaging and to whom they compare themselves, and of course, they rarely "measure up." Weight issues may be showing because this young person, like any other "normal" young child or preteen, is eating poorly, and the body is responding with excess weight. But that's not what gets focused on.

A 2015 study as reported by Common Sense Media, revealed that 80 percent of ten-year-old girls have been on a diet. The authors of the study stated, "Furthermore, this horrifying new research found that more than half of girls and one-third of boys ages six to eight want thinner bodies. These statistics are far from new."[42] According to NOW.org, 40 to 60 percent of elementary school girls are concerned about their weight or about becoming "too fat." Moreover, 46 percent of nine- to eleven-year-olds are "sometimes" or "very often" on diets, and 82 percent of their families are '"sometimes" or "very often" on diets. NOW.org further states that by the time these girls reach their teens, 50 percent are "self-conscious" about their bodies and another 26.2 percent reports being "dissatisfied."[43]

So many studies have been made similar to the above, and the results interpreted in many ways, many concluding that diets don't work (we

What Is Food Addiction?

lose weight and then gain back what was lost and more) and that we live in a culture that is distorted and damaged by our pursuit of thinness.

In the 1970s and 1980s, University of Toronto psychologists Janet Polivy and C. Peter Herman studied dieters who had learned to view eating as a lifelong exercise in restraint. Polivy and Herman concluded that dieting not only taught their subjects to ignore physical feelings but disrupted their ability to normally handle emotions. Their subjects could not tell when they were hungry and when they were anxious or sad. They ate when they were anxious and ate when they were disappointed; they used food to express—and suppress—their feelings. "The upshot of such misuse of food...seems to be not only losing touch with internal signals for behavior," Polivy and Herman wrote," but in some sense, with oneself."[44]

So, the questions become—Why do we set our children up for this misery? Why do we allow them to hurt themselves with food—to end up feeling unacceptable? Why are *we* caught up with eating in a way that our bodies respond with unwanted and unnecessary weight? The answer, as you can guess, is food addiction! It has made us lose all reason when it comes to eating—for ourselves and our children.

For every mother who has a daughter and looks in the mirror and judges/criticizes her own body, there's a young girl standing behind her, learning to do the same. This has been going on for generations. Children who have negative body images don't love and accept themselves as they are, and often, they learned this from Mom and Dad. This unhealthy attitude doesn't allow for the exploration of important aspects of growing up, such as developing good friendships, growing more independent from parents, and challenging themselves physically and mentally.

FAT IS NOT A FEELING

When a woman says, "I feel fat," she's basically saying, "There's something wrong with me" or "I'm defective!" Our society's message about thinness being the only acceptable standard leads to the mindset that a woman's worth is in her appearance—that it's her most important aspect. And if her body doesn't measure up to the cultural ideal, then she must devote much energy to pursuing the ideal. This pursuit of thinness perpetuates the belief that weight is the issue and that losing it is the solution. This results in attempts at starving/restricting—and if successful, moving into the arena of anorexia, and if not successful, maybe moving into the arena of bulimia (vomiting, laxatives, excessive exercising, enemas, crazy eating patterns/restricting and bingeing). And if none of the above is an option, the medical establishment provides "solutions" in the form of gastric bypass surgery, the sleeve, or lap-band. All of this thinking and focusing on the weight as the problem keeps everyone's attention off the true problem: food addiction.

A recent study found that many women would rather have cancer than be fat. How crazy and sad is that?! Again the problem here is that we are only focusing on the symptom, not the cause. The weight is the symptom—*not* the problem. We live in a society that tells us to take a pain reliever if we have a headache, antacids if we have heartburn, Alka-Seltzer for a hangover, and Metformin for type 2 diabetes. We are taught to deal with symptoms not the problem. If we're always treating the symptom(s), we aren't looking for the cause.

It's easier to say, "I feel fat" than experience what the real feelings are. If I "feel fat," my go-to is another diet; with any other feeling (scared, disappointed, angry, etc.), I might have to deal with another person—too scary! More proof that fat is not a feeling is that feelings are on the inside, and fat is on the outside.

A Disturbed Sense of Self and Inability to Identify Feelings

A disturbed sense of self can leave a person without a sense of identity, so the food addiction *becomes* the identity. Food addicts can wear their addiction like a shield to keep themselves from being overwhelmed by everyday life stressors and/or painful memories. The addiction is all consuming and leaves no room for the emergence of the individual's personality and potential. However, it does have its purposes. It satisfies certain needs:

- **Power and control**—Since food addicts feel powerless in the world, eating behavior becomes an area in their life they can control. Food can be used to set boundaries with others: "*You can't control me, I will overeat (or not eat at all).*" The food-related behavior can be used to manipulate the behavior of others.

What Is Food Addiction?

- **Numb feelings**—The family environment was the "classroom" in which the food addict learned that painful feelings must be avoided. The child learned to pretend that everything was fine, while hiding their true feelings. They learned not to trust others and to get rid of feelings by bingeing, purging, or restricting food.

- **Approval and attention**—Food addicts are often perfectionists and will go out of their way to please others. In surrendering their sense of self, they use food to obliterate their "self."

DOES FOOD ADDICTION DIFFER FROM EATING DISORDERS?

Is there a difference between food addiction and eating disorders? *Eating disorders* is a term that was created to describe a set of extreme eating behaviors that are on the far ends of the spectrum of eating behavior, occurring due to faulty brain feedback circuitry. One end sees the restriction of eating (anorexia) and the other end sees overeating (binge-eating disorder) and overeating with purging (bulimia). A set of criteria as described in the *DSM-V,* the diagnostic manual for psychiatric disorders, has been developed to determine if the eating behavior belongs to these described conditions:

- **Anorexia nervosa** requires that an individual refuse to maintain body weight at or above a minimally normal body weight for age and height; that there is an intense fear of gaining weight even though the person is underweight; there is a disturbance in the way one's body weight or shape is experienced by the individual and, in postmenarcheal females, there is an absence of at least three menstrual cycles. (The more weight the anorexic loses, the more their mind becomes distorted and they can't see themselves clearly. They see themselves as being overweight and continue their commitment to limit their intake of food or starve completely.)

- **Bulimia nervosa** involves recurrent episodes of binge eating, a sense of lack of control, overeating during the episode, and recurrent compensatory behaviors to prevent weight gain, such as self-induced vomiting, misuse of laxatives, diuretics, enemas, overexercising, etc. This cycle of behavior must occur, on average, at least twice a week for three months. In addition, the individual's self-evaluation is unduly influenced by body shape and weight.

Finally, there are variations of the above eating disorders that may meet criteria under the category of "**Eating Disorders Not Otherwise Specified.**" *Compulsive overeating* involves the binge behavior with the absence of compensatory behaviors, and thus fit diagnostically in this category. This applies to both males and females.

When one initially attempts to describe an eating disorder, topics such as weight, physical symptoms, and food intake or the lack thereof are discussed. It is imperative that the term *addiction* comes to mind and enters into the discussion. However, eating disorders are not actually about food. They are about an unhealthy relationship between an individual and a mood-altering process involving food. Eating disorders are addictive illnesses and are progressive in nature.

Food addiction can take several forms: anorexia, bulimia, and compulsive overeating. People with these disorders engage in behaviors such as bingeing, purging, restricting, overeating, calorie counting, excessive exercise, abuse of diuretics, etc., in order to feel "normal" and/or to alter their moods. Physiologically, "pleasure foods" such as sugars, sugar substitutes, starches, and fats can temporarily alter one's mood and outlook on problems. Thus, the food addict tends to gravitate toward these types of food, which can include cake, candy, cookies, bread, pasta, nuts and cheeses.

Please note that whenever a discussion of any of these eating problems notes "a mood change" or "alter their mood"—they are talking about brain chemistry. Mood is a function of chemicals in the brain being stable with even mood or the brain being provoked by a triggering substance(s)—sugar, substitutes, flour, carbs that quickly raise blood sugar levels, wheat, volume, caffeine, excess fat, alcohol/drugs/nicotine, etc.

It's useful to think of the **"Coin Principle of Food Addiction."** Eating problems all exist on the same "coin"—but take different sides. The food addict who overeats lives on one side of the coin, while the anorexic (who starves) occupies the opposite side. The bulimic, who can be thought of as the failed anorexic (wanting to not eat, but unable to stave off the rule of her cravings and finding the taking in of the food intolerable—purges)

What Is Food Addiction?

79

and lives on the edge of the coin between the two sides. But, in the final analysis, it's all food addiction.

Historically, the term *eating disorders* was used to encompass anorexia *and* bulimia. Binge eating was not considered a *DSM-III* diagnosis disorder until 1994. The concept of food addiction, as it is used here, differs from the concept of eating disorders because the addiction dynamic is considered causal. A disorder may occur independent of an addiction. This is determined by deciding whether loss of control over food intake is the precipitating factor. If, for example, the motivation for the disorder is fear of fat, then this fear translates into uncontrolled limitation of food intake, then food addiction is said to be present. As discussed by Dr. Dena Cabrera in *Thin to Win:*

> "If the psychiatric disorder of Anorexia Nervosa had to be reduced to one word, it would be starvation. Those with this disorder starve themselves to dangerously thin levels, at least 15% of what would be considered a normal weight. Often, anorexia starts innocently enough: an adolescent or young woman wants to lose a few pounds, so she starts dieting. Unfortunately, she probably does not embark on a "smart" course of action: eat a little less, move a little more. Instead, influenced by the multi-billion-dollar diet industry, she opts for the latest fad diet that guarantees amazing results with very little effort. She starts the diet and probably loses weight fairly quickly; the fact that it is undoubtedly water weight isn't the issue. She feels good about the results and even starts receiving compliments about how good she looks."[45]

Cabrera goes on to describe the girl's descent into starvation—and, before she knows it, she is genuinely compulsive about the behavior.

People with anorexia may eventually develop a true lack of appetite, but for the most part, the illness entails not a loss of appetite, but rather a strong desire to control it. Anorexics deny their bodies of food even when driven by hunger pangs, and they obsess about food all day long. Anorexics are afraid of food as well as of themselves. What begins as a determination to lose weight continues and progresses to a morbid fear of gaining back any lost weight and becomes a relentless pursuit of thinness. Being thin, which translates to "being in control" becomes the most important thing in the world. The operative belief is "never thin enough"—but for what?

Anorexics fear that they will become fat, weak, undisciplined, and unworthy. With the progression of the illness, eventually there are no longer fattening foods, but simply the idea that any food is fattening. Dieting/starving becomes a purpose and a "safe place to go." It's a world created by the anorexic to cope with feelings of meaninglessness, low self-esteem, failure, and the need to be successful, unique, special, and in control.

The problem is that this description and understanding of eating problems excludes what we've been talking about—biology, biochemical changes, and withdrawal symptoms (which are grounded in/hallmark of addiction).

This way of looking at food addiction, as "eating disorders," excludes people who suffer from out-of-control eating behaviors but do not fit the established criteria—e.g., someone who restricts eating during the day but eats volumes at night or someone who finds the "answer" in "grazing" all day long. Food addicts often experience different phases of the three eating disorder behaviors. Some with anorexia become compulsive eaters or begin purging; some with bulimia fall into anorexic patterns; still others may move completely through all phases of food addiction over a period of time. Some food addicts maintain average weight, never binge eat, but purge after meals, or starve/restrict, but not to the point of being anorexic. Additionally, food addicts may experience some form of alcohol or other drug abuse as part of the eating-disordered process. As I have discussed and will discuss further on, food addicts also suffer from distorted body image and low self-esteem, and a significant percentage have experienced sexual abuse in their childhood.

Food addictions are about being thin and feeling fat . . . or being overweight and minimizing it, telling oneself, "I'm not all that fat." Food addictions are about what society tells us we ought to be, that there's no such thing as "too thin," so we're always falling short of the mark. Food addictions are cunning, baffling, and powerful. They control our lives, even when we feel we're in control. The problem is, we're never "thin enough" but for what we don't know. Or there's never enough food to fill the emptiness inside us.

Food addictions are about what we're afraid of, how inadequate we feel, how much pressure we're under, and how overwhelmed we get.

What Is Food Addiction?

81

They're about the pain we push away with food or the depriving of ourselves of healthy eating. They're about shame, about anger, about all the other feelings we refuse to face. They're about filling a void by avoiding the real issues.

But before we can get to the reasons we became food addicts, we have to arrest our self-destructive behavior. We have to change our relationship with food, so it won't continue to rule our lives. Thankfully, there is a solution, which I discuss in Part Two.

ANALYSIS OF FOOD ADDICTION BEHAVIORS

- An **anorexic** experiences a Secret Sense of Pride (power, control, which is why it's so difficult to treat).
- A **bulimic** experiences a Secret Sense of Shame.
- An **overeater** experiences a Secret Sense of Hopelessness.

Even if they went unnoticed before, eating problems eventually begin to interfere in various aspects of a person's life. As the addiction progresses, the problem eater socializes less frequently with family and friends, and may begin to lose time from work or school. She becomes preoccupied with thoughts of food and body image, which may eventually reach a point where these thoughts utterly dominate the day. Left untreated, the addiction leads to serious physical and emotional complications. The following table is a helpful way of seeing the physical, psychological, and medical implications of the symptoms of food addiction.

TABLE 2.1. ANOREXIA, BULIMIA, AND COMPULSIVE OVEREATING OVERVIEW

ANOREXIA	BULIMIA	COMPULSIVE OVEREATING
Definition		
Marked by a refusal to maintain a body weight at or above a minimally normal level for age and height. Characterized by at least 15% below normal body weight, an intense fear of fat, becoming obese; repeated claims of "feeling fat" even when obviously underweight. Characterized by an obsession with thinness that results in self-starvation. Weight loss due to severe fasting and/or vomiting. May include abuse of diuretics*, laxatives*, amphetamines, thyroid medication, exercise, and running.	Characterized by repeated cycles of out-of-control eating followed by attempts to control weight/prevent weight gain through purging behaviors in forms of vomiting, diuretics*, laxatives*, enemas* cathartics*, amphetamines, cocaine, diet pills, insulin, over-exercising, running, dieting/fasting.	Characterized by eating binges, rapid eating, inconspicuous eating, and secret eating. There are feelings of loss of control, the inability to terminate the binges, and episodic binge eating. Diets and fasting cycles to control weight. Some abuse of amphetamines and over-the-counter weight control drugs, laxatives*, enemas*, diuretics*. Compulsive overeating may occur with or without bingeing. Continuous eating may go on all day long, sometimes becoming more intense in the evening hours. This is the most common type of eating problems
Onset		
Any age, often at puberty (12) to late adolescence (18). Can continue indefinitely. Predominately female but does occur in males.	Any age, often during early adolescence to mid-twenties. Can continue undetected indefinitely. Often after weight loss or dieting attempts.	Appears in all ages, often not recognized until adulthood. Starts in childhood although symptom of overweight may not appear until the person is older. Can continue indefinitely.
Onset sometimes associated with stressful life situation.	Feeling guilty and ashamed of bingeing can cause the food addict to purge to avoid weight gain. This starts the cycle of bingeing and purging that becomes an addiction. Predominately females but occurs in males more often than has been previously reported.	Affects females and males equally, but sports may conceal the weight issue in young males.

Physical Signs

Small, consistent weight loss progressing to severe unrelenting weight loss—25% to 50% of body weight.	Often, but not always, maintain "ideal" or slightly less than ideal body weight or overweight.	Usually overweight or obese.
Dry Skin and hair.	Brittle hair/nails.	Progressive weight gain with periods of weight loss.
Cold hands and feet.	Acne-like skin, dry, flaky.	Menstrual cycle may be present, irregular or absent (amenorrhea).
Thinning hair/hair loss.	Difficulty sleeping.	Having difficulty exercising because of excess weight.
General weakness, fatigue, reduced energy expenditure due to malnutrition.	Vomiting blood.	
Fainting spells.	Tiredness and apathy.	
Hyperactivity.	Hypothermia.	
Modified sense of taste, leading to changes in appetite.	Brachycardia (slow heartbeat).	
Constipation due to low-calorie and low-fiber intake.	Hypotension (low blood pressure).	
Digestive problems—slower emptying of food from the stomach, which can cause bloating and early satiety during a meal.	Lanugo (fine, soft body hair).	
Complaints of nausea, bloating, or constipation after eating normal amounts of food.	Low body temperature.	
Insomnia/sleep disturbance/interrupted sleep patterns.	Tooth decay, erosion of tooth enamel, leading to cavities, toothaches, swollen gums, gum disease (gingivitis) caused by acid in the mouth from vomiting.	
Loss of menstrual periods (amenorrhea)—related to overall malnutrition.	Receding gums.	
Development of soft body hair (lanugo) on face, arms, legs, stomach), grayish skin.	Physical harm to self.	
Sunken eyes, dark circles under eyes.	Tremors.	
Brittle hair.	Stomach pain.	
Leg cramps.	Constipation—long-term problems with bowel movements because of laxative abuse.	
	Indigestion.	
	Muscle weakness, fatigue, exhaustion due to malnutrition.	
	Split lips, cold sores, mouth sores.	

ANOREXIA	BULIMIA	COMPULSIVE OVEREATING
Physical Signs (continued)		
Frequent headaches.	Sore throat.	
Impaired concentration.	Swollen glands in neck and cheeks (parotid glands)—"chipmunk look."	
Loss of muscle, body fat, and other body proteins due to inadequate calorie and fiber intake.	Calluses on backs of hands.	
Heart tremors.	Broken blood vessels.	
Shortness of breath.	Harsh/hoarse voice.	
Depressed immune system resulting in increased susceptibility to infections.	Frequent weight change (loss or gain).	
Water retention.	Menstrual cycle may be present, irregular or absent (amenorrhea).	
Stress fractures.		
Ketosis (severe chemical imbalances).		
Weakness of the heart muscle that can lead to death.		
Psychological Signs		
Wish to reduce weight by all means.	Excessive concern/preoccupation with weight, body image, shape, eating/food.	Excessive concern about weight.
Preoccupation with food, calories, nutrition, and/or cooking, exercise.	Compulsion to reduce weight by all means.	Often eats alone because of shame or embarrassment.
Obsessing about food but not eating.	Expressing guilt or shame about overeating.	Feelings of depression, disgust, shame, or guilt after eating/overeating.
Low self-esteem.	Secrecy-dishonesty-sometimes leading to stealing.	Becoming secretive about binges.
Denial of hunger.	Increase in impulsive behavior.	Planning binges or opportunities to binge.
Social withdrawal, depression, moodiness.	Feeling out of control.	Feeling out of control.
Emotional withdrawal.	Depressive moods.	Being profoundly unhappy with body image and may avoid even pleasurable activities.
Perfectionism, obsessive thinking, anxiety and shyness.	Mood swings.	Stealing food.
Refusal to admit eating patterns are abnormal.		

Views issues in polarities—black-and-white thinking.	Loneliness, shame, feelings of emptiness and self-deprecating thoughts following the eating binges (although may pretend to be cheerful).	Lying about food.
Depression, anxiety. Distorted body image (seeing oneself as fat even when emaciated).	Most commonly, depression is secondary to feeling out of control and helpless.	Use of food to relieve uncomfortable feelings. Uneasiness and irritability in situations where food is not available.
Intense fear of weight gain.	Primary depression usually occurs when the binge/purge cycle is interrupted.	Obsessive thoughts about food.
Extreme concern with body weight and shape.	A tertiary interaction is possible; interrupting bulimic symptoms may uncover a depressive state.	Feeling ashamed. Antisocial behavior.
Frequent mood swings.	Avoiding social invitations because of food that might be served.	Preoccupation with the thoughts of food and eating or not eating, dieting, body weight.
Social isolation—from family and friends.	Isolation from friends and family.	Experiences hunger, but binge-eating behavior often unconnected to this feeling.
Overly perfectionistic attitude. The "model child."	Possible drug and alcohol abuse.	Feeling irritable when withdrawing from a binge or trying to diet, and depressed and sleepy immediately after overeating.
Feelings of helplessness and hopelessness.	Purging after a binge (vomiting, laxatives, diet pills, diuretics, excessive exercise or fasting).	Accompanied by an awareness that the eating pattern is abnormal and fear of not being able to stop voluntarily.
Separation/individuation problems between mother/daughter or father/son.	Extreme concern with body weight and shape and appearance; feelings of self-worth based on weight.	Depressed mood and self-deprecating thoughts following the eating binges.
Frequent mood swings.	Preoccupation with the thoughts of food & eating or not eating and dieting.	Feelings of loss of control, the inability to terminate the binges, and episodic binge eating.
Avoids adult responsibilities and perpetuates child-like dependency.	Bingeing accompanied by an awareness that the eating pattern is abnormal and fear of not being able to stop voluntarily.	Distorted body image. Frequent mood swings.
Less sexually active. Avoids sexual relationships.	Feeling out of control when eating and unable to stop binges.	Less sexually active. Sexual relationships are consciously desired, but seem to be unconsciously avoided.
Often does not act out or abuse drugs or alcohol.	Intense fear of fatness. Great concern about body weight.	Drug and alcohol abuse, compulsive spending, gambling is not uncommon.
Avoids decision making/indecisiveness.	Feeling uncomfortable eating in front of others.	Eating to escape from emotions (anxiety, worry, or emotional pain).
Believing that others are judging them based on their control of food, they frequently feel anxious about eating when people are around.		
Making judgments about themselves based on how well they control what they eat.		

ANOREXIA	BULIMIA	COMPULSIVE OVEREATING
Psychological Signs (continued)		
	Preoccupation with body image and appearance. Distorted body image. Extremely focused on how others perceive them. Life dominated by conflicts about eating. Low self-esteem. Sexually active. Sexual relations tend to be short term and have a superficial quality. Suicidal thoughts and often attempts. Kleptomania, gambling, drug and alcohol abuse, self-mutilation is often present. Believing that others are judging them based on their control of food, they frequently feel anxious about eating when people are around. Make judgments about themselves based on how well they control what they eat. A vulnerability and inability to express emotions, esp. anger, which tends to surface in adolescence due to demands of that period.	Low self-esteem. Self-esteem based on weight and control of eating. Fantasizing about being happier, more out-going when thin. Believing that others are judging them based on their control of food, they frequently feel uncomfortable, anxious about eating in front of others. Avoiding social invitations because of food that might be served. Trying to avoid physical activity or anything that might call attention to or increase own awareness of one's body. Make judgments about themselves based on how well they control what they eat. Intense fear of rejection related to weight. Putting off taking risks in life until thin. Feeling tormented by eating habits. Professional failures attributed to weight. Weight becomes focus of life. Intense fear of anger and conflict.
Food & Exercise Habits		
Dieting with relish when not overweight. Excessive exercising, being overly active. Frequently weighing oneself.	Strict dieting followed by eating binges. Frequent overeating, especially when distressed.	Eats much more rapidly than normal. Eats to the point of feeling uncomfortably full. Strict or frequent dieting followed by eating binges.

Use of laxatives and/or vomiting to control weight.	Eats very large meals, but without gaining weight.	Losing and regaining weight (weight cycling) or chronically dieting without losing weight.
Disappearance after meals, usually into bathroom (secret vomiting).	Disappearing (to bathroom) after a meal (secretive purging).	Frequent overeating or eating when not hungry especially when distressed.
Prefers to eat alone.	Becoming secretive about (hiding) binges and vomiting.	Hiding food from others.
Refusal to maintain body weight at or above a minimally normal weight for age and height.	Large quantities of food missing.	Recurrent episodes of binge eating (consumption of large amounts of food in short periods of time [15,000 calories in 1–2hrs.] often several times a day).
Purging (bulimic episodes).	Planning binges or opportunities to binge.	
Binge eating.	Repeated episodes of bingeing and purging.	
Preparation of elaborate meals for others.	Frequent dieting followed by bingeing.	Eating to the point of extreme discomfort.
Hoarding food.	Experiences hunger but eating behavior often unconnected to this feeling.	Night eating, secret eating, hurried eating, lying about eating or eating only small amounts when with others.
Hiding food.		
Throwing food away.	Recurrent episodes of binge eating (consumption of large amounts of food in short periods of time [15,000 calories in 1–2 hrs.] often several times a day).	
Rigidly avoiding specific foods or whole categories of food (dairy, meats, fats, etc.).		Eating little in public.
Refusing to eat, denying hunger, eating tiny portions of food.		Food is used for reward, nurturing and excitement.
Possessing in-depth knowledge of calories and fat in foods.		Concern over not having a specific food.
Consuming odd food combinations or large amounts of low-calorie condiments (e.g., mustard, vinegars).		
Exhibiting ritualistic eating behaviors, such as cutting foods into tiny bits or using special utensils or places each time when eating.		
Avoiding social invitations because of food that might be served.		
Frequently weighing oneself.		

ANOREXIA	BULIMIA	COMPULSIVE OVEREATING
	Family Patterns	
Often obesity in parents. Frequent preoccupation with food. Emotionally absent father. Mothers are rejecting, ambivalent, or overinvolved. Frequent denial. Enmeshed family—leads to a lack of privacy. Boundary problems—weak family boundaries. Need to appear as the perfect family: • Perfectionistic home in which questioning of parental authority or diverging from parental values is negatively reinforced. • Near obsessive attention is paid to social appearance and to the protection of the outside image of "the perfect family." Overprotective family. Rigid family system. Conflict avoidance. Separation – individuation problems: • Failure to develop autonomy from parents, especially the mother, due to parental intrusiveness and overcontrol. Parents rewarding the dependency of the child so that she develops a compliant false self—"a good girl"—as a defense against parental intrusiveness. Parental control constantly redefining the children's feelings and emotions to stay consistent with the family's values. High expectations and fostering of ambitions for external achievement.	Often obesity in parents. Frequent preoccupation with food. Frequent substance abuse. Frequent denial. Enmeshed family—lack of privacy. Boundary problems—weak family boundaries. Need to appear as the perfect family: • Perfectionistic home in which questioning of parental authority or diverging from parental values is negatively reinforced. • Near obsessive attention is paid to social appearance and to the protection of the outside image of "the perfect family." Overprotective family. Chaotic family—no rules. Frequent sexual abuse. Separation—individuation problems: • Failure to develop autonomy from parents, especially the mother, due to parental intrusiveness and overcontrol. • Parents rewarding the dependency of the child so that she develops a compliant false self—"a good girl"—as a defense against parental intrusiveness. Parental control constantly redefining the children's feelings and emotions to stay consistent with the family's values. Food is used for reward, nurturing and excitement. Alcohol or drug use.	Often obesity in parents. Frequent preoccupation with food. Frequent substance abuse. Frequent denial. Enmeshed family –lack of privacy. Boundary problems—weak family boundaries. Chaotic family—no rules. Frequent sexual abuse.

What Is Food Addiction?

Medical Consequences		
Shrunken organs. Bone mineral loss, leading to osteoporosis. Low body temperature. Low blood pressure. Slowed metabolism and reflexes. Irregular heartbeat, which can lead to cardiac arrest. High blood cholesterol levels (in this situation this does not signify a cholesterol problem and does not warrant a low cholesterol diet or medication). Fluid and mineral abnormalities.	Damage to the esophagus. Edema. Thyroid conditions. Lung irritation. Ulcers. Gastrointestinal disorders. Seizures. Stomach rupture. Diabetes. Damage to bowels, liver and kidneys. Electrolyte imbalance, which can lead to irregular heartbeat, and in some cases, heart damage and failure/cardiac arrest. Sleep disorders. Dehydration, which can lead to weakness, fainting, or kidney damage. Fainting or loss of consciousness, usually because of low blood pressure. Inflammation or tears of the esophagus, which may cause bloody vomit.	Diabetes mellitus/hypoglycemia. High cholesterol. Coronary artery disease/heart disease. Cerebrovascular disease. Fatigue. High blood pressure (hypertension). Hypothyroidism. Pulmonary disease. Asthma. Gastrointestinal (digestive) disorders. Gall bladder disease. Mobility problems. Degenerative joint disease. Joint disorders. Hormonal imbalances. Endocrine disorders. Fertility problems. Sleep apnea/sleep disorders. Sleep deprivation. Nutritional deficiencies. Cancer. Cushing's syndrome. Polycystic ovarian syndrome.
Death occurs primarily from consequences of starvation. Anorexia is one of the deadliest of these addictions—leading to death in up to 20% of those with the condition.	Death occurs primarily from electrolyte imbalance or hemorrhaging.	Death is due to weight gain, heart disease, stroke, diabetes.

* See "The Truth About Laxatives, Diuretics, and Ipecac Syrup" on page 90.

THE TRUTH ABOUT LAXATIVES, DIURETICS, AND IPECAC SYRUP

Laxatives appear to move food rapidly through the body and seem to relieve distention after bingeing. However, they do *not* prevent the calories in food from being absorbed by the body. Water and mineral losses are the only losses that immediately show up on the scale, but they will be regained when the behavior stops—the body replenishes them. Abuse or misuse of laxatives is dangerous because they leave the body dehydrated and upset the mineral balance; they damage the lining of the gastrointestinal tract and cause the bowels to get lazy. If the large intestines are not active, constipation results and laxative use increases, which is why laxatives can be habit forming.

Diuretics, aka water pills, also cause sudden weight loss by increasing urine output. Someone who believes this water loss is loss of fat may begin to use diuretics for the purpose of weight loss. In truth there is no fat loss, but rather dehydration, which is a serious condition, develops. Water pills also increase the loss of calcium, potassium, magnesium, and zinc from the tissues and blood. These trace elements are critical to the proper functioning of the body and their loss may cause cataclysmic organ failure. In the end, diuretics cause a rebound retention of sodium and water, which sensitizes the body to dietary changes even more.

Ipecac syrup, which is used to induce vomiting, has been linked to death in people with eating problems. The active ingredient, emetine, builds up in body tissues and can cause muscle or cardiac muscle weakness. Whether taken as a single large dose or repeated small doses, Ipecac is toxic and dangerous.

People with food addiction can experience a wide variety of symptoms, and many of the symptoms overlap. People with eating problems may deny they are hungry and may be preoccupied with thinness. They may base their self-esteem and self-respect on how much they weigh. The may engage in periodic eating binges, followed by feelings of guilt or remorse, and they may purge through vomiting, laxatives, diuretics, or excessive exercise or running.

What are the consequences of food addiction?

- Some will recover completely.

- Some will lead a borderline existence—marginal life.

- Some will die.

CHAPTER 3

Little Food Addict in Training
An Illustration of How
Food Addiction Develops

In this chapter, we'll explore the typical experiences the young food addict has with regard to her family system and demonstrate how deeply rooted the origins of food addiction are. We'll also touch upon the biological factors and underpinnings at work to unequivocally establish that a recovery approach (which you will learn about in Part 4) is *the* solution to food addiction. One's family system always plays a major role in the development of food addiction. Most people who suffer from food addiction report that they don't feel like they fit into their family unit. This is not to say that the family is to blame, but it sets the stage. The experiences in the family and how the child perceives those experiences is an important part of establishing the food addiction foundation.

> *"But such is the way of family: We are what they tell us we are,*
> *and part of life's great struggle, it seems,*
> *is to know oneself despite that imposing collective definition."*
> —ELIZABETH POLINER,
> *AS CLOSE TO US AS BREATHING*

So how does a person develop issues around eating—i.e., inappropriate eating, overeating, undereating, or purging—and issues with weight and appetite? Let's go back to the beginning and see how it happens. Let's "grow" a food addict. The only assumption we must make is that the person has a genetic predisposition to addiction as a result of the development of faulty feedback circuitry in the brain, as discussed in Chapter 1. When we experience pleasure, we want more; there is no "off switch."

CHARACTERISTICS OF A NEWBORN

First, let's assume that the baby is fed, dry, warm, and generally healthy. Now, let's take a look at an organic list of this newborn's characteristics:[46]

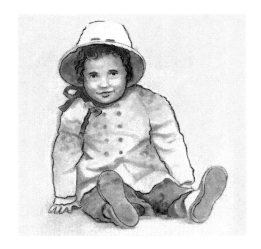

Precious/valuable	Loving	Curious/inquisitive	Undamaged
Imperfect	Loyal/Faithful	Outgoing/friendly/ gregarious (social)	Untarnished/unjaded
Trusting	Enthusiastic/Optimistic/ Positive/Hopeful	Natural relationship with food	Unexploited
Open			Pure/untainted
Receptive	Energetic/Spunky	Filled with feelings	Unstressed
Vulnerable/fragile	Has expectations	Lovable	Present/living in the moment
Safe	Eager	In touch with feelings	
Dependent	Clear-brained	Self-centered	Attention-seeking
Defenseless	No worries	Comfortable with self	Authentic/genuine
Alert/Focused/ Observant	No guilt	Unself-conscious	Resilient
	No resentments	Uninhibited	Persistent
Unguarded/ Uncensored	Non-judgmental	Sense of self	Instinctual/intuitive
	No prejudices	No fear/fearless	Impatient/impulsive
Demanding	No responsibilities	Adventurous/bold	No impulse control
Sensitive	Honest about feelings	Risk taker	No sense of time
Innocent/naive	Direct/straight-forward	Reckless	No sense of consequences
Impressionable/ Spongelike	Expressive/ Communicative	Happy/Joyful/Playful/	
Accepting	No masks	Carefree/Free- Spirited	Unique
Willing	Transparent	Infantile—childlike	Sense of wonder(ment)
Giving	Copycat	Perceptive	No boundaries
Adaptable	Teachable	Many needs and wants	Creative
Spontaneous	Responsive		Huge potential
Stubborn			

These characteristics are altered by genetic predisposition and family dysfunction, as we will begin to discuss. But first, let's look at the needs of a newborn.

BASIC CHILDHOOD NEEDS

Psychologist Abraham Maslow developed the psychological theory Maslow's Hierarchy of Needs in his 1943 work *A Theory of Human Motivation*. This theory suggests that people are motivated to fulfill their basic needs before they move on to other, more advanced needs. This hierarchy is often shown as a pyramid (see the graphic to follow), with the lowest levels representing the most basic needs, and the upper levels representing the more complex needs.

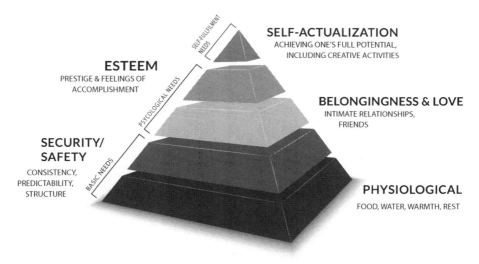

As we progress up the pyramid, needs become increasingly psychological and social. Soon, the need for love, friendship, and intimacy become important. Further up the pyramid, the need for personal esteem and feelings of accomplishment take priority. Maslow emphasized the importance of self-actualization, a process of growing and developing as a person in order to achieve individual potential. While there has been criticism of his theory that needs develop in a "hierarchy," the model does offer a useful way to categorize our needs. The list below includes general needs and those needs specific to childhood.

Physiological Needs

Basic physiological needs include breathing/air, food, water, clothing, good grooming, shelter, sleep, exercise, excretion, and other factors toward homeostasis (e.g., regulation of temperature, pH balance).

Security/Safety Needs

Physical security, environmental security, resources, health, stability, consistency, predictability, structure, routine/traditions (when a child knows what to expect in terms of routine, she feels safe)—all of these are necessary for any child to feel safe, to live without dramatic, traumatic negative surprises that cause incalculable stress.

Being touched and held allows a child to feel safe, as does eating regularly on a schedule. Many of us got these cues confused early in our lives because our needs for routine and for being touched and held were not met. So when we need to be held, it may come through the filter of "I'm hungry—I want something to eat!"

ASK YOURSELF

What were some of the routines you grew up with? What was your bedtime routine? Bath time? Brush teeth? Change into pajamas? Have a story read to you? Say prayers? Get tucked in? Get a goodnight kiss? You carry part of the discipline of this process with you to today (i.e., brushing your teeth before bed, bathing/showering, changing into sleepwear, and going to bed at an appropriate time).

What was mealtime like? Did you ever hear something like: "We're waiting for you" or "We're not starting without you," or "Make sure your hands are clean"? Maybe the demand was delivered harshly, but there was an underlying message that you are part of the family, you are important to the group, you matter, and they don't function without you.

What were your family traditions? Holidays, birthdays, religious observances, Sunday dinners, weekend activities? All these come with repetition that a child can look forward to and know what to expect.

Little Food Addict in Training

With regard to protection, a child needs to be protected by their caregivers by honoring their right to personal space, privacy, and control of her own body. As different situations develop at various ages and stages, a child needs to know that she doesn't have to be subjected to "sloppy kisses," lap sitting, and other forms of unwanted attention to please the adults in her life.

Part of safety and security is gentle discipline, which demonstrates respect and empathy. By emphasizing empathy and respect, gentle discipline nurtures these same qualities in the child. The goals of gentle discipline should be:

- to provide good care that allows the parent(s) to nurture the human elements in their child

- to help the child develop an ability to meet her own needs

- to help the child feel safe with parent(s), who are to be a trusted resource(s)

- to forge a positive relationship between parent(s) and child

By emphasizing empathy and respect, gentle discipline nurtures these qualities in the child.

Belongingness and Love Needs

- Attachment—Connection/feeling a part of/belonging; the child needs a "heart" connection with others. Therapists discuss it in terms of attachment. Healthy or unhealthy attachment starts at an early age. (See "Attachment Theory" on page 97.)

- Attention/to be attended to

- Affection, touching, and holding—appropriate touching, hugs, holding. This normal biological need lays the groundwork for developing a secure, self-affirming identity later. (See "Did You Know?" on page 96.)

- Nurturing—encouragement, love, support, caring, kindness, cherishing, tenderness, to be looked after, taken care of. All of these needs can all be classified as "nurturing," but it's important to examine and detail the specifics to identify the benchmarks of a healthy family as a measurement of how much the little food addict did not receive.

- To love and be loved
- Trust in people around her and in the surroundings
- Emotional safety
- Guidance
- Reassurance
- Relationship/being wanted—the child comes to feel that she is wanted and special. The rejection of a child can be overt or covert. The child may be the wrong gender or perhaps the parent didn't want a child. Maybe the child is seen as being damaged because the child didn't "look like" what they had hoped for (e.g., left-handed, not cute, not "right"). The child in these circumstances will feel blamed. It is important that the parent be there for the child, not vice versa.

DID YOU KNOW?

Do you know what happens if a baby is not touched? It dies. It's called "failure to thrive," and it won't survive. This has been seen in situations like wartime—when babies are left in orphanages, with feeding but without affection. That tells us how critical affection is to a child. For this reason, foundling homes* seek volunteers (preferably women) just to hold and cuddle the babies.

*A children's home offering shelter, care, and education for children who have been abandoned or exposed and left for the public to find and save.

The next four needs were brought to my attention during a long-ago therapy session, when my therapist of long standing "offhandedly" noted, "*Oh, Dianne, you mean you weren't . . .*

- *listened to*
- *understood*
- *heard*
- *taken seriously.*"

This was an epiphany because it summed up so much of my childhood and the reason that I was sitting in front of this therapist. What a setup for living life defensively and adaptively.

ATTACHMENT THEORY

Attachment theory is based on the belief that the mother-child bond is the essential and primary force in infant development, and thus forms the basis of coping, negotiation of relationships, and personality development. If the mother is absent or unavailable, a primary caregiver serves the mother's role. *Attachment* can be defined in both behavioral and emotional terms. From the behavioral perspective, attachment is represented by a cluster of instinctive child behaviors that serve to create the attachment bond, protect the child from fear and harm, and assist in the safe exploration of the world. These behaviors include reaching, clinging, sucking, and locomotion, and all facilitate maximum physical and emotional development.

From an emotional perspective, attachment is the creation of a mutual bond in which the mother shapes infant development through her interactions and the relationship with her child. Not born with the ability to decode and decipher meanings and emotions, the baby relies on the mother to help her navigate the world, both internal and external. This relationship allows for the formation of "internal working models" that function as scripts or templates by which babies can then gauge their own emotions and those of others. As the baby begins to create these internal working models, the mother acts as a "secure base" that is used for explorations, learning, and developing the necessary skills of self-protection and intimacy.

Psychologist John Bowlby, known for his pioneer work in attachment theory, described *attachment* as "a lasting psychological connectedness between human beings."[47] He believed that the earliest bonds formed by children with their caregivers have a tremendous impact that continues throughout life. Attachment theory tells us that mothers who are available and responsive to their infant's needs establish a sense of security in their children. The infant knows that the caregiver is dependable, which creates a secure base for the child to explore the world.

Failure to form normal attachments to primary caregiving figures results from early experiences of neglect, abuse, abrupt separation from caregivers, frequent change of caregivers, excessive numbers of caregivers, or lack of caregiver responsiveness to the child's communicative efforts.

Attachment Styles

Children develop and display distinct attachment styles, loosely defined as either "secure" or "insecure." Insecure styles are hallmarked by traits of instability, including ambivalent behavior, preoccupation, avoidant responses, and a lack of cooperative communication in the mother-child bond. Secure attachments, on the other hand, show a child consistently connected to the mother, with a firmly established sense of trust and an unwavering, nurturing response.

Close attachment to the mother remains crucial to children through the toddler and early childhood years, and even in adolescence. At each developmental point, the infant must have a close attachment with a consistent caregiver to ensure protection in the face of both internal changes and environmental stimuli. Put another way, attachment is, quite simply, key to survival. This need for "secure" attachment can be described as the need to:

- be known and loved, no matter what
- feel important; have a sense of personal value
- have a safe place to land
- feel secure enough to be different
- have one's own opinions
- be comfortable with one's sexuality
- have a feeling of "home"

Further belongingness and love needs include:

- Friendships/socialization

- Intimacy

- Having a supportive and communicative family

- Language/communication (including being read to)

- Education (e.g., being taught about nature/life/customs/coping)

- Boundaries—like fences, they are necessary, and built by the way parents talk to and treat their child.

Healthy boundaries are built when parents correct with love, show respect, and give guidance and support to their children. Children with firm boundaries can distinguish their own ideas, problems, and feelings from those of others. They know what they like and dislike and have little

Little Food Addict in Training

trouble describing themselves to others. They know where they end and others begin.

Conversely, parents who abuse their children emotionally, physically, or sexually "teach" the child that there are no such things as boundaries. As a result, the child becomes confused and cannot distinguish her own thoughts and feelings apart from those of others. The child will find it hard to describe herself, who she really is, and to identify and defend her own likes, dislikes, opinions, and ideas.

Children too fearful to be part of life hide behind the "wall" they build for protection. Parents who criticize, control, and create tension-filled homes "teach" their children the need for protective walls. Since usable information about who they are cannot penetrate their wall, children without these needed boundaries seldom know what they like or dislike, and they have usually encased or frozen most of their feelings.

What's the job of a two-year-old? To test boundaries. They test boundaries so often that I sometimes think they might begin to think their name is "No." But that presupposes a tolerant, patient, and empathic caretaker to teach the child boundaries and help her learn delayed gratification, or frustration tolerance. The child also begins to experience rules as limits. According to Dr. Laura Markam in her book *How to Set Effective Limits for Your Child*:

> "What I learned by watching kids is confirmed by research findings in neurology. As children get faced with the necessity to rein in their impulse toward something they want (e.g., to grab a toy from the baby), so they can have something they want more (a warm, happy connection with you); they learn self-control.
>
> "Research shows that children develop optimally when we set limits as necessary, but do so with empathy. Empathy makes your limit more palatable to your child, so she doesn't resist as much. That's what allows her to internalize it. Kids need appropriate limits, but it's how you do it that counts. Because studies show that when we try to control kids, especially punitively, they react with anger and resistance, as all humans do. Unfortunately, limits are perceived as punitive by the child, unless they are offered with empathy."[48]

Parents need to model/exhibit good boundaries themselves, respect the child's need for privacy, and support the child when she is in unappealing situations and defenseless to help herself.

PARENTING STYLES

Sociologist Reuben Hill conducted a study of thousands of teens and parents in Minnesota. He found that different parenting styles produced different responses among children:

- **The Permissive Parent**—high in love, but low in discipline. Produces children with very low self-esteem plus feelings of inferiority. Though the parents express a lot of love, the lack of boundaries leaves their children with a high level of insecurity.

- **The Neglectful Parent**—not much expression of love and doesn't care enough to discipline. The children tend to grow up with little or no lasting relationship with Mother or Father. These children grow up with deep emotional scars.

- **The Authoritarian Parent**—doesn't express love and affection well but is very high on discipline. Their children are provoked to rebellion. Communication between parent and child takes the form of arguing and fighting, especially when the child is old enough to fight back. These parents squeeze their kids until the kids can't wait to leave home, and as soon as they do, they rebel.

- **The Authoritative Parent**—best combination of love and discipline. This kind of parent is authoritative—not an overbearing authoritarian, but a compassionate yet firm authority. They have clear boundaries but are also very loving. Everyone knows who the boss is, but there's also a connection between parents and child. The result is a child high in self-esteem and equipped with good coping skills.

This study found that the parent who balances love and discipline, without compromising either, produces well-adjusted offspring, who maintain a positive relationship with Mom and Dad.[49]

Belongingness and love needs also encompass the need for:

- Identification—The need to identify is a strong biological need. Identification carries the essence of connectedness and rootedness. It is through the natural human desire to identify with others, to belong to something greater than ourselves, that we learn to be a fully integrated person. It is in our families that, through identification, we know rootedness.

Little Food Addict in Training

Through mirroring, the parent allows the child to identify with her. If this identification is done via shaming, we identify ourselves as shameful beings. If this identification is affirming, we identify and accept ourselves as okay in our human being-ness. Through identification with the parent and internalization of the parent's view of us, the relationship of the self with the self is developed. This is identity. Identity is either a self-affirming one or a shaming one.

- Separation—This need must be supported through each developmental phase and starts as soon as the child becomes mobile. To allow for, and to support, good skills for separation is to teach the child how to handle life on life's terms. Separation is necessary to feel mastery over life. Absolutely the only way to individuate (become an individual) is through identification and separation. Overprotective or overly possessive parents can greatly hinder the need to differentiate, by shaming the process: "You must think you're better than we are."

  Separation-individuation is a term Margaret Mahler, MD, psychiatrist, gave to the process by which internal maps of the self and others are formed. These internal representations are built up through interactions with caregivers during the period from birth to three years of age and consist of both positive and negative aspects of experience within the relationship. According to Mahler, it is the ability to integrate frustrating and pleasurable aspects of experience with another person that leads to a stable sense of self that can tolerate fluctuating emotional states within the self and others. The inability to integrate these aspects of experience can lead to maladaptive thinking and behaviors, a distorted view of oneself and the surrounding world.[50]

Esteem Needs

It has only been since the early nineteenth century that our society started viewing children (and women) as independent beings of value and worthy of respect. Up until that time, they were considered the chattel/property of men. There were no child labor laws. However, children and women are now regarded as valuable individuals with worth and appropriate needs of their own, worthy of regard and attention.

Childhood needs that relate to esteem are:

- Praise/admiration/approval/recognition
- To be valued, treasured, prized
- Consideration
- Confidence
- Respect
- Achievement
- Affirmation—This is crucial to avoid people-pleasing later in life. Through having this need met, the child can slowly, over time, decide what values and truths have importance to her.
- Validation/acknowledgment/acceptance
- Positive reinforcement (giving rise to feelings of satisfaction and fulfillment). To applaud or acknowledge (with words, hugs, and maybe a reward [not food!]) that the child has achieved something difficult or worthwhile or something that took effort. It's saying to the child, "Good job," "That's great," or "I'm proud of you."

If you have ever been to a 12 Step meeting and watched participants raise their hands and say: "I have thirty [or however many] days" and everyone applauds—on the surface it appears to be a silly demonstration, but it feels so good to experience that acknowledgment. That's positive reinforcement. (Actually, everyone, whatever their age, needs it.)

Maslow considers the first four layers of the pyramid to be **"deficiency needs"**—those of survival, safety and security, love, belonging, and esteem. He believes that if these needs are not met, a person will feel anxious and tense but the body gives no psychical indication of it.

Self-Actualization Needs

The determinant of a healthy self is dependent upon the level of fulfillment of the following needs:

- Compassion/forgiveness
- Creativity
- Honesty
- Independence
- Learning manners and politeness

Little Food Addict in Training

- Morality/values
- Play/fun/toys
- Problem-solving
- Recognition

- Responsibilities
- Solitude
- Spontaneity
- Stimulation

For a child to experience the fulfillment of the self-actualization needs listed above, she requires the following:

- Healthy role models (especially those who model healthy, nonaddictive eating behavior) who are committed to providing healthy nurturing and caring

- An established, secure base from which the child can grow and develop a sense of self/identity, morality, virtue, and, of course, whole, mature, available, consistent, healthy, supportive, loving, caring, tolerant, and patient caretaker(s) to fulfill these needs.

We know there is no ideal, so it's fair to say that the extent to which we are missing these things determines our own dysfunction.

THE FOOD ADDICT'S FAMILY

Going through any developmental phase alone—whether due to family food addiction, substance abuse, physical or mental illness, financial problems, neglect, or physical/emotional/sexual abuse—can set up a pattern of facing all of life's turbulence alone. Believing that the need for support and affirmation is somehow wrong, bad, or shameful predisposes us to seek comfort in ways that don't require us to acknowledge our human needs (e.g., other people). Again, this isolation makes it so clear why *using* food from a tender age becomes a "solution" to the pain of living in an unhealthy family. (This is discussed in greater detail in Chapter 15: Family and the Food Addict.)

Developmental Process Leading to Food Addiction

Before we examine the little food addict's family, a brief discussion of developmental stages as they relate to the development of food addiction is important in order to understand that food addiction doesn't "occur in a vacuum"; it is an organic evolutionary process.

- Infancy—The major developmental task of the infant is to develop trust and security. This is enabled by the parents' attunement to feeding the child and their ability to respond appropriately to the child's needs. If the parents do not properly nurture and care for the child, the infant is left insecure about whether her dependency needs will be met or will she be abandoned. In most individuals with food addiction and addiction in general, this primary task is not met successfully.

- Childhood—If parents read and respond to a child's hunger accurately, the child learns to identify and respond correctly to her own hunger cues. However, when a parent uses food frequently as a pacifier or reward and/or punishment, food becomes a tool to control the child. If the child is shamed about her other emotional needs (need to cry, to feel anger), she learns that food can be more reliable as a source of comfort than people can. (See the discussion about shame in Chapter 14: Self-Esteem and Family Systems.) At this stage, parents are also modeling eating behaviors for their children. And if they are "using" food for comfort, connection, soothing, and so forth, the child is primed to mirror the behavior.

- Adolescence—An adolescent must struggle to discover and find her own identity while negotiating and struggling with social interactions and "fitting in." This is the time of emerging self-image and greatest body changes, and the task now is to combine one's sense of self, one's body image, and one's sexual sense, and to separate from one's parents. Attempts to control food and body shape as a source of identity and self-esteem is often seen in adolescents whose sense of self is fragile.

- Adulthood—By this stage, the disease is cemented; those with food addiction are well established in using food to cope with the challenges and conflicts present in developing committed relationships, discovering meaningful work, balancing play, negotiating differences, losses, and disappointments and being comfortable with success and achievement.

Now that we have a more complete picture of the little food addict's characteristics and needs, let's bring her home. In other words, let's take a look at her family dynamics and home life.

Common Dynamics of the Food Addict's Family ("The War Zone")

Our relationships within our family of origin are our most powerful ones, yet for many of us, these relationships were contaminated by dysfunction and filled with tension. Often, we've been shaped and influenced by critical, shaming, abandoning, neglecting, and possibly blatantly abusive parenting.

With various types of dysfunction within the little food addict's family, as you will see, there is a lack of respect shown in personal interactions, including various forms of abuse, physical, mental, emotional, sexual, or spiritual. Implicit in any form of abuse is the message to the child that she is abusable, worthless, and unworthy of having personal boundaries. This, of course, builds the foundation of shame.

According to John Bradshaw in an interview on *Recovery Networker* in September 1992, we've all come out of patriarchal families where we've been taught blind obedience.[51] We've basically been taught to suppress all emotions except fear. We've had our wills crushed at an early age. If you don't have a will, you don't have willpower (you can't say no) and you've suppressed all your emotions (you're set up to be an addict). Bradshaw affirms that a child has a right to say no, a right to change her mind, and a right to say, "Stop." But most children don't know that they have these rights because we as a society don't teach them that they do. In fact, we teach them just the opposite—that they don't have rights when it comes to their parents. Who hasn't been taught that you must obey your parent at any cost? Who hasn't heard, "Do it because I said so"? Bradshaw says this is pure patriarchy, and there is compliance because of the fear of mental, verbal, and/or physical abuse.

How Dysfunctional Parenting Styles Play Out in Families

There are different types of dysfunction in families. Some parents under-function, leaving their children to fend for themselves. Other parents over-function, never allowing their children to grow up and be on their own. Others are inconsistent or violate basic boundaries of appropriate behavior. Think about your early experience in your family. Maybe you'll relate to some of the circumstances on this list, if not all, especially if you grew up amid alcoholism, drug or food addiction, mental illness, divorce, single parenting, gambling, rage, high stress, or with parents who were emotionally or physically unavailable due to a variety of circumstances such as Holocaust survival, criminal justice issues, and the like.

In the following sections, let's look at the various types of dysfunctional parenting and examine how each supports/influences/sets up the genetically predisposed child to become a food addict.

Alcoholic/Chemically Dependent/Food-Addicted Parents

As explained later in Chapter 14: Self-Esteem and Family Systems, these parents tend to be chaotic and unpredictable. Rules change on a whim. Promises are broken or not even remembered. From one day to the next, expectations change and parents' behavior runs the gamut from strict to indifferent. Feelings are taboo, as is any discussion about parental drug use, drinking, or eating behavior. The overriding message is to keep family problems a secret and never seek help. In these families, the children believe that they caused their parents to behave this way, that something is wrong with the child. These children carry into their adult lives mistrust of others and difficulty with emotional expression and intimate relationships.

Deficient Parents

These parents hurt their children more by omission than by commission. Frequently, chronic mental illness or a disabling physical illness contributes to parental inadequacy. Children tend to take on adult responsibilities from a young age in these families. Parental emotional needs tend to take precedence, and children are often asked to be their parents' caretakers—overtly or covertly—thus becoming parentified. Children are robbed of their own childhoods, and they learn to ignore their own needs and feelings. Because these children are simply not up to the task of playing an adult role and taking care of their parents, they often feel inadequate and guilty. These feelings continue until adulthood.

Controlling Parents

These parents fail to allow their children to assume responsibilities appropriate for their age. These parents continue dominating and making decisions for their children well beyond the age at which this is necessary. Controlling parents are often driven by a fear of becoming unnecessary

Little Food Addict in Training

to their children. This fear leaves them feeling betrayed and abandoned when their children become independent.[52] These children, on the other hand, frequently feel resentful, inadequate, and powerless. Transitions into adult roles are difficult, as these adults frequently have difficulty in making decisions independent from their parents. When they act independently, these adult-children feel very guilty, as if growing up were a serious act of disloyalty.

Abusive Parents

As explained later in Chapter 14: Self-Esteem and Family Systems, abuse may be verbal, emotional, physical, or sexual. Abuse is any action or inaction by a major caregiver that is less than nurturing or is experienced as shaming. Abuse exists along a spectrum, from the most nonthreatening form of abuse—neglect—to verbal abuse, which creates emotional and mental trauma, to physical abuse, to the most severe form of abuse, which is sexual. Abuse is shaming to the child, giving the message that the child is worthless and doesn't matter and is abusable.

TYPES OF ABUSE

Abuse takes many forms, some of which may be more obvious than others but still fall under the heading of abuse.

Overt abuse is out in the open, obvious, and abject.

Covert abuse is hidden, less obvious; it may be masked as humor, tone of voice, crazymaking (manipulation—e.g., "You didn't see" what you know and saw).

Disempowerment occurs when power and value are taken away. A child having suffered too many putdowns, verbal attacks, and/or physical beatings grows up to act out of a victim mentality. False empowerment is not teaching the child accountability and limits. The child becomes grandiose, is taught that she is better than others, feels special, and does not have humility. Often this is not intentional, but it is still abusive.

Verbal abuse, such as frequent belittling, can have lasting effects, particularly when it comes from those entrusted with the child's care. Criticism can be aimed at the child's looks, intelligence, capabilities, or basic value. Some verbal abusers are very direct, while others use subtle putdowns disguised as humor. Both types are damaging.

Physical abuse has a broad definition. Many parents, at one time or another, have felt the urge to strike their child. With physically abusive parents, however, the urge is frequent, and little effort is made to control this impulse. The Federal Child Abuse Prevention and Treatment Act defines *physical abuse* as "the infliction of physical injuries such as bruises, burns, welts, cuts, bone or skull fractures caused by kicking, punching, biting, beating, knifing, strapping, paddling, and so on."

Striking a child has more to do with meeting the parent's emotional needs than with concern for the child; parents often erroneously justify the abuse as "discipline" intended to "help" the child. Physically abusive parents can create an environment of terror for the child, particularly since such violence is often random and unpredictable. Abused children often feel anger. Children of abusive parents have great difficulties developing feelings of trust and safety, even in their adult lives.

While parents may rationalize verbal or physical abuse as discipline aimed at somehow helping the child, there is no rationalization for sexual abuse. Sexual abuse is the most blatant example of an adult abusing a child purely for that adult's own gratification.

Sexual abuse can be any physical contact between an adult and child, where that contact must be kept secret. Demonstrations of affection—such as hugging, kissing, or stroking a child's hair—that can be done openly are quite acceptable and even beneficial. When physical contact is shrouded in secrecy, however, then it is likely inappropriate. It is also any instance of someone taking advantage of a position of trust, age, or status to lead a child into a situation of real or perceived powerlessness around issues of sex and humiliation. In other words, when children must passively submit to the will of another, rather than having the choice to defend themselves or to tell someone—whether or not they are "forced"—that constitutes sexual violation or assault.

Responsibility for sexual abuse, as with all abuse, rests entirely with the adult. No child is responsible for being abused. Most sexually abused children are too frightened of the consequences for themselves and their families to risk telling another adult what is happening. Even if not admonished (or threatened) to keep the assault secret, children often do not tell due to embarrassment, shame, and guilt, or the intrinsic knowledge that it is "wrong" or "bad" and that they are to blame. In their naiveté, children mistakenly assume that they themselves are "bad." They carry the shame that belongs to the molester. As a result, they grow into adulthood with feelings of self-loathing, shame, and worthlessness. They tend to be self-punishing and have considerable difficulties with relationships and ordinary sexuality. They carry the belief that the only thing they have to give is sex.

Little Food Addict in Training

> Sexual abuse steals a child's innocence and affects her self-worth, personality development, socialization, achievement, and, later, intimacy in adolescent and adult relationships. In addition, these children are prone to somatic symptoms, such as physical rigidity, awkwardness, or using food for comfort, relief, control, stuffing of feelings, and to disconnect, resulting in excessive weight gain/loss born of a conscious or unconscious attempt to "lock out" others and not be in one's own body and also to make oneself unattractive. Also common are tendencies to live in a fantasy world, to have issues with attention ("spacing out" and daydreaming) and to dissociate to compartmentalize the awful experiences. (See the discussion of survival skills, beliefs, and behaviors of the young food addict on page 132.)
>
> The eating-disordered self contains the dissociated trauma-related needs, emotions, and beliefs. Because people cannot be trusted, the traumatized child turns to food to meet primary relational needs. A very compelling substitute for many reasons, food is a first medium for the transmission of soothing and comfort. It is also a symbolic language for relationships. The individual can express anger through vomiting, rebellion, and control by refusing to eat, or quell feelings of deprivation by binge eating.

Common Family Characteristics
Resulting from Dysfunctional Parenting

Here are some examples of how dysfunctional parenting styles play out in families:

- Drama

- Chaos—Studies suggest that bulimic females may be more likely than nonbulimics to come from a chaotic family environment that either encourages the development of an eating disorder or maintains already existing eating-disordered behaviors.[53]

- Yelling, fighting, anger, and/or violence

- Danger

- Extremes in conflict—Either too much fighting or insufficient arguing between family members

- Lack of consideration, empathy, understanding, and sensitivity toward family members, and expressing extreme empathy toward one or more members (or even pets) who have real or perceived "special needs." In other words, one family member constantly receives far more attention than that person merits, while another is often marginalized—which sets up high levels of jealousy, which then leads to unhealthy competition (see Chapter 14: Self-Esteem and Family Systems for more on this). Sometimes the little food addict feels guilt when there's an accomplishment and then "dumbs down" to protect herself due to jealousy and competition.

- Denial—A refusal to acknowledge abusive/inappropriate behavior or addiction; this is also known as living with the "elephant in the living room." In this family, the child may have been taught that what they know to be real isn't accurate. Maybe Mommy screamed at her and then said she really wasn't angry or maybe Daddy was drunk and Mommy said he was "just tired" or "not feeling well." To survive this "minefield," the little food addict must deny what she knows and accept the myths of the dysfunctional system. As an adult, she depends on others to tell her what is real because she can't trust her own sense of reality. Often, the mentality of family members is, "If you just ignore it, maybe it won't hurt; if you ignore it, it may go away."

- Boundary issues—Inadequate or missing boundaries for self (e.g., tolerating inappropriate treatment from others; failing to express what is acceptable and unacceptable treatment; tolerance of physical, emotional or sexual abuse) and/or disrespect for others' boundaries (e.g., physical contact that another person rejects or dislikes; breaking important promises without just cause; purposefully violating a boundary another person has expressed).

- Conflict influenced by marital status: between divorced or separated parents, usually related to or arising from their breakup; between parents who remain married, often for the "perceived" sake of the children, but whose separation or divorce would, in fact, remove a detrimental influence on those children; parents who wish to divorce but cannot, due to financial, societal (including religious), or legal reasons.

- Fear—children are afraid to talk (within or outside the family) about what is happening at home, or otherwise fearful of their parents.

- Sexual behavior, abnormal familial behavior—e.g., adultery, promiscuity, or incest.

- Secrets—Family system is censored and closed.

- Lack of time together, especially in recreational activities and social events ("We never do anything as a family").

- Family members (including children) disown each other and/or refuse to be seen together in public (unilaterally or bilaterally).

- Manipulation—Use of kids as pawns (by destructively narcissistic parent[s] who rule by fear and conditional love and rage); occurs when a parent manipulates a child to achieve some negative result in the other parent, rather than communicating with them directly. Examples include verbal manipulation, gossip, trying to obtain information through the child (spying), or causing the child to dislike the other parent. There is no concern for the damaging effects this has on the child(ren).

- Unrealistic expectations.

- Conditional love—Conditioned on performance.

- Perfectionism—Fixating on order, prestige, power and/or perfect appearances, while preventing their child from failing at anything.

- Glorification and pursuit of thinness and the practice of chronic dieting may be a part of this family's values.

- Emotional intolerance—Family members not allowed to express the "wrong" emotions. This child may have been feeling excited, happy, sad or fearful, and an agitated parent or adult, without patience or insight-fueled ability to deal with the child, squashed the emotions. Often the children are told (verbally or nonverbally) not to feel what they feel or that it is wrong somehow to feel the way they do. So early in life, they learn to move into their heads and not feel in life or in relationships because it is safer to avoid exposure.

- Social dysfunction (e.g., parents unwilling to reach out to other families—especially those with children of the same gender and approximate age—or to do anything to help their "friendless child").

- Dogmatic or cultish—Harsh and inflexible discipline, with children forbidden, without reason, to dissent, question authority, or develop their own value system, which has the effect of denying the child an inner life.

- Rigid family system with inflexible rules that keep changing. (See Chapter 14: Self-Esteem and Family Systems for more on this.)

- Inequitable parenting—Unequal or unfair treatment of one or more family members due to their gender, age, birth order, familial role (mother, provider and so on), and/or abilities. May include frequent appeasement of one member at the expense of others, or an uneven enforcement of rules.

- Deprivation—Control or neglect by withholding love, support, necessities, sympathy, praise, attention, encouragement, supervision, or otherwise putting the child(ren)'s well-being at risk.

- Silent treatment—Punishment by not speaking to the child, shutting the child out of the family circle (the "violence of silence"—since the child is terrorized by experiencing what she senses is behind the silence—rage! Silence is also a form of abandonment).

- Abandonment by a parent who willfully separates from their child(ren), not wishing any further contact and, in some cases, without arranging alternative long-term parenting arrangements, leaving them as orphans. Sheer negligence, too, is another form of abandonment. There are parents who, in their desire to force discipline as easily and quickly as possible, will wield the threat of abandonment, overtly or subtly, to achieve this control. The message they give to their children: "If you don't do exactly what I want you to do, I won't love you anymore, and you can figure out for yourself what that might mean." Such withdrawal means, of course, abandonment and death. So it is that such children, abandoned either psychologically or in actuality, enter adulthood lacking any sense that the world is a safe and protective place. On the contrary, as they perceive the world as dangerous and uncertain; they are not about to forsake current gratification or security for the promise of later gratification or security, since for them the future seems dubious. (See the discussion of self-care on page 342.)

Little Food Addict in Training

- Peace at any price, or appeasement—Parents who reward or ignore bad behavior and inevitability "punish" another child's good behavior to maintain the peace and avoid temper tantrums.

- Loyalty manipulation—Giving unearned rewards and lavish attention, trying to ensure that a favored yet rebellious child will become loyal and well-behaved, while subtly ignoring the wants and needs of their current loyal child.

- Helicopter parenting—Micromanaging child(ren)'s lives and/or relationships among siblings—even minor conflicts.

- Deception—Deceivers may be well-regarded parents in the community, likely to be involved in local charitable/non-profit works, but who abuse or mistreat one or more of their children.

- Public image managers—Sometimes related to deceivers above, with children warned not to disclose any fights, abuse, or damage that occurred at home, or face severe punishment ("Don't tell anyone what goes on in this family").

- Paranoia—Parent has persistent and irrational fears, accompanied by anger and false accusations that their child is up to no good or that others are plotting against them.

- "No friends allowed"—Discouraging, prohibiting, or interfering with their child from making friends, often of the same age and gender.

- Role reversal—Parents who expect their minor children to take care of them instead, thus causing their children to become parentified.

- "My baby, forever"—Parent who will not allow one or more of their young children to grow up or begin taking care of themselves. (See the discussion of self-care on page 342.)

- "The cheerleader"—One parent "cheers on" the other parent, who is abusing their child.

- "The politician/liar"—A parent who repeatedly makes promises or agrees to a child's request with little intention of following through.

- "It's taboo"—Parents rebuff questions the child(ren) may have about sexuality, pregnancy, romance, puberty, areas of human anatomy, nudity, etc.

- "The identified patient"—One child, usually selected by the mother, forced into going to therapy, while the family's overall dysfunction is kept hidden.

- Being under- or overprotective.

- Hypocrisy ("Do as I say, not as I do.").

- Unforgiving ("Saying 'sorry' doesn't change anything.").

- Giving "mixed messages" by having a dual system of values (i.e., one set for the outside world, another in private, or teaching divergent values to each child).

- Discussion and exposure to sexuality: either too much, too soon or too little, too late.

- Faulty discipline (i.e., punishment by "surprise") based more on emotions or family politics than on established rules.

- Unpredictability/mood swings—Creating and manifesting unpredictable reactions in parents, arising from addictions, mental illness, personality disorder(s), stress, gambling, etc.

- Inconsistency of mood, behavior, reactions.

- Frequent withholding of consent ("blessing") for culturally common, lawful, and age-appropriate activities their child wants to take part in.

- Older siblings given either excessive authority or none over younger siblings with respect to age differences and level of maturity.

- Rules imposed mandated by religious fervor.

TOXIC STRESS

Here is some interesting commentary on life-long consequences to a child who is a victim of a toxic family. In the January 2012 article "A Poverty Solution That Starts With a Hug," which appeared in the *New York Times*, Nicholas D. Kristof states:

> "Perhaps the most widespread peril children face isn't guns, swimming pools or speeding cars. Rather, scientists are suggesting that it may be 'toxic stress' early in life, or even before birth. This month, the

> American Academy of Pediatrics is issuing a landmark warning that this toxic stress can harm children for life. This is a 'policy statement' from the premier association of pediatricians, based on two decades of research. Toxic stress might arise from parental abuse of alcohol or drugs. It could occur in a home where children are threatened and beaten. It might derive from chronic neglect—a child cries without being cuddled. Affection seems to defuse toxic stress—suggesting that the stress emerges when a child senses persistent threats but no protector. Cues of a hostile or indifferent environment flood an infant, or even a fetus, with stress hormones like cortisol in ways that can disrupt the body's metabolism or the architecture of the brain. The upshot is that children are sometimes permanently undermined."[54]

A LOOK AT SHAME

Shaming is an act of abuse. I'll discuss this in more depth in Chapter 14: Self-Esteem and Family Systems, but for now, it's being examined because it is a large part of the dynamic in a dysfunctional family. When a parent shames a child (e.g., by telling the child she is worth less than others, crazy, stupid, doesn't measure up, defective, a loser, hopeless, and so on or by inflicting corporal punishment or by ignoring or rejecting the child), Dr. Morton Schatzman calls that "soul murder."[55]

Shame tells a child that who she is wrong, while guilt tells a child that what she did is wrong. Here's an example: a parent calls their kid's action of chasing an errant ball into the street dumb because they could've been hit by a car. The child can think, "Okay, if I don't do that again, then I'm not dumb." The criticism was for an act; it had nothing to do with the child's core identity. However, if a parent attacks the child's "being" and says, "You are too dumb to make smart choices," the child hears, "You are defective." And that becomes the child's definitive lifelong struggle against a judgment about who and what she is.

Shame numbs self-esteem, creativity, and spirit. A person who is shamed feels as if they are unacceptable; therefore, despair sits where the soul used to be. People who see themselves as bad or defective develop low self-worth. This process, of course, starts at an early age and follows them into adulthood. And a poor self-image affects the way they act, react, think, feel, and relate to others.

Shaming Words and Actions

- Physical punishment: "the belt," punching, kicking, hitting, slapping, arm twisting
- Shame ("Shame on you!")
- Punishing
- Belittling ("You can't do anything right!")
- Patronizing
- Ridicule
- Humiliating
- Degrading
- Disgracing
- Inflicting guilt
- Saying "If only…"(e.g., "If only you were better or different.") or, "You should…(e.g., "You should be better or different.")
- Joking about the child
- Laughing at another's expense
- Mimicking
- Teasing
- Sarcasm
- Manipulating
- Deceiving
- Tricking or misleading
- Lying
- Pretending
- Breaking commitments/ promises
- Canceling plans

- Betraying
- Hurting
- Being cruel
- Hiding
- Intimidating
- Threatening
- Inflicting fear
- Overpowering or bullying
- Controlling
- Bribing
- Lecturing
- Limiting
- Disrespecting; especially contempt
- Apathy ("I don't care." = "You don't matter.")
- Raising hopes falsely
- Responding inconsistently or arbitrarily
- Stifling speech (children banned from dissent or questioning authority)
- Bitterness (using a bitter tone of voice, regardless of what is said)
- Withdrawing
- Withholding love
- Silent treatment
- Not taking seriously
- Invalidating
- Discrediting
- Disapproving

- Comparing ("Why aren't you more like … ?")
- Excessive criticism
- Making light of or minimizing the child's feelings, wants, or needs
- Saying, "You shouldn't feel such and such [emotion]" (e.g., anger)
- Religious infliction
- Judgmental statements or demonization (e.g., "You are a liar!")
- The absentee, unavailable/passive parent (seldom available for their child due to work, alcohol/ drug abuse, gambling or other addictions; the message is that the child is not worth being around for)
- Unfulfilled projects, activities, and promises affecting the child (e.g., "We'll do it later.")
- Unfairness—Giving to one child what rightly belongs to another.
- Gender prejudice— Treating one gender of children fairly, the other unfairly.
- Scapegoating— Knowingly or recklessly blaming one child for the misdeeds of another.

Little Food Addict in Training

- The "know-it-all"—Has no need to obtain child's side of the story when accusing or to listen to child's opinions on matters which greatly impact them.

- Either being miserly ("a Scrooge") in totality or selectively allowing child's needs to go unmet.

- Nature vs. Nurture—Parents, often non-biological, blame common problems on child's heredity, where faulty parenting may be the actual cause.

Shaming words and actions build the foundation for the struggle the little food addict has with development of self-worth.

My early childhood environment was not a safe place to voice feelings, assert power, or express needs that challenged the status quo of family functioning. My mother's struggle with alcoholism and depression, coupled with my father's fear of self-assertion, created a family environment where I had to suppress how I actually felt and what I genuinely experienced to survive the chaos. The oppressive forces within my family kept each member detached from authentic and genuine connections with one another. Chances are you can relate.

CHAPTER 4

Little Food Addict in the "War Zone"
Damaged Characteristics and Resulting Adaptation

All of the circumstances I discussed in the previous chapter have a powerful impact on the little food addict in training. Let's now return to the characteristics listed on page 92 and see what effect these "War Zone"–style family dynamics have had on this vulnerable being. After this experience, does the little food addict still feel or does she now feel . . .

Precious? Valuable?	No.
Imperfect?	Yes, but now feels shame because of it. (See the discussion on survival skills on page 133.)
Trusting?	No! Most children begin life thinking that adults—their parents, other relatives, family, friends, and even strangers and older children—will protect them or keep them safe. When that trust is broken, either because a child is physically, emotionally, or sexually abused, or abandoned, or neglected, that trust is violated. As a result, the child may have lost the ability to trust anyone and may have a hard time developing close relationships, or even knowing what a close or intimate relationship is and lives with chronic disappointment. (Were there any instances in your childhood when your trust was betrayed by a parent or adult caretaker? Looking back, did you view the situation different when you were a child versus today? For example, did you blame yourself for the abuse, neglect or abandonment? What judgments did you form about the world around you from this instance where trust was broken?)
Open?	No. Because they've been shut down or shut off too often.
Receptive?	Maybe, but walls (defiance) may also have been established to hide behind to feel safe. Little addict may be shut down and hostile.

Little Food Addict in the "War Zone"

Vulnerable? Fragile?	Maybe, the little food addict may become a bully or harass others or be an easy victim thereof, possibly taking a dual role in different settings.
Safe?	No. Little addict has learned that she cannot depend on the family for protection.
Dependent?	Yes. (See the discussion on survival skills on page 134.)
Defenseless?	No. Now has developed various defenses, including using food, to not feel. Denial becomes a major defense, which is used by the entire family.
Unguarded/ Uncensored?	No. Now very guarded. Now the little food addict has a filter that supervises her expression.
Demanding?	Maybe, but finds answers elsewhere.
Sensitive?	Yes, very sensitive, although trying to have a thick skin.
Innocent? Naive?	No. Abuse is the thief of innocence.
Impressionable? Sponge-like?	Yes, continues to absorb information.
Accepting?	Maybe.
Willing?	Maybe.
Giving?	Yes, still with hope of receiving love, kindness, consideration, approval, validation, etc.
Adaptable?	Yes, it's a survival strategy.
Spontaneous?	No, the family system is too inflexible/rigid and there are too many rules to allow for spontaneity.
Stubborn?	Maybe, as a way to be safe.
Loving?	Maybe. While being in the "War Zone" that is this family, may have mixed feelings of love-hate toward certain family members.
Loyal/Faithful?	Yes, the bonding is established early on; the family is this child's anchor, dysfunctional as it may be. May rebel against parental authority, or conversely, uphold their family's values in the face of peer pressure, or even try to take an impossible "middle ground" that pleases no one. Maybe loyal/faithful out of fear.
Enthusiastic? Optimistic? Positive?	No, this family system is not offering a positive future
Hopeful?	Yes. Always hoping for a different result.
Energetic? Spunky?	No, this family system is a heavy weight on this little person and draining of positive energy.
Has Expectations?	No, because of living with the family's dysfunction, this child gives up. Spirit is broken. (See "Feelings This Child Is Now Having" on page 125.)

Eager?	In time, eager to get out of the house!
Clear brained?	No, all is chaos and confused.
Alert? Focused? Observant?	Yes, has to be vigilant for survival; must be on guard to dodge landmines.
No worries?	No, now many worries.
No guilt?	No, now feels responsible for family's problems and receives blame for many problems.
No resentments?	No, resentful of other family members or others who are more favored or held up as better human beings.
Non-judgmental?	No, outgrowth of being shamed and copying the critical and judgmental attitudes of other family members, especially the addict/dependent.
No prejudices?	No, influenced by the biases and blaming behavior/attitudes of older family members.
No responsibilities?	No, often given responsibilities beyond her age appropriateness, or maybe tries to get praised by taking on responsibilities beyond her age or feels the weight of feeling responsible for the dysfunction of the family.
Honest about feelings?	No, absolutely not! Little addict learned early on that her feelings were invalid and not valued and should be eliminated.
Direct? Straightforward?	No, the family operates with mixed messages, protective alliances, denial of reality, secrets, criticism and judgments—not a safe environment for open and direct communication.
Expressive? Communicative?	No, that's gone. The rule of "Don't talk" is well established. The other negative rules and messages that serve to rob the little food addict of her voice are: • "Don't think or talk; just follow directions." • "Don't ask questions." • "Be seen and not heard." • "No backtalk." • "Don't contradict me." • "I'm always right; you're always wrong." • "You're so stupid." Maybe the family only talked to each other during mealtimes. (See more family rules listed in Chapter 14.)
No masks? Transparent?	No. Now the little food addict knows she has to hide true feelings and finds a way to "present well."
Copycat?	Yes, most likely continues since copying others is a learning strategy.
Teachable?	Maybe not. The shaming message is the expectation that the little food addict "should know; why don't you know?" Little addict's confidence is weak/damaged.

Little Food Addict in the "War Zone"

Responsive?	Maybe, in a cautious way, and maybe not as despair/hopelessness sets in.
Curious? Inquisitive?	Maybe, but since family rules dictate "Don't talk, don't ask questions, don't feel," that natural curiosity is stifled.
Outgoing/friendly/ gregarious?	Maybe, the little food addict has become more cautious in her interactions since now doesn't feel good about herself. Socially, this child has difficulty forming healthy relationships within her peer group (usually due to shyness or a personality disorder) and spends an inordinate amount of time alone watching TV, playing video games, surfing the Internet, listening to music, and engaging in other activities which lack in-person social interaction. Or she socializes with other addicts, gangs, internet chat rooms, Facebook (where they pretend to be someone else)—places to feel free, powerful. "Looking for love in all the wrong places."
Natural Relationship with food?	No! Now is beginning to use food to manage the stress that comes from living in this dysfunctional family as well as mirroring the eating behaviors in the family. Also, as the problematic eating/non-eating behaviors increase, tends to minimize the behaviors and its consequences.
Filled with feelings?	Yes, but can't/won't express them.
Lovable?	After experiencing the "War Zone" that is this family, most likely feels angry (especially toward herself), anxious, depressed, isolated from others, and/or unlovable.
In touch with feelings?	No, works hard to get rid of feelings, complying with the family message of "You don't feel that way" and the family rule of "Don't feel!"
Self-centered?	Yes, uncomfortable in her own skin and consumed with herself.
Comfortable with self?	No, because of the shaming messages, the little food addict wants to "leave" herself.
Unselfconscious? Uninhibited?	No, now very self-conscious and is cautious about how she thinks she appears to others.
Sense of self?	No, this child feels worth less than others. John Bradshaw explains that the symptoms of codependency result from developmental deficits, which are the consequences of abuse and neglect. He further explains that developmental deficits refer to unmet developmental dependency needs. These needs must be met in order for a person to develop a solid sense of self and emotional literacy; these needs depend on source figures for their fulfillment. A child's needs cannot be met without reliance on a functional adult. Emotional literacy is characterized by the ability to think about and contain feelings, using them for self-soothing and expressing them with appropriate intensity. With a solid sense of self, a person has good boundaries. This little food addict was denied caretaking by a functional adult(s).

Sense of self? (continued)	At this point, adult little food addict lacks a solid sense of self-identity being rooted in "toxic shame" (Bradshaw) or "carried shame" (as described by Pia Mellody).
No fear/fearless? Adventurous? Bold?	No, now filled with many fears; may be bold to get attention or not, too dangerous.
Risk taker? Reckless?	May continue as a way to act out, to get attention.
Happy? Joyful? Playful? Free Spirited? Carefree?	The negative messages and negative rules generated in this family create a cloud over this child's ability to experience pleasure.
Infantile?	The child lacks the ability to be playful or childlike, and may "grow up too fast" (may need to act grown up because it's safer). Conversely she may grow up slowly, or be in mixed mode (e.g. well-behaved, but unable to care for herself).
Perceptive?	Yes, has to be to survive in this family's landscape.
Many needs and wants?	No, now this child has become needless and wantless because of the basic message that "You're not good enough," and "Your needs are not all right with me." (See "What Happened to the Child's Needs and Wants" on page 123.)
Undamaged? Untarnished/ Unjaded? Unexploited? Pure/ Untainted?	No, now wounded! Becomes cynical.
Unstressed?	No! Now filled with stress.
Present/Living in the Moment?	No. Now the little food addict ruminates about yesterday and worries about tomorrow. To deal with painful/abusive experiences, the little food addict dissociates (see discussion of "Dissociation" in "Survival Skills" on page 134).
Attention seeking?	Maybe yes, if it's not dangerous or scary to seek the attention. (See the discussion of "Lost Child" in the Chapter 15: Family and the Food Addict.) Would rather get out of the chaos and not be focused on because it's safer. Looks for attention elsewhere.
Authentic/ Genuine?	No, everything is now shrouded in masks, filters, façades, people pleasing.
Resilient?	Yes, that's what's amazing; you're still here, with the opportunity to recover and heal.
Persistent?	Yes, to a limit. The thinking is "Maybe this time it will be different," then the little food addict gives up.
Instinctual/ Intuitive?	Yes, developing good radar but doesn't trust it. (See Feelings This Child is Now Having" on page 125.)

Impatient?	Yes, no patience nor tolerance.
Impulsive with no impulse control?	Yes, caregiver failed to teach delay of gratification—must grab whatever while it is available.
No sense of time?	Either not concerned with time at all or over-concerned with time.
No sense of consequences?	Yes.
Unique?	No, doesn't feel special.
Sense of Wonder(ment)?	No, that's gone. No "Oh Wow!"
No boundaries?	Yes, that continues. The family members don't respect each other's boundaries; there is no role modeling for having healthy boundaries.
Creative?	Yes, but the creativity maybe impaired by criticism and lack of reinforcement.
Huge potential?	Yes, that exists and waits for the little food addict to find recovery and healing for her potential to be realized.

WHAT HAPPENED TO THE CHILD'S NEEDS AND WANTS?

By not having needs met, the child assumes it must be wrong to have them and they must be eliminated. To want is defined as "to desire, to promise one's self, set one's heart on, aspire, and dream of." This child had her ability to want stolen by their parents. If she wanted to be a policeman, superman, princess, or doctor, and she heard, "That's silly," or, "You'll never be that with those grades," this child's attempt at aspiration has been stolen. It is the learning to aspire that matters, more so than the child's aspiration itself.

When parents show little or no interest, support, or encouragement in the things the child thinks they want, their "wanter" gets stunted or stolen. When parents pay little attention to what the child really wants yet pour into their lives things the parent wants vicariously through the child, the child's "wanter" gets run over. The child learns that what they want matters less than what others want.

Parents who meet all of their children's needs and wants are not teaching the children to meet some of those needs themselves. The children may grow up expecting others to meet all of their needs. (See the later discussion regarding self-care on page 342.)

> Children who are attacked for having any needs may grow up to be anti-dependent. They learn that it is unsafe to ask for any needs to be met. Children who are neglected and abandoned may grow up with issues of feeling needless/wantless. They learn at a young age to "turn off" their needs as they learn that they are not important enough to have them.
>
> The food connection is easily seen in this context: Food needs were met, but not emotional needs, and the little food addict, early on, confuses the two. When in need of nurturing (i.e., being held, talked with, kindness), the little food addict experiences "I'm hungry." Also, how we feed and care for ourselves is a reflection of how our family and our culture cared for us. As children, when we are fed good care, our sense of self grows, our capacity to play and symbolize/think abstractly develops, and we learn how to recognize and deal with various need states.
>
> In contrast, when there are difficulties in the bonding between mother and child (due to neglect or infringing on an infant's unstructured states of being) during early development, the self withdraws and fragments. Children become alienated from their needs and are unable to safely experience them. They then project their needs onto food, the body, and relationships, searching for a way to feel self-worth and a way to manage that which feels so out of control. Unfortunately, these projections function only to reproduce the internal world of seduction, attack, and abandonment. Along with becoming needless and wantless, feelings of deprivation are experienced (See "Feelings This Child is Now Having" on page 125).

So, at this point, what is developing in this little innocent being, who now is very wounded? What do you think? Does this child want to break out? Is the little food addict so angry/enraged that she wants to EXPLODE? Ah, but that couldn't happen; the little food addict would get killed if she blew up. So, instead of *ex*ploding (which is too dangerous), this child . . .

* IMPLODES *

Just like a building that's being razed, she caves in on herself. And just for reference, what do we, in the treatment profession, call *depression*? Anger turned INWARD!

Little Food Addict in the "War Zone"

FEELINGS THIS CHILD IS NOW HAVING

Now that the little food addict has experienced the trauma ("implosion") of this "War Zone," let's look at some of the feelings she is now experiencing:

- **Disappointment:** Little addict comes into the world needing, hoping for, and expecting love, understanding, attention, appreciation, care, encouragement, recognition, and affection. These are needed for emotional survival. When these needs, hopes, and expectations are not met and realized, this child feels massive disappointment. Little addict now begins to live below the emotional poverty line. She hopes that these wonderful gifts will arrive "at the doorway of her heart," but it never quite happens. So the little food addict lives in constant disappointment. This chronic disappointment is overwhelming, so this young person eats to avoid the hollow, sinking, empty feeling.

- **Deprivation:** It's possible that in the little food addict's family, food was plentiful, but love was not. As with disappointment, the little food addict learned to substitute food for the deep pain of the lack of love, attention, affection, understanding, tenderness, recognition, or warmth. So she begins the conflating of food needs with emotional needs. (I recently had a client who, upon starting the Realization Center Food Plan for True Recovery, complained that she felt "deprived." As we explored her family history and her lifelong efforts to not experience the ambient feelings of emptiness by using food, it made perfect sense that, as she placed boundaries around her eating, she would experience those feelings she had spent her life avoiding with the substitution of food. As the patient began to follow the food plan and get support for her ABSTINENCE,[56] she began to identify her real feelings of deprivation. She also realized that she had to allow herself to experience the feelings that she had buried for so many years if she were going to achieve recovery.)

- **Self-doubt:** Every child has the power of intuition. They're born with it and, if nurtured, they grow up accurately perceiving their environment and those in it. Children intuitively know how to keep themselves and their environment safe, even though they often lack the ability to make it so. Intuition is the act or faculty of knowing or sensing without the application of rational processes; a perceptive insight, a sense of something not evident or deducible; an impression. This dysfunctional family stole our little food addict's ability to intuit her environment, as it is—her sense of reality. By family denial, minimizing, and blaming, the little food addict was "taught" that what she sensed was not consistent with family myths. Therefore, her perceptions were discounted and nullified. Little addict then eventually abdicates her power of intuition. Recovery is a process of attaching the "gut" to the head, which is key to building trusting relationships. Without the ability to trust her intuition, the little food addict never really learns to trust anyone. The adult little food addict either enters relationships naively, as if wearing blinders, or she never really develops trusting relationships. As long as the little food addict is "using" food in this way, she won't be able to listen to and hear her "gut" and be in sync with her emotional intelligence.

Learning to trust her intuition allows this person to step back from control and surrender to others the responsibility of earning that trust, then listen to her intuition and watch the actions of those with whom she is in relationship—or decide if she wants to be in a relationship. Have you ever had the experience of meeting someone, and your heart started to pound with fear? Your head said, "Oh no, no, this is a nice, an okay person—you're wrong," so you dismissed your gut reaction. And before you knew it, you got involved, either with a friendship or something more serious—in a "romantic" relationship. And in a short time, you discovered that you had made a serious mistake; this person has turned out to be a crazy person—rageful, shaming, maybe mean, narcissistic, rejecting, demanding, abusive (like your parent[s]). And now you're stuck! You can't get out!—either emotionally or perhaps even physically. Awful, wasn't it? Do you know what happens in this scenario when the little food addict is well into recovery? When the adult little food addict meets someone and her heart starts to pound with a danger signal, she says to herself, "It's okay, sweetheart, we're out of here!"

- **Insecure/unsafe:** Little addict has no anchor and feels unmoored, with nothing and no one to attach to.

Little Food Addict in the "War Zone"

- **Fear:** The little food addict is afraid of people and authority figures.

- **Timid:** The little food addict is frightened by angry people and any personal criticism.

- **Overwhelmed:** This is all too much for the little food addict who has no one to protect them.

- **Hurt/Pain:** The little food addict is hurt and/or in pain.

- **Powerless(ness):** The little food addict has no control to make it all stop and be nice.

- **Hopeless(ness)/Despair:** This is never-ending.

- **Nightmares:** The little food addict can't escape the "War Zone" even in sleep.

- **Lost; loss of self:** The little food addict doesn't trust herself and can't rely on her own judgment.

- **Not comfortable being in own skin:** This is where the little food addict experiences the desire to not be with herself, wanting to be someone else because it's too painful to be herself (see page 139 for further discussion).

- **I'm broken/I'm defective/I'm the problem:** The little food addict has come to believe that these are true.

- **It's my fault/guilt:** In some respects, by the little food addict's feeling responsible for creating the craziness/abuse/ neglect/abandonment/ drama/dysfunction in this family, then maybe she can figure out a way to be different to make it stop—it's a futile attempt at feeling that she has some control.

- **Alone, lonely, abandoned/left out/isolated:** The little food addict has learned there's no one to rely on.

- **Anger/rageful:** The little food addict has these feelings but can't show them.

- **Anxious/nervous/having panic attacks:** The world, as modeled by the little food addict's family, is not a safe place, and the little food addict is not equipped to navigate it.

- **Frustrated/helpless/impotent:** Nothing the little food addict attempts as a solution succeeds.

- **Confused:** The little food is confused by mixed messages, broken promises, inconsistencies, and unpredictability within the family unit.

- **Inadequate/incompetent:** The little food addict believes she is not good enough, that she is a disappointment.

- **Low self-esteem:** The little food believes that she has no value, no worth, that she doesn't matter and is disposable.

- **Sadness, depressed mood:** The little food addict has lost her spirit because the "War Zone" is a dark place.

- **Shame:** Because of the shaming messages that say she is flawed and defective, the little food addict has internalized the belief that she is worthless and valueless. She has developed a "core of shame."

- **Tortured/Tormented:** Living in this family, this "War Zone," experiencing neglect, abandonment, shaming, and various forms of abuse is tantamount to being in a major war conflict with similar resultant consequences.

All of this leaves this sensitive and vulnerable person:

Depressed or Dysthymic

Dysthymia is a chronic type of depression in which a person's moods are regularly low (low-grade depression) or irritable for an extended period of time. However, unlike major depression, the person can function, but struggles with feelings of hopelessness, sleep issues (too much sleep or insomnia), indecisiveness, low energy/fatigue, low self-esteem, poor concentration, and eating issues. Psychiatrist Atilla Turgay says, "Chronic unhappiness in childhood and adolescence may represent a significant risk for serious depression and an increased risk for self-injurious behavior and attempted or completed suicide. These clinical features may also be an associated risk factor for the development of alcohol and substance use. Most patients with Dysthymic Disorders have co-morbid problems, the common ones being major depression, anxiety disorders, attention deficit hyperactivity disorder, oppositional defiant disorder, conduct disorder, and substance-abuse."[57]

THE ATTACHMENT ISSUE

Throughout this process, the little food addict is the victim, with no choices. This child (at five, six, seven, or eight years old) can't say, "You're all crazy and toxic; you're not treating me well; you're hurting me, and I'm leaving and moving in with that kind, caring, nurturing and sane family down the street. Or I'm getting a job, getting my own apartment, and moving out of this insanity!"

The little food addict feels trapped and *is* trapped, because she is bonded/attached to the very people who are inflicting the harm and creating the profound wounds. Little addict loves the people who are hurting her, and the little food addict is being hurt by the very people she loves.

The little food addict has lived and grown up with addiction or similar disabling emotional extremes.

Neuroscience explains that emotions are experienced in the body and processed by the limbic system. The body does not know the difference between physical danger, like an oncoming car, or emotional danger, like a drunk and raging parent. The limbic system will react either by pumping out enough stress chemicals, like adrenaline, to give the spurt of energy needed to flee to safety or stand and fight.

The dysfunctional dynamic of the family follows the child into adulthood. The "COA" (child of an addict) becomes the "ACOA" (adult child of an addict). In Dr. Tian Dayton's book *Emotional Sobriety: From Relationship Trauma to Resilience to Balance,* she states:

> "But what happens when the family itself becomes the proverbial saber-toothed tiger? Children cannot flee; where would they go? They cannot fight; they would lose. So they shut down, they freeze, they flee on the inside. But without somehow processing what's going on for them, that numbed and frozen pain can lie dormant within the self-system, an emotional accident waiting to happen, in what is now called a post-traumatic stress reaction. That is what being an ACOA (Adult Child of Trauma and Addiction) is all about. Years after the stressor is removed, the ACOA lives as if it were still there. As if some emotional threat lurks just around the corner. This is the dilemma of the adult child of addiction and/or trauma. Unresolved pain from childhood gets recreated and acted out in adult relationships."[58]

In other words, the little food addict is attached to her tormentors. Attachment is an emotional bond to another person; it does not discriminate as to how sensible it may be. Children will, must, and do attach to adult caretakers, who most often are the biological parents. The problem in a severe trauma family is that there is a chronic pattern of abuse, neglect, abuse, kindness, neglect, abuse, etc., in a cycle that goes on forever. While a child fears, flees, avoids, and shuts down, the child must also simultaneously (or sequentially) attach if he or she is to survive. A failed attachment system exposes the child to extreme levels of unmodulated stress, isolation, and inner emptiness. Such stress can drive the urge to restrict, overeat, or both.

LOCUS OF CONTROL SHIFT

Another perspective of the little food addict's experience in this "War Zone" is the locus of control shift. All children think in a way that is self-centered: *I am the center of my world, everything revolves around me, and I cause everything that happens in my world.* On top of that, *I have magical power to make things happen.*

In the severe, chronic trauma family, the young child shifts the locus of control from where it resides inside the adults to inside the child. The child thinks: *Hey, I am not powerless, helpless, and trapped. I am making this abuse happen; the cause of it is inside me. So therefore, I am in control and have hope for the future. It is happening because I am bad. How do I know I'm bad? Because I have bad feelings about my parents.* (In the child's mind, the parents have to remain safe, consistent attachment figures.) *Also, I know my parents are good. Good parents would not abuse a child unless she/he was bad and deserved it. Also, I know that if I decided to be good, the abuse would stop, so the fact it hasn't stopped proves I am bad for not deciding to be good.*

The traumatized child is trapped, overwhelmed, and helpless, and unable to control, predict, or escape the abuse and neglect. When the person who cares for her is perceived as dangerous, the child experiences anxiety, depression, uneasiness, and disequilibrium.

As an adult, the thinking is the same: *Only by being bad can I maintain control, holding onto the illusion of power, control, and mastery.* This protects the adult child from experiencing the real truth: *I loved the people who hurt me and I was hurt by the people I loved.*

A trauma history is often seen in food addicts. To deal with traumatic experiences that create emotional distress and alienation from one's self, a

Little Food Addict in the "War Zone"

child is often drawn to using food to self-soothe. It certainly does work to help soothe the pain. What was the solution, however, is now the problem.

The great British psychiatrist D.W. Winnicott said that two things can go wrong in childhood: That which shouldn't happen but does happen, and that which should happen but doesn't happen. When people think of trauma, it's usually some specific bad event, not the absence of a parent who was attuned to the child's needs. *Attunement* is what allows the child's brain circuits to develop without chronic anxiety and fear.

Attunement is a term used to describe parents' reactiveness to their babies' moods and emotions. Well-attuned parents detect what their babies are feeling and reflect those emotions back in their facial expressions, voices, and other behavior.

Dr. Gabor Mate explains that when something should happen for a child but doesn't, it's usually attunement that is missing.[59] That's when two people, parent and child, are sharing an emotional space and fully communicating. We all need that to become fully ourselves, and its loss is hurtful. And when it is absent, we are not fully ourselves. We develop addictions. To avoid this deepest level of sadness and grief, food addicts hold on to the "badness" of the self. And they reinforce it with negative self-talk, by treating themselves and their bodies badly, and by contracting with outside people to abuse and neglect them in word and deed.

Accepting this truth provides the basis for the fundamental work of recovery, which is mourning the loss of the parent(s) the child never actually had. This can't happen unless the food addict is abstinent and allows herself to experience these feelings.

The parents the little food addict never had were reasonable, consistent, loving parents who, once in a while—when she needed it—disciplined her. The deepest trauma is not the bad things that *did* happen, but the good things that *didn't* happen. It is the errors of omission by the parents, not the errors of commission, that hurt most deeply.

Of course, the preoccupation with eating/not eating and associated behaviors serves the attempt to cope with the intense, deregulated emotions and confusion regarding identity and self-esteem. Unable to establish a stable identity base, the food addict in effect says, "I don't know who I am," "I feel like an imposter," or "I'm really bad, but I pretend to be good."

At the core of any individual's capacity to bond lies self-empathy and the related capacity for self-care. Without a caretaker to mirror and validate the little food addict's real self and her feelings and to protect the little food addict in overwhelming situations, the child is left with feelings of profound shame. So what has been happening is the following:

Survival Skills, Beliefs, and Behaviors of the Little Food Addict

- The child becomes a caretaker; it's a way to feel some control and not so vulnerable/powerless. Taking care of others keeps the focus outward, and thus the little food addict doesn't have to experience her feelings. As adults, many abused children go into the helping professions—nursing, social work, and so on—trying to give the world the love they never received. (See the discussion of the role of the "Hero" in Chapter 15: Family and the Food Addict.)

- The child has a need to control or be controlled.

- The child becomes an actor, telling everyone what they want to hear and doesn't let anyone know how she really feels.

- The family and survival rules of "Don't feel, talk, or trust" become entrenched early, as well as:
  - ➤ Anger
  - ➤ Avoidance
  - ➤ Humor
  - ➤ Isolation
  - ➤ Blame
  - ➤ Secretiveness/dishonesty—Following the family rules, the little food addict never reveals true feelings or needs and prefers that no one know about what she is doing. This can be cloaked by being too open about other things.
  - ➤ Becoming manipulative—Little addict actually develops skills as a master manipulator, since this family system is not open and communication is not direct, and rules are inflexible, this child learns alternate ways to get some needs met.
  - ➤ Becoming passive-aggressive
  - ➤ Always putting others first—Fixing everybody else in the hope that if they are okay, they'll reach back to the little food addict; not feeling or showing anger or sadness, or both
  - ➤ Looking put-together

Little Food Addict in the "War Zone"

➤ Keeping everybody happy—people pleasing

➤ Being ultra-responsible

➤ Not making mistakes

➤ Not troubling others—can't ask for what she needs from others

➤ Being brave

➤ Being invisible

- Keeping feelings under control at all times

- The child is unable to identify and express feelings in compliance with the family rules. Little addict stuffed her feelings inside from her traumatic childhood. (And the food [eating/restricting] puts a lock on the door to the feelings "room.") Because of this basic denial, the little food addict has lost the ability to feel or express her true feelings, either bad and good, because to feel at all has been so filled with pain. By not allowing herself to feel, the little food addict protects the self from pain. This can be described as "emotional constriction." As Dr. Bessel van der Kolk explains emotional constriction in his book *Psychological Trauma:*

  > "Emotional numbing is a natural response to trauma, and can last anywhere from a few hours to many years. Emotional constriction refers to a restricted range of feelings or a lack of expression of authentic emotion. The kinds of sharing that are part of therapy and 12-Step programs slowly and over time counter this numbing and constriction as the addict learns to safely feel and share strong feelings in the presence of others."[60]

- The child becomes perfectionistic/has a fear of failure. Because this child was shamed for being imperfect (which is human), she looks for an answer in perfectionism. And pressure to achieve is perceived as criticism for mistakes. The little food addict expects flawless performance from herself in every area of life. In the little food addict's family, she had to do things "right" to receive approval from her parents. "Right" meant perfectly. Mistakes or less-than-perfect were not acceptable. That translated into the little food addict not being acceptable. Little addict's parents placed unrealistic expectations on her, which the little food addict internalized. Then this child attempted to gain approval but learned that, no matter what she did, "It's never good enough." Little addict became obsessive/compulsive in the process.

- As the little food addict becomes older, she has difficulty with authority figures, and finds it particularly difficult to deal with anger or criticism.

- She is self-punishing; works harder and stays in uncomfortable situations longer than is good or sensible to do.

- She tends to isolate (see "Little Addict's Fortress" on page 138). People who have been traumatized may have a tendency to isolate and withdraw into themselves when they are feeling vulnerable. Isolation is also a feature of depression.

- The little food addict develops high tolerance for inappropriate behavior, for pain and suffering.

- The child withdraws to fantasy.

- This person dissociates. Dissociation is used to escape from uncomfortable situations, feelings, or traumatic events, such as sexual, physical, mental, spiritual, emotional, or verbal abuse. In dissociation, thinking (one's head) detaches from feelings (one's body). You may, as an adult, have been accused of "living in your head," experiencing life intellectually, not emotionally. This translates as shortchanging yourself, living in a limited way. Forms of dissociation include:
  - ➤ Daydreaming/withdrawing to fantasy
  - ➤ Having imaginary friends
  - ➤ Dissociative episodes—during traumatic events, extreme stress or overwhelming emotions, the person may "blank out" or even fall asleep.
  - ➤ Out-of-body experience—during traumatic events, the person has the sense of being outside of their body and feel that they are viewing themselves from a completely different vantage point.

- The little food addict as an adult looks and acts independent but feels dependent; the veneer of independence hides long-standing unmet dependency needs (those that an individual cannot provide for themselves—can only be met by another person). Childhood was when this child was supposed to be dependent and get her developmental dependency needs met, but because the parents defaulted, the little food addict had to take care of herself before she had enough experience and training to handle it. Compensating, as the little food addict

Little Food Addict in the "War Zone"

grows older, she becomes fiercely independent/self-sufficient or contrarily overly dependent. Also, because this child has had the ability to think independently stolen from her by being told what to think or not to think and was shamed when she voiced a thought that an adult thought was silly, wrong, or childish (of course; it's coming from a child), the little food addict begins to believe that something is wrong with reality—or at least something someone else says is reality. Little addict is now shamed into giving up her views and submitting to someone else's imposed way of thinking. The potential consequence is that the little food addict often gravitates into systems, relationships, even marriages she allows to think for her or ordain for her what to think. As a result, she remains dependent on those contingent relationships and systems to think for them. In effect, the little food addict is a dependent personality, desperate to hold on to a relationship to avoid the pain of abandonment felt when the original parents weren't there emotionally. Growing up in a symbiotic family structure, the little food addict feels unable to live an independent life.

- She tends toward impulsivity—Important decisions are made with little thought or research.

- She has low frustration tolerance, trouble coping with stress. When things go wrong, the adult little food addict often turns to food (an ongoing coping mechanism), alcohol or other painkilling drug or medicine (anodynes), and/or violence—even child abuse.

- She has excessive anger, especially toward herself.

- The addict ends toward all-or-nothing thinking. All-right or all-wrong attitudes; judges self or others harshly.

- She minimizes problematic eating/non-eating behaviors and their consequences.

- She experiences low self-esteem—Little addict still thinks she is "bad" or worthless, and that she deserved abuse then and now therefore needs the approval of others (approval-seeker). Is a people pleaser and loses her identity in the process; puts others' needs first and bases her behavior/feelings on others' behavior or feelings to her own detriment (co-dependence). "If I perceive that you like me/approve of me/won't be angry with me, then I'm okay (and feel good about myself), and I'll do anything to get you to feel that way about me."

- She has an overdeveloped sense of responsibility.

- Concern for others instead of herself enables the little food addict to not look too closely at herself and her problems (displacement).

- She can't be assertive (has never developed her "voice"); gets guilty feelings when standing up for herself instead of giving in to others.

- Her fears change. Old patterns of living and relating to others feel familiar and "safe," even if they're clearly destructive.

- She doesn't act, instead reacts.

- She becomes hyper-vigilant. Always on guard for perceived threats; suspicious.

- She is more aware of others' needs and feelings than of her own.

- She has poor/no boundaries. One effect is the impaired ability to discern the difference in identity between self and other. This may express as enmeshment with another, where the little food addict adopts thoughts and feelings of another person and any semblance of boundaries is blurred, if not altogether lost.

- She is inconsistent in behavior.

- She experiences loneliness, even in a crowd.

- As the little food addict ages and begins to live like a victim, she is attracted to that weakness in friends and lovers.

- She confuses love and pity. Wants pity for herself and tends to love people she can pity and rescue.

- She has troubled relationships. Because of the "War Zone" experience, the adult little food addict is unable to form close bonds. Often she allows herself to be abused again, because the role feels familiar and secure—and it's the only one the little food addict knows.

- Sometimes, paradoxically, the little food addicts become abusers themselves.

- Inability to play, have fun, be spontaneous, she finds it difficult to relax and enjoy the moment.

Little Food Addict in the "War Zone"

- She becomes addicted to excitement, after years of living in the midst of heightened traumatic and often dangerous family soap operas.

- She may experience nightmares.

- She has difficulty concentrating.

- She develops phobias.

- As the little food addict advances, develops passive/aggressive personality as a result of growing up in an environment where it was not safe to express frustration or anger.

- Families in which the honest expression of feelings is forbidden tend to teach children to repress and deny their feelings and to use other channels to express frustration.

- She becomes obsessive/compulsive.

- She may develop a personality disorder.

- She may have suicidal thoughts or attempts.

- If the little food addict becomes a parent, she will often have problems raising children:

  - Doesn't know what to expect from children at different ages. For example, she might assume that an infant can be toilet trained, or that a five-year-old thinks like an adult.

  - Abuse her children, because she was taught it's okay to abuse the ones you love.

  - Can't cope well with the stress that raising children can bring.

  - Can't feel close to her children, although the little food addict wants to. If the little food addict was physically or sexually abused as a child, she may be loath to touch or hold her own children.

THE JOURNEY OF FOOD ADDICTION CONTINUES

What has been developing in this "Little Food Addict in Training" are the general characteristics of an addict:

- Lack of trust (believing that it's dangerous to trust people or their own feelings, or may be loyal beyond reason to people who don't deserve trust).

- Poor social skills/isolation (difficulty being able to relate intimately with at least one other person. Not able to share any meaningful information about themselves, fears, dreads, aspirations, hopes).
- Low self-esteem
- Poor impulse control
- Isolation

THE LITTLE ADDICT'S FORTRESS

As the addict grows, she builds a virtual fortress to protect herself from the scary, unmanageable world: This fortress has turrets on each corner with guns mounted on each to block out the world. It has a moat around it, filled with hungry alligators so no one dares to enter. The drawbridge is always in the "up" position with rusted chains from lack of use. The fortress is stocked with everything the food addict needs: refrigerator, TV, computer, and phone. There is a side door with a secret path over the moat—for the food delivery man (and the alcohol or drug dealer).

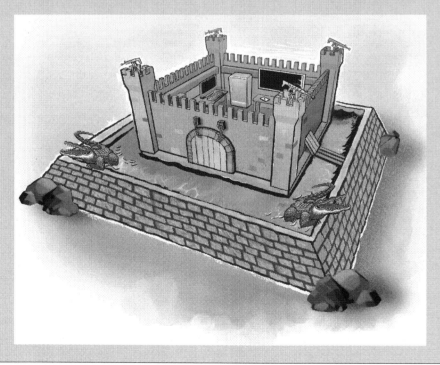

The fortress represents the internal life of a person who was raised in the "War Zone." Shame has been the building material of this fortress designed to keep at bay all dangerous relationships, while maintaining the safety of the addict. She has everything she needs inside and doesn't have to confront the feelings that manifest as a result of shame. The setup is that the family becomes shame-bound, and because the little food addict is being neglected, controlled, or abused, her personal needs become shame-bound. Gershen Kaufman (as quoted in Bradshaw's *Healing the Shame That Binds You*, page 102) states: "When one feels empty inside, hungry to feel a part of someone, desperate to be held close, craving to be wanted and admired—but these have become taboo through shame—one turns instead to food."

FOOD IS NOW THE DRUG

Because of the circumstances we've been discussing, this young person is not comfortable in her own skin and needs to detach, distract, numb, mood-alter, escape—disappear. What this is all meant to explain is that the actual seeds of food addiction are sown at a very young age. Seven- and eight-year-olds get societal messages that their personal worth depends upon their physical appearance. They respond to these messages by adopting complaisant opinions, attitudes, dieting, and other behaviors that are the symptoms of food addiction (over/under-eating, purging) in its early stage.

Various studies have shown that, by age nine, fully 85 percent of females are dissatisfied with their body size and shape and over 59 percent have begun dieting. Many who go on to develop anorexia were labeled "finicky" eaters in childhood. Remember, however, the symptoms of food addiction are found on a continuum, and many addicts shift their eating behaviors from one symptom to another during the course of their progression. Many female food addicts who have come for treatment at the Realization Center (see page 483) for their out-of-control eating (or eating-and-purging) report starting at a young age with dieting, leading them to anorexia.

Not only is the little food addict using the eating behavior to help her manage her feelings, but added to that is the pressure of society's values about body image and weight. Young girls particularly, growing up with the effects of shaming and already dealing with issues of low self-esteem, low self-confidence, and confusion about themselves, are placed in a school environment that plunges them into a tailspin of self-doubt, body hatred, indecisiveness, and a lack of assertiveness. David and Myra Sadker's book *Failing at Fairness: How America's Schools Cheat Girls* explains:

> "Girls are systematically denied opportunities in areas where boys are encouraged to excel. They are taught to sit quietly, defer to boys, avoid math and science, value neatness over innovation, and value appearance over intelligence. Boys are complimented more for their academic acumen, girls for their appearance, social skill and docility."[61]

The little food addict is beginning to experience lack of control over eating behaviors: eating when not physically hungry, isolating to eat, becoming preoccupied with eating behaviors and/or weight, body size, and shape, and experiencing cravings for sugars, starches, and/or fats. Most likely, other members of the family also use food to cope with the histrionics, chaos, shame, and stress of the family environment. Little addict's family has set the stage for her to employ overeating, undereating (anorexia), or eating and purging (bulimia) when dealing with suppressed feelings of intense inadequacy, vulnerability, and fear.

These eating behaviors provide a temporary "solution" that blocks out and minimizes the anxiety and uncertainty that would accompany going ahead with life's challenges and dilemmas. However, as time goes on, this same "solution" entraps the little food addict in a demanding, medically compromising, and tyrannical relationship.

When sex abuse is also present, the child experiences that her body is not her own and that her life is beyond her control. But with food, the child can control the frequency and amount of food that is eaten. The child may binge and purge to exercise that control, to feel "cleansed," or to punish herself. The child may overeat to become physically overweight in order to become "unattractive" to the abuser. Or, if a girl, she may starve herself to lose or reduce the physical characteristics she believes might be the reason she was abused (developing breasts, for example). These strategies may temporarily relieve the emotional stress or pain, but eventually they take on a life of their own. What began as a way to get or maintain control is now very much out of control. The temporary food abnormality no longer serves as a way to deal with a problem or to sidestep a problem—it is the problem.

FOOD ADDICTION BEHAVIORS

Food addiction exists on a continuum. We can think of anorexia at one end of the spectrum, binge eating on the other, and bulimia as somewhere in between. Some food addicts shift from one to the other during the course of the progression of their illness. (This was discussed in Chapter 2.)

If the little food addict is a girl and finds comfort in food, she begins to put on weight and her appearance is commented upon (most likely negatively) by family or peers, or she is unavoidably and deeply affected/influenced by society's "standard of beauty" as reflected and dictated by the media, celebrities, etc. What began as a determination to lose weight continues and progresses to a morbid fear of regaining any lost weight. It becomes a relentless pursuit of thinness. Being thin, which translates to "being in control," becomes the most important thing in the world.

Boys are not immune to using food to deal with their feelings. Because boys are often involved with sports, their eating issues are not so much evidenced by weight gain or loss. They too are being influenced by mass media messages on physical appearance. "The physical standards are becoming just as impossible for men as they are for women," says Arnold Andersen, MD, one of the nation's experts on male eating disorders.[62] He is Professor of Psychiatry at the University of Iowa College of Medicine and is the coauthor of *Making Weight: Men's Conflicts with Food, Weight, Shape & Appearance* and three other books on eating disorders.

The reigning male standard is a svelte, buff body with clearly articulated muscles. If a boy is teased for "being on the chubby side," he can begin to equate thinness/fitness (being muscular) with confidence and happiness. He suffers the same damage to his emerging self, as does a girl. Dr. Andersen's research on boys reveals that some 80 percent are dissatisfied with their bodies: "Half want to bulk up, and half want to lose."

The way women go to weight-control groups/programs, men go to the gym, where the incentive to compulsively over-exercise as a weight control/reduction method is noted.

Dieting is a major starting point for all the problem behaviors with eating—anorexia, bulimia, binge/obsessive eating. Diets are used initially by anorexics and bulimics, who soon abandon them and move into other, more extreme weight-loss measures. The overeater is likely to have been a chronic dieter.

Self-starvation is the fantasy of internal control. Individuals with anorexia find this internal control virtuous. They have managed to escape feeling fat, weak, undisciplined, and unworthy.

With the progression of the illness, eventually there are no longer *fattening foods*, but now simply the idea that any food is fattening. Dieting becomes a purpose and a "safe place to go." It's a world created by the anorexic to help cope with feelings of meaninglessness, low self-esteem, failure, and the need to be successful, special, and in control. This is a world where they can be "good," "successful," and "safe" if they deny themselves food, making it through the day eating little, if anything at all. (Many anorexics ultimately end up binge eating and purging food to the point where approximately 30 to 50 percent develop bulimia nervosa.) Also, the little food addict has learned that, rather than relying on people, it is best to rely on her ability to control her intake of food to overcome desperation, frustration, disappointment or abuse.

If the little food addict is not able to restrict her food/caloric intake sufficient to be "thin enough," but instead ends up bingeing as a rebound to the attempts at restricting/starving, she suffers weight gain, with the family's snide comments or her own increased self-loathing. Often, this person will discover, out of anxiety and desperation, purging through self-induced vomiting, laxatives, fasting, over-exercise, or similar behaviors to make up for the binges. According to Shaindy Holtzman in the *Jewish Press* article "Anorexia and Bulimia: Deadly Illnesses":

> "Purging often serves to calm down the [food addict] and ease their guilt and anxiousness about having consumed too much food or gained weight. As the disorder progresses, the [food addict] will purge or compensate for eating even normal or small amounts of anything they consider 'bad' or 'fattening' and maybe eventually—any food at all.
>
> "Bulimia [purging] eventually becomes a means of mood regulation in general. The food addict finds solace in food and often in the purging itself. The act of purging becomes powerfully addictive, not just because it controls weight, but because it's calming or serves as a way of expressing anger."[63]

The cycle starts with using the food to stuff negative feelings down in the body, and when they throw up the food, they throw up the feelings. By contrast, anorexics, who deny themselves food, feel that eating may be the one thing in their lives they can actually control.

Other coping behaviors are also developing—smoking cigarettes, perhaps stealing (shoplifting), alcohol, and so on. Peers may introduce the little food addict to marijuana, and sex may serve the purpose of feeling wanted, cared about, acceptable, and even lovable. The little food addict may also be introduced to other drugs that serve to further numb her pain, offer pleasure and, if she discovers that these substances control appetite, then this person has invited in another problem: addiction to alcohol or drugs. This may happen anywhere from preteen to young adulthood, depending on opportunity or family circumstances.

These youths will begin drinking or using out of peer pressure, to be a part of a social group, to gain a sense of belonging. Kids start to experiment, and many simply like the feeling that these behaviors bring about. Some find that alcohol and drugs are a plausible way to anesthetize or medicate the pain of life. Alcohol and drugs momentarily allow fears, angers, and disappointments to disappear. For some, it produces a temporary sense of courage, confidence, and even power.

As the eating behavior continues (and if alcohol/other substances are involved) this person eventually crosses the invisible line: she stops being a "cucumber" and becomes a "pickle" and progresses to addiction (see the illustration below). So, our little food addict marches inextricably toward the invisible line, which is "loss of control" (see page 145).

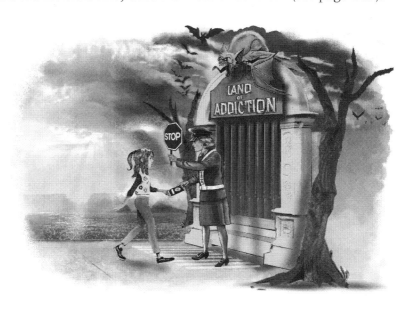

The Land of Addiction

The problematic invisible line has a "guard" in front of the entryway, attempting to dissuade the little food addict from continuing the trajectory—even as her family argues with her to stop. Of course the little food addict, finding the food lure too powerful (for purposes of relief, numbing, comfort, mirroring her peers, perhaps appetite control—certainly, brain reward) to stop, turns a deaf ear, cannot see what is happening, and doesn't want to see what is happening. Denial is entrenched. So the little food addict goes through the ONE-WAY door—because once she goes through this door, there is no way out—and she enters the "Land of Addiction."

There are two states in this "Land of Addiction." The first is the "Active" state, which is where the little food addict first entered. The second state is "True Recovery."

One day, the little food addict (probably much older now) says, "I can't stand this anymore. I hate my life. I am sick and tired of being sick and tired." And she remembers that when she originally entered the "Land of Addiction," the guard handed her a booklet titled *Passport*, which the little food addict is now reading. To the little food addict's surprise, it contains instructions on how to enter the "other" state in this "Land of Addiction." It says that to leave the "Active" state, the addict must go through the "DMZ."[64]

The "DMZ" for our the little food addict is "Detox." Little addict must go through a withdrawal process (for sugar, sweeteners, flour, wheat, volume, caffeine, purging, starving) to enter the other "state." If this person has managed to become sober and clean from alcohol and/or drugs, she has already experienced a withdrawal process, but she has to do it with the food and additive substances just mentioned all over again.

There are two doors between the two states representing the potential to jockey between them—i.e., the relapse/recovery dance. Once this detox is done, the little food addict enters the other state: "True Recovery/ Discovery," and decides to be abstinent (by following the food plan in Chapter 11).

Little addict understands at this point that she must work hard on herself to live in this privileged place. She realizes that she must discard the Band-Aids of food, alcohol, and drugs so that healing can take place from the inside out.

Little Food Addict in the "War Zone" 145

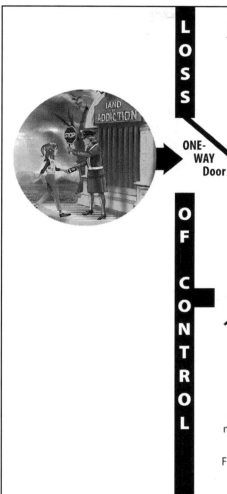

L O S S

O F

C O N T R O L

LAND OF ADDICTION

ACTIVE STATE
Bondage

Enslavement

Cravings that must be
continually satisfied

Shame

Vagueness

No Clarity

No Self-Esteem

Hopelessness

Progression

ONE-WAY Door →

*The doors swing both ways: Little Addict can
go back & forth between the two States*

IN **DMZ (DETOX)** OUT

TRUE RECOVERY
Abstinence (following food plan)

Sobriety (in full measure) / No cravings

Normalized blood sugar levels
(resulting in optimized energy, stabilized
mood, normalized weight, sleep, digestion,
optimized brain function)

Freedom / No longer in bondage to cravings

Energy / Full access to intelligence

Elimination of the shame that
comes from overeating, purging

Self-esteem / Clarity

Much less self-criticism
(particularly regarding body image)

Integrity, which gives rise to dignity

Creativity / Real feelings

Passion / Hope

The beginning of feeling whole/real **Healing**
(of all the wounding that set all this
in motion in the first place)

Copyright © 2013 Dianne Schwartz.
All Rights Reserved.

HEALING FROM THE INSIDE OUT

Becoming **abstinent**—that is, relinquishing the option to use food (and alcohol/drugs) as Band-Aids to cover up the hurts of her inner child—and working a program of recovery allows the little food addict, who grew up with distorted mirrors to begin to learn to trust her own perceptions. Recovery requires a persistent quest for authenticity, to accept and appreciate oneself for the individual one is in an effort to stop trying to change oneself into something one is not. Being with others who are involved in a recovery process helps the little food addict see that the aspects of herself that she most wanted to be rid of are the very characteristics that make her who she is, that have helped her survive. Healing from addiction happens when:

- Foods that promote obsessional thoughts and compulsive eating are eliminated.

- New behaviors around food are developed.

- The commitment to abstinence requires the little food addict to find new ways to manage feelings.

- Unfinished business is resolved. That's going back to the source of the wound and, through therapy, 12 Step work, allowing it to be "cleaned out" so that there can be real healing from the inside, while staying committed to not using the food as a Band-Aid over one's feelings.

The reasons for being and staying abstinent and living in recovery are many, with the overriding one being: **Taking the power back from your history.**

Functioning under the coping strategies developed during childhood requires a high price in terms of integrity, authenticity, wholeness, and sense of spiritual connectedness. You must unravel your history so it ceases to rule, so you no longer have to run from it. Take back your power from the food, so you can find your voice. In an article in *Recovery Today* titled "Our Families, Ourselves," John Bradshaw writes:

> "Childhood is over with. We have to be healed. We have to learn to face our pain and feel it and get through it. One of the first steps is to recognize our lost-child self and grieve for the pain. We have to learn to grieve—for ourselves, for our families, for our wasted lives [and for

Little Food Addict in the "War Zone"

the substance]. Because grieving completes the past. And the end of grieving is to be reborn."[65]

A vital aspect of recovery is in knowing and honoring our feelings, desires, and ideas, and expressing them in healthy ways. Most of us have lost years avoiding, numbing, using food, drinking, drugging, acting out sexually, or whatever else we could to avoid owning our feelings. But here we are now as adults with the potential to deal with feelings and people in far more mature and adaptive ways.

The key to recovery is the little food addict's ability to feel her feelings and begin to honor them. Why that's important is not that we are our feelings, but our feelings show us more about who we are. Each feeling state contains literal information regarding our truest identity, what's important to us and what's not, and what it is that we need to express and share with our world.

No one is placed here by mistake. Everyone has something unique to share with the world. What a loss it would be to self and others if we were not expressing our truth in the world. Are you willing to stand in your truth, take healthy risks, and express your feelings and heart's desires more readily and more directly? Are you willing to become the person you were meant to be?

To do the work of healing, we must have access to our feelings, whatever they may be. And that means being abstinent. Otherwise, the healing work becomes an intellectual exercise. These very feelings serve as the "threads" that lead us back to when we were abandoned as children. We have had to develop survival skills to bear the pain to "get through" our childhoods. When we chose to survive, instead of what felt like drowning in pain, our adapted child states took over the reins from our more authentic, raw child states. We survived the best we knew how, but we paid the price by forgetting who we were and what we really felt.

The ability to identify the feelings attached to our discomfort is a powerful tool to help us recognize our inner selves. Being abstinent allows our increasingly strong functional adult to deal appropriately with our feelings and in a manner that allows us to flourish. These feelings are actually golden invitations to freedom.

CHAPTER 5

Food Addiction
The Precursor/Gateway
to Chemical Dependency

Food addiction and chemical dependency are two sides of the same coin—in fact, cross addiction of food addiction with alcohol and drug addiction is high. Both are biologically based, affecting the reward pathways of the brain, and both are addictions that make a life unmanageable. Moreover, it is also common for addicts to switch back and forth between the addictive substances and behaviors. This chapter presents the relationship between food addiction and drug and alcohol dependence.

FOOD AS THE FIRST DRUG

Most addicts start on the path to addiction using food as the first drug. The addict "to be" starts life with a genetic predisposition, as we discussed in Chapter 1. At its very core, addiction stems from faulty feedback circuitry, that is, the inability of the addict's brain to experience satiety—"enoughness," and "No thank you, I don't need any more."

Whatever was happening in the future addict's life to set her on the addiction journey (with this genetic vulnerability) happened at an early age. The little food addict in training couldn't tell her family, "You're not meeting my needs, you're abusive or absent or crazy, so I'm packing my bags to live with the Jones family down the street. They seem like a nice, warm, loving, open, nurturing, supportive, functional family." Since the child couldn't leave the situation, she needed a coping mechanism—and food was there! And it worked to distract, numb, comfort, and fill the emptiness. And, most likely, the rest of the family was also using food (or some other substance) for the same reasons.

Unlike drugs or alcohol, food is readily available to a young child. Some clients report that from the time they were two years old, they have had an abnormal relationship with food—for example, stealing food to make sure there would be enough in a crisis. These clients often started with food addiction at an early age and then experimented with

148

Food Addiction

substance abuse as they matured. As the addict grows and finds "better living through chemistry," the food may or may not take a backseat. But it is always there.

For some food addicts, the lure to find "better living through chemistry," i.e., alcohol and drug use, is ever present if there was addiction in the family. Claudia Black, MSW, Ph.D., a renowned author and lecturer on the subject of family systems and addiction, explains that most children raised with addiction vow to themselves and often to others, "It will never happen to me. I will not drink like my father, or use drugs like my mother."[66] Certainly, that was my vow—I was not going to be like my mother!

Peer pressure to drink or use is difficult for a child to resist, as well as the need to be a part of a social group, to have a sense of belonging. Kids will experiment just to see what it's like, and many simply like the feeling. Some discover that alcohol and/or drugs are a wonderful way to anesthetize or medicate the pain of life (of living within their dysfunctional families). Albeit momentary, fears, angers, and disappointments can be made to virtually disappear with alcohol and drugs. And, for some, it produces a momentary sense of courage, confidence, and maybe even power. Also, these children are vulnerable to being triggered by early alcohol/drug use because of the genetic influence on their brain chemistry; they can quickly demonstrate addictive behavior. And then the food may not be so important. It gets put on the "back burner" to be "revisited" when and if the adult child comes into recovery.

IT'S ABOUT "USING" A SUBSTANCE

Food addiction is not about weight, as I've been explaining. It's about "using" a substance for distraction, for numbing feelings, for comfort, and for a mood change. However, many food addicts "wear" their addiction—with extra weight—but not *all* food addicts do this. Some struggle with eating issues but are able to maintain a relatively normal weight.

Food addiction involves biological, psychological, and social factors, as does alcoholism. When an addict enters recovery and puts down their major coping tool—alcohol and/or drugs—food addiction (especially for sugar and refined carbohydrates) still remains. In fact, food has most likely played an important supporting role for that addict to be able to begin to and continue to abstain from their primary coping tool and deal with (that is, continue to medicate) the emotional pain lurking underneath. The addict views herself, as does the lay population and the treatment and recovery world, as now *switching* to food, when in reality, the addict is returning to or continuing to medicate with their number-one substance—the one that has been there the longest and is most deeply rooted. Those with alcohol dependence and/or drug addiction commonly hit bottom with drugs and/or alcohol before hitting bottom with their food addiction.

If you are in recovery from drugs or alcohol, it's important to answer the following questions:

- "Now that I'm sober and clean, is my eating out of control?"

- "Am I concerned that I behave with food as I did with alcohol and/or drugs?"

- "Am I preoccupied with eating?"

USING FOOD TO SATISFY THE CRAVING

If you've ever gone to an AA meeting, you are familiar with their offerings: coffee and sugar-laden bakery items—i.e., cookies, cakes, pastries, etc. Eating sugar in the form of candy or chocolate is actually recommended in *The Big Book* of Alcoholics Anonymous.

As discussed in Chapter 1: The Disease Concept of Addiction, the phenomenon of craving is the scourge of any addict. To deal with and satisfying the cravings, the addict uses sugar in any form to avoid turning to drugs or alcohol. As explained in Chapter 7: The Culprits and Triggers, the sugar satisfies the craving by affecting the brain's reward circuitry in the same way as alcohol and/or drugs do. But the problem is that eating these sweets satisfies the cravings only to have them return when the body's glucose levels start to plummet; the addict then has to get more sugar or other quickly absorbed refined carbs to bring their blood sugar levels back up again. That's why addicts gain weight in recovery (unless they start to purge with vomiting, laxatives, exercise, or restricting). They are looking to the food to help them feel okay.

Studies are now backing up what we know empirically with regard to sugar and its satisfying effects on the addict's craving. One researcher, Bart Hoebel, Ph.D., professor of psychology at Princeton University, explained that the sweetener (sugar) seems to prompt the same chemical changes in the brain seen in people who abuse drugs such as cocaine and heroin. He further concluded from his findings that a "sugar addiction" may even be a "gateway" to later abuse of drugs such as alcohol.[67]

WHAT ABOUT CIGARETTE SMOKING?

Cigarettes present a double whammy. Nicotine suppresses appetite and provides an alternative oral activity to eating. But nicotine is a drug and the tobacco leaves, in the processing to become cigarettes, are cured with sugar. Certainly smoking a cigarette satisfies the brain's craving for reward, but it actually also gives the smoker the "hit" of sugar. Besides the strong addictive qualities of nicotine, it's no wonder many smokers are resistant to stopping smoking because they fear weight gain. The "food" (sugar and its relatives) are waiting to "replace" the cigarettes, just like with alcohol and other drugs.

UNWILLINGNESS TO SEEK 12 STEP FOOD RECOVERY FELLOWSHIPS

Many people with solid sobriety who are actively recovering in Alcoholics Anonymous (AA) or Narcotics Anonymous (NA) are unwilling to seek help in treatment or attend 12 Step food recovery focused fellowships (FAA, OA, GreySheeters, CEA-HOW) because the key "rationale" is that their compulsive eating (overeating, binge eating) is not thought of as an addiction or a serious medical disease. Often, even as those alcoholics and drug addicts celebrate recovery, there is an ongoing denial (on their part as well as others) that using food to deal with their lives is a serious problem. Their "disordered" eating behavior is justified, rationalized by the thoughts of *It's better than picking up a drink or a drug*, or *My weight is fine*, or *It's just a Twinkie, a candy bar, a soda, etc.* or *I'm not doing anything illegal*. For others, suffering is dealt with more secretively and silently—adding to the unmanageability and shame they already feel as a result of having food addiction.

There is also the general attitude in AA and NA, as in society in general, that those who have eating problems should just exercise a little more willpower. That is, there is an unwillingness or inability to apply the principle of Step One (powerlessness and honesty) to their relationship with food: "Surely I'm powerless over drugs and alcohol, but eating is something I *should* be able to control."

Again, there is much more denial within our society about the dangers of food addiction (eating disorders, especially compulsive overeating). It is much easier to blame fatalities on coronary artery disease or heart attack rather than on food addiction—a disease that requires a recovery solution to keep it in remission, one day at a time. The evidence of this denial is found in the volume of diet books on the market. These books focus on weight issues—lose "10 pounds in 10 days"—and ignore the real problem.

If food addiction is not concurrently treated with the other addiction, the addict is vulnerable to relapse and is short-changed in achieving a level of self-esteem in recovery that only emerges when a person is not "using" any substance to deal with life.

From One Substance to Another

A dramatic demonstration of food addiction "morphing" into alcohol abuse/alcohol dependence is the food addict who undergoes gastric bypass surgery, which prevents them from eating a sufficient amount of sugar to satisfy their brain's demand for "more." Since the gastric bypass didn't create a "bypass" for the reward pathways of their brain (which is the seat of their addiction) nor did it address the resultant obsessional thinking, they find that alcohol does the trick.

At Realization Center, we have seen a number of individuals with late-onset drinking problems who have had bariatric surgery. This is not to say that all who have the surgery develop into alcoholics, but it makes sense to think about the idea that the surgery is like a diet—only a permanent one—but it does not address the food addiction. The patient continues to experience cravings, and since they physically cannot eat enough to feed their "addiction," they find alternate methods.

Contemporary research has shown that a high number of alcohol-dependent and other drug-dependent individuals have a preference for foods with a high-sugar concentration. And both human and animal studies have demonstrated that, in some brains, the consumption of sugar-rich foods primes the release of euphoric endorphins and dopamine within the nucleus accumbens (being one part of the brain's reward system; the pleasure circuit), in a manner similar to some drugs of abuse. The neurobiological pathways of drug and "sugar addiction" involve similar neural receptors, neurotransmitters, and hedonic regions of the brain. Craving, tolerance, withdrawal, and sensitization have been documented in both human and animal studies.

We know that food addicts—more often women, but men are now quickly catching up[68]—who, as part of their illness, are preoccupied with their weight and body image and attempt to control their weight by

Food Addiction

dieting and, in some cases, purging. Some of these women, maybe starting in adolescence, as a form of purging, find and use alcohol, speed (amphetamines), cocaine, or other stimulants, which causes them to lose their appetite and lose weight. What magic! But now they have another problem—alcohol dependency and/or drug addiction! (That's what happened to me; it launched me into a twenty-year addiction to amphetamines.) In some cases, these individuals jockey back and forth—using alcohol and/or drugs to not eat, and sometimes using the food to not drink or use drugs. What a trap! Realization Center once treated a woman who ate cocaine to numb her "insides" so that her appetite would also be numbed.

According to Nancy Fiorentino and Katie Regan in the publication *Facts On: Food Addiction,* one-third of food addicts are addicted to alcohol or other drugs, and one-third of cocaine addicts are anorexic or bulimic. These proportions reflect several times the rate of these disorders in the general population.[69]

Most observers of alcoholics and drug addicts and addicts themselves believe that when they put down the alcohol and drugs their eating becomes more significant—less controllable—more important. I agree with this view, but I disagree with the idea that the addict has now "switched" to food as her substance. I believe that all addicts start on the road to addiction by using food as a substance before they find "better living through chemistry (alcohol and drugs)." I don't believe that when they put down the alcohol and drugs, they *then* begin using food. The food has been there from the get-go and maybe took a backseat position when the addict discovered drugs and/or alcohol.

When the addict comes into recovery and embraces sobriety, the food is there—and has been waiting patiently to be called to the forefront of the addict's need to deal with cravings and feelings. Insofar as addiction is an issue of brain chemistry imbalance (see Chapter 1: The Disease Concept of Addiction and ASAM's latest definition of addiction), poor diet, deficient in essential nutrients, prevents the body from adequately producing important neurotransmitters. That's what precipitates the onset of anxiety and increases the urge to self-medicate.

THE MISSING LINK IN RECOVERY

A healthy diet,[70] which tends to be overlooked by many traditional treatment programs and 12 Step fellowships, is one of the most crucial aspects of holistic recovery. Studies show that improper nutrition perpetuates the cycle of addiction. In addition, chemical dependency combined with poor diet can wreak havoc on the immune system and lead to emotional turmoil. To restore healthy brain function, it is imperative that harmful junk foods, sugar, caffeine, and starches be removed from the person's diet.

A growing number of experts readily agree on the fact that biochemical intervention (proper diet along with supplements, i.e., vitamins, minerals, essential fatty acids, and other essential nutrients) has the power to heal the root symptoms of chemical dependency (i.e., craving, depression, anxiety, sleep problems, mood swings, etc.). There is much evidence that biochemical repair leads to a dramatic drop in the addict's symptoms and diminishes the likelihood of relapse—which is common among recipients of traditional treatment approaches. Biochemical repair is increasingly being identified as the "missing link" in successful addiction treatment.

Also, it important for the "recovering" chemically addicted person to know that often her symptoms of craving, depression, anxiety, mood swings, low energy, and sleep disturbances will, in time, abate with abstinence from alcohol and drugs, abstinence from over/undereating by following a structured food plan that normalizes blood sugar levels, moderate exercise, sufficient sleep, and supplementation with essential nutrients. Often these symptoms are direct biological consequences of the alcohol/drugs rather than symptoms of an underlying psychological condition.

It's a sad reality that the brain is being damaged during drug/alcohol use. But the brain has an amazing ability to repair itself—with the help of good self-care. Experience and research simply reinforce the importance of good nutrition as a recovery tool for repairing the brain and rebalancing the neurochemical systems.

Clinicians agree that compulsive behaviors for both chemicals and food must be addressed for a person to achieve and maintain recovery from chemical dependency. Most also agree that the chemical addiction must be tackled first, unless the eating problems are so severe that the person requires immediate medical attention.

"Most people think the best way to treat someone with both problems is to address the problems concurrently," says Elke Eckert, M.D., professor of psychiatry and director of the Eating Disorders Clinic at the University of Minnesota. "Yet you can't treat the eating disorder without

Food Addiction

155

first dealing with the chemical issues. It doesn't work. If people are using substances, they are not cognitively aware enough to deal with their eating disorder. If they are still using chemicals, that [the work involved in food recovery] all goes out the window."[71]

At Realization Center, clients focus on their chemical dependency first, but they also begin learning about how their chemical use and food addiction are connected—that they affect the same regions in the brain that cause the phenomenon of craving. Food addiction does not cause chemical dependency, nor does chemical dependency cause food addiction, but the two aggravate each other and may contribute to dual relapse. Our clients learn that for "True Recovery," their eating behaviors, their food addiction, must be addressed with abstinence being the goal.

Even though there have been "advances" made in treating addictions, the long-term success rate of treatment programs historically has been around 15 percent. Whether alcoholism, drug addiction, "eating disorders," or any combination of these, most programs treat the mind but completely ignore the body. 12 Step programs such as Alcoholics Anonymous (AA) emphasize a three-pronged approach to recovery: physical, mental, and spiritual; however, emphasis is given to mental and spiritual recovery while the physical aspect is generally limited to abstaining from the drug of choice.

The biological focus of addiction treatment often ends at the withdrawal management stage for acute intoxication and treatment of any serious medical problems. What gets ignored is the fact that the substance abuser's body has adapted over the years to the effects of chronic intoxication. The body needs energy, good fuel, and nutrients to repair all the systems of the body.

According to Joseph D. Beasley, M.D., an expert in addiction treatment, "There can be no full recovery without attending to the body's needs."[72] When a traditional program is combined with an intensive nutritional regimen, success rates can rise to as high as 80 percent.

Bringing focus to the (malnourished) physiological condition of the alcoholic/drug addict with education about food addiction and the encouragement to incorporate "abstinence" as part of their recovery along with basic nutrient supplementation is what makes Realization Center a unique "holistic" treatment program and what makes the information in this book so invaluable.

CHAPTER 6

Understanding Metabolism and the Development of the Disease of Food Addiction

We don't connect symptoms with substances. For example, if we develop a headache in the afternoon, we don't think it's from dehydration (not drinking enough water) or from eating chocolate, drinking coffee, or consuming aspartame. We are clueless to the fact that we're having an allergic reaction. So we don't treat the problem; we treat the symptom with a pain reliever like aspirin. We don't stop and ask ourselves, "Why do I have this headache?" But rather, "What can I take to quickly get rid of it?" Our entire society is focused on treating symptoms while the causes go unrecognized and, therefore, unresolved. My goal is to "revolutionarily" connect causes (food addiction), symptoms, and the solution.

Do you love sugar—sweet, sugary foods? Do you have to have sugar every day? Or is your preference flour, i.e., bread and pasta? Or are you doubly blessed (actually cursed!) with loving them both? Do you have to have a cup of coffee to wake up or some (diet) cola?

If you answered yes, you're certainly not alone. Most likely you're reading this book as a result of not being able to control your intake of these substances despite many diets, diet programs, exercise programs, diet pills, using alcohol or other drugs (like smoking [tobacco], cocaine, amphetamines, opiates) to get control.

Even if you don't think you have a sweet tooth, you may be a sugar addict without realizing it. It's hard to live in the United States and escape our sugar-soaked diet, courtesy of the $28 billion American sugar industry. Sugar, in the form of high-fructose corn syrup, dextrose, fructose, or honey, is added to thousands of processed products—ketchup, baby formula, soup, peanut butter, canned vegetables, breakfast cereals, and barbecue sauce, to name just a few. I always point out to my clients that

Understanding Metabolism

157

this "love" they have for these foods/drugs is actually addiction. Our amazing major emotion of love is meant to attach to many things but not, I believe, to sugar, flour, wheat, pizza, doughnuts, cookies, lasagna, etc. Actually, the experience is bliss (reward and pleasure). That's what we "fall in love" with: the reward. And that's entirely brain-driven and biochemical. It's biochemically seductive, which is why we keep going back for more. (Take a moment to reread pages 35–43 in Chapter 1: The Disease Concept of Addiction.)

HOW DOES EATING AFFECT BLOOD SUGAR LEVELS?

Every cell in your body depends on blood sugar for the energy to stay alive and perform its function. Without a steady supply of blood sugar (aka blood glucose), your brain couldn't think, your heart couldn't beat, and your feet couldn't walk. Before we continue on, we need to understand how eating affects blood sugar levels. We'll take a look in this section.

Glucose Metabolism

The fuel of the body is blood sugar. Blood sugar is to your body what gasoline is to your car. It's the fuel that makes it go. If your car ran out of gasoline, it would sputter, cough, and come to a stop. If you ran out of blood sugar, you would soon go into a coma and die. But, as you will see, our bodies have a built-in mechanism to prevent that from happening—at great cost to our health if we ignore good nutrition.

When we eat, proteins, carbohydrates, and fats are digested and broken down into smaller parts. Once broken down, these parts will affect blood sugar differently depending on how they are absorbed and how the body uses them. Almost all carbohydrates eaten and a portion of protein and fat will be converted into a simple sugar called glucose, the body's energy source, and transported into the bloodstream. This process is called glucose metabolism. The only carbohydrates not changed to glucose are those that cannot be digested, like fiber.

Right after a meal, the body's glucose levels rise. In response to the elevated blood glucose levels, the pancreas (an organ located behind the stomach) releases the hormone insulin. Insulin regulates the uptake of glucose into the cells—it takes the glucose from the bloodstream (thereby lowering blood glucose levels) and sends it into the cells—the muscle, fat, and the liver cells to be used as fuel. In this way, glucose becomes available to the cells to be metabolized into energy.

The cells that need glucose have specific insulin receptors on their surface so that insulin can bind to them, encouraging glucose entry and utilization in the cells.

Insulin also stimulates the liver and muscle tissue to store excess glucose; the stored form is called glycogen, a starch, readily available for energy use. If blood glucose levels are low, the hormone glucagon and epinephrine are secreted, having an effect opposite to that of insulin, forcing the conversion of glycogen in liver cells to glucose, which is then released into the blood.

If all the glycogen storage areas are filled, and there is still more glucose in the blood beyond that which the body needs to function, insulin will convert the excess to fatty tissue called triglycerides, which we carry in our bodies as the main chemical constituent of adipose tissue.

Most people know what can happen to a diabetic when they have too high levels of blood glucose—the diabetic can have a seizure, heart attack, stroke, go into coma, or die. In knowing that, we understand that the body is not made to sustain high levels of glucose in the bloodstream.

If blood sugar levels rise unrestricted, the result is: first feeling "good," then hyperactive, then irritable, agitated/angry, anxious, drowsy, and possibly stupor/coma/death. The pancreas is the organ responsible for maintaining even levels of glucose in our bloodstream—given normal/healthy conditions. The whole system is a very carefully orchestrated symphony.

When refined carbohydrates (see page 193 for a list) are eaten, blood sugar levels spike rapidly. Basically, once carbs are refined, their structure is broken down and the body doesn't need much time to convert them into glucose—see Figure 6.1 on page 162. In response, the pancreas floods the blood with insulin—to take the body out of danger, triggering cells to quickly take up large amounts of glucose—so much in fact that blood-sugar levels plummet. Then you're in a hypoglycemic (low glucose) episode or CRASH!

To explain "crash," we should know that the brain is the busiest organ in the body. It receives 15 to 25 percent of the body's blood supply. If any component of the brain's fuel supply (glucose and oxygen in the bloodstream) slip, the brain's functioning is dramatically affected.

Understanding Metabolism

159

Remember, the brain is the "air traffic control center" for thinking, feeling, mood, judgment, decision-making, analyzing, interpreting, creativity, cravings, instincts (hunger, thirst, sleep, sex, fight/flight).

As you read the following section, refer to Figure 6.1. on page 162.

Understanding Blood Sugar Swings

Let's say we eat a food addict's breakfast—or any meal—comprised of the following or any combination of these foods (see #1 on Figure 6.1):

- 4 ounces of orange juice. This is the equivalent of 6 to 8 oranges, which translates into 10 teaspoons of sugar; that's the amount in a 10-ounce can of Coke. (Any other fruit juice is about the same.)

- Doughnut or bagel. There is really no difference between these two.

- Muffin. This is basically the same as eating a cupcake.

- Any cold cereal. Cereal is flour, a refined carb. It doesn't matter if it's stamped into O's or flakes and laced with some form of sugar, including "fruit juice sweetened." This category includes granola, which sounds healthy but actually contains a lot of sugar.

- Pancakes/waffles. These breakfast cakes must be served with syrup (sugar); otherwise, they are basically deemed inedible.

- Pasta. These strings of flour—including artichoke and spinach that are milled into flour—are too quickly absorbed by the body.

- Candy, cookies, cake, or ice cream

- Fruit. This is too much of a sugar "shot," and this is why we never eat fruit by itself—always with a protein.

- Leftover pizza or Chinese food.

- Bread. Toast, roll, rye, whole-grain. It doesn't matter. It's all flour.

- Soda. This is sugar or sugar substitutes and may contain caffeine.

- Coffee with sugar or artificial sweetener (which is basically "Red Bull").

Any of these foods or a combination of these foods will overwhelm the body with sugar. Caffeine has a different effect in the body, so we'll discuss that one separately in the section titled "Caffeine" on page 183.

As the body begins to digest these foods and convert them into blood glucose—quite quickly since they are all so refined/processed (broken down) the body doesn't need much time to do the job, glucose levels in the blood start to rise dramatically. As that happens, we start to feel energy and feeling "good" (see #2 on Figure 6.1).

The pancreas is always on "duty" working to manage/regulate blood glucose levels with the production of insulin. However, in this situation with the spike in glucose, it becomes an emergency since the body now is in danger with the rising glucose levels in the blood, so it goes to work to take the body out of danger by producing massive amounts of insulin (see #3 on Figure 6.1). There is no gauge or "governor" on the pancreas to make it stop when the blood sugar levels reach the "normal range" (about 2 teaspoons of glucose circulating in the bloodstream at any one time is optimal—but in this example, the intake from the meal could be upward of 10-plus teaspoons).

As the insulin is being pumped out, blood sugar levels start to nose-dive; this could be an hour (more or less) after the intake of the sugary/floury meal. As the glucose levels rapidly descend, you start to feel the effects of "**crash.**" This is familiar to all of us—we have all experienced some of the symptoms of low blood sugar—and most of these are the result of the brain being starved of fuel (glucose) being delivered by the bloodstream (see #4 on Figure 6.1).

SYMPTOMS OF LOW BLOOD SUGAR

• Feeling tired; fatigue, low energy	• Craving
• Irritability/grumpiness	• Agitation/anger
• Frustration	• Anxiety
• Hunger	• Palpitations
• Poor focus/concentration	• Depression
• Lightheaded	• Nausea
• Headache	• Drowsiness/can't keep eyes open

Additional symptoms are listed under "Hypoglycemia" on page 163.

Understanding Metabolism 161

If blood sugar keeps being removed from the bloodstream, the result is coma and death, but the hormone cortisol, which is discussed on page 164, offers protection.

Maybe you don't often feel the effects of "crash" because you keep yourself "jacked up" with sugar every day, which keeps you on an artificial high and in a Neptunian fog you won't know you're in until you eliminate the culprits.

Important note: If you are an alcoholic or drug addict trying to recover, a day at a time, this is a very dangerous experience for you. Low blood sugar events create a big vulnerability to relapse. You brain is not functioning to help you "think through the drink or drug"; you just want to feel better and your emotional memory kicks in (from the primitive part of your brain) reminding you what will make you *feel* better—a drink or some drug and, bingo, now you've relapsed—and most likely it won't stop at "one"! In the state of crash, extreme behavior, rage, violence, and even crime are not out of the realm of possibility.

At the point of crash, you are feeling really awful, and you will look to some food/drink to make you feel better. *You will not want broccoli!* (Hence, the subtitle of this book.) Most likely you will turn to something sugary/floury, such as candy or a candy bar, cake, ice cream, coffee, juice, soda, Red Bull—something that will quickly bring your blood sugar up again (see #5 on the figure).

So the cycle starts all over again.

Important note: If this is your pattern and you have seen a psychiatrist for help with your up and down or mostly depressed and/or anxious mood, the psychiatrist will most likely *never* ask you, "What do you eat for breakfast?" trying to assess the influence of cycling blood sugar levels on your mood. Instead, you will most likely be diagnosed as being bipolar, or diagnosed with ADD, ADHD, depression, dysthymia (low-grade depression), or an anxiety disorder, and be given strong meds to manage your depression, agitation, anxiety, and/or hyperactivity. And, most likely, these meds won't work as effectively as they are supposed to because your mood swings are coming from cycling blood sugar levels and not from a true imbalance of chemicals in your brain.

I strongly believe that you first have to normalize your blood sugar levels by following the food plan presented in Chapter 11 before you really know how you feel and before anyone can accurately assess your mental state. Eliminate the substance (sugar and other refined carbs and poor eating behavior), and you will probably eliminate any potential medical diagnosis!

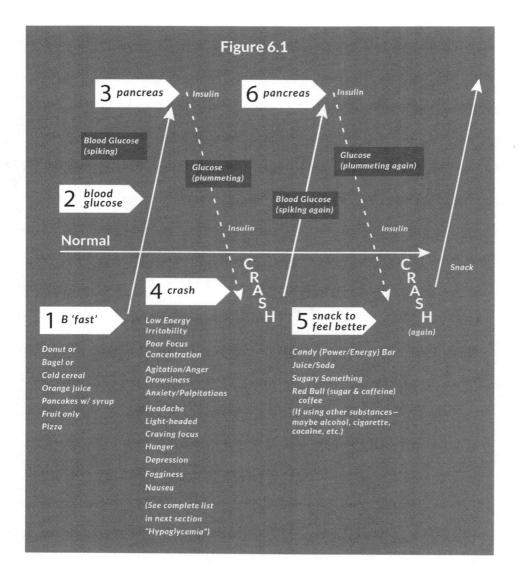

Understanding Metabolism

163

A LOOK AT CARBOHYDRATES

All carbohydrates are made up of "sugars." The type of "sugar" is determined by the length of their molecule, as follows:

- Simple (or sweet) sugars consist of lots of short-stranded molecules hooked together.

- Complex sugars (plant foods) are similar strands of molecules hooked into very long strands.

All carbohydrates are broken down into a one molecular sugar the body can use, glucose.

Table sugar or sucrose (cane sugar) is simply a very short-chained carbohydrate. Because it is such small molecule, it can be digested or broken down into glucose very quickly and moves into the blood at a very rapid pace. The more complex the carbohydrate, the longer it takes to be broken down into glucose and enter the bloodstream.

If your style of eating includes a lot of refined/processed carbs (sugars and flour) resulting in blood sugar swings during each day, you are inviting hypoglycemia, syndrome X, prediabetes, and type 2 diabetes into your life. These diseases are "invited" because they would not occur if one were eating in a way that allowed blood sugar to be level. (That's the food plan you'll find in Chapter 11.) These diseases are discussed in this chapter.

HYPOGLYCEMIA

Hypoglycemia means low (hypo) blood sugar/glucose (glycemia). It can be the result of too much insulin or oral medications used to treat diabetes, hormone deficiencies, organ failure, alterations of metabolism associated with disease, or as we're discussing here, excessive insulin produced by the pancreas to reduce the spiking of glucose from eating quickly absorbed carbs.

Hypoglycemia can also be caused by a prolonged period of not eating (aka restricting or starving). Not eating all day will cause blood sugar to descend. It can also produce a variety of symptoms and effects, but the principal problems arise from an inadequate supply of glucose to the brain (because the excessive insulin has removed a lot of the glucose from the bloodstream), resulting in impaired function. The signs and symptoms of hypoglycemia, which happen quickly, in the approximate order they manifest, can include:

- Shakiness/tremors
- Altered mood and thinking
- Sudden moodiness
- Weakness/fatigue/tiredness/exhaustion
- Personality change
- Nervousness or anxiety/panic attacks
- Sweating, chills and clamminess
- Irritability/negativism/impatience/combativeness
- Fogginess/spaciness/difficulty paying attention
- Confusion/impaired judgment
- Rapid/fast heartbeat/palpitations
- Lightheadedness or dizziness
- Sugar/refined carb craving
- Hunger
- Nausea
- Abdominal pain
- Sleepiness/drowsiness
- Blurred/impaired vision
- Tingling or numbness in the lips or tongue
- Headache
- Hot flashes
- Cold extremities
- Anger, rage, stubbornness
- Sadness/depression
- Crying
- Lack of coordination
- Nightmares or crying out during sleep

There is no consistent order to the appearance of the symptoms, if symptoms even occur. Specific manifestations may also vary by age, by severity of the hypoglycemia and the speed of the decline. In the absence of true physiological problems, these symptoms are often attributed to other causes (like lack of sleep, mood disorder, aging, tainted food, etc.) rather than to a person's intake of sugar, flour, or other refined carbs.

Cortisol's Response to Low Blood Sugar

To keep us from dying as a result of glucose being entirely removed from the bloodstream, the "orchestrated symphony" of our metabolism has a built-in mechanism to release glucose into the bloodstream when blood sugar is nosediving. Cortisol, a steroid hormone, which is produced by the adrenal glands, increases blood sugar levels in the bloodstream in response to low blood sugar levels. Cortisol is also a "stress hormone"

Understanding Metabolism

165

released in response to fear or stress as part of the fight-or-flight mechanism. For the most part, the release of cortisol is to protect you from imminent life-or-death danger.

The release of cortisol in response to a nosedive in blood sugar due to eating quickly absorbed carbs (sugar, flour, refined carbs) and insulin's protective response to high levels of glucose become a problem when these responses continue for prolonged periods of time. Persistent and sustained elevated levels of cortisol (which may also be due to chronic stress) can lead to damage to the cells in the hippocampus, resulting in impaired learning and memory. Additional effects of too much cortisol include the following:

- Adrenal glands start to get depleted, which raises levels of the hormone prolactin in the body, thereby increasing the body's sensitivity to pain, such as backaches and muscle aches. Depleted adrenal glands predispose you to chronic fatigue/weakness.

- Poor sleep/insomnia; this is because cortisol levels are supposed to drop at nighttime, allowing your body to relax and recharge. But if cortisol levels are too high, you might notice that, even if you've been tired all day, you get a second wind right around bedtime. Then you toss and turn all night and feel tired again the next day.

- Reduces bone formation, increasing the risk for long-term development of osteoporosis.

- Lowers immune function by deactivating the body's natural self-repair mechanisms.

- Muscle and bone loss

- Thyroid imbalance

- Skin problems

- Hair loss

- Increased weight gain, especially around the abdomen

- Lower sex drive

- Nausea, heartburn, abdominal cramps, diarrhea, or constipation

- Increased blood pressure

- Increased cholesterol

- Increased heart disease

- Increased risk for depression/moodiness; cortisol suppresses the production of serotonin.

- Increased risk for mental illness

- Lower life expectancy

- Shuts down the reproductive system

SYNDROME X, INSULIN RESISTANCE SYNDROME, METABOLIC SYNDROME

Metabolic syndrome is not a disease in and of itself. It involves a cluster of symptoms that predispose you to diabetes and heart disease. These symptoms include:

- Obesity, particularly excessive fat in the waist and stomach area

- High levels of triglycerides (type of fat found in the blood), reflecting problems metabolizing carbohydrates

- Low HDL ("good") cholesterol

- Although LDL ("bad") cholesterol is usually within normal range, the size of the LDL particles tends to be the small, more dangerous type, which can attach to artery walls and form plaque

- High blood pressure

- Elevated blood glucose

- Insulin resistance

- Chronically elevated inflammation

- Abnormal blood vessel function

As previously discussed, insulin is a natural hormone secreted by the pancreas, which oversees the utilization of glucose. Insulin's job as a "carrier" or "mediator" is to bind to specific insulin-receptors on body cells and help transport glucose into the cell to be utilized for energy or stored for later use. In many cases, muscle cells are the ones most in need of glucose, since muscle movements caused by physical activity frequently

Understanding Metabolism

167

deplete the muscles' energy supply. Circulating glucose that is not utilized by the cells may be stored as fat throughout the body.

What happens over time with the consumption of refined carbohydrates is that the cells develop a resistance to the body's own insulin. With insulin resistance, the body produces insulin, but the insulin is unable to bind to the insulin receptors on the cells so the cells are left without the glucose they need. In effect, muscle, fat, and liver cells do not respond properly to insulin and therefore cannot easily absorb glucose from the bloodstream. So the glucose remains in the bloodstream—leading to hyperglycemia (high blood sugar), as well as elevated levels of insulin.

As a result, the body needs higher levels of insulin to help glucose enter cells. The pancreas tries to keep up with this increased demand for insulin by producing more. As long as the pancreas is able to produce enough insulin to overcome the insulin resistance, blood glucose levels stay in a healthy range. But if the extra insulin still cannot bind to the cells, it causes high levels of insulin to circulate unused in the body. If you have too much insulin, you are likely to experience an energy "crash," and your cells quickly learn to ignore the hormone altogether. High insulin levels can also be dangerous because they can lead to serious health problems (in no particular order):

- Hypoglycemia

- Diabetes

- Increased risk of polycystic ovary syndrome (PCOS)

- Hypertension (high blood pressure)

- Damage to the walls of arteries—leading to coronary artery disease or cardiovascular disease

- Accelerated age-related health concerns. (This is because insulin increases the amount of the stress hormone, cortisol, in the body.)

Or, over time, the pancreas fails to keep up with the body's increased need for insulin. In either scenario, the resulting condition is insulin resistance. Without enough insulin, excess glucose builds up in the bloodstream, leading to the development of prediabetes (a condition in which blood glucose levels are higher than normal but not high enough for a diagnosis of diabetes), type 2 diabetes, cardiovascular disease, and stroke.

Note: Major contributors to insulin resistance are obesity, especially around the waist (belly fat), and physical inactivity.

Diabetes 101

Diabetes has reached epidemic proportions, with approximately 347 million cases worldwide, as a result of the global pandemic of obesity, a major risk factor according to *The Lancet*. In the United States almost 26 million fight the disease—more than 8 percent of the population.

Diabetes is a metabolic disorder in which the body cannot regulate the level of blood sugar/glucose in the blood and the levels are above normal. In people with type 1 diabetes, the pancreas doesn't produce insulin; in type 2 diabetes, a condition often associated with obesity, the body does not produce enough insulin or the cells become insulin resistant, in effect, the body can't seem to use the insulin the pancreas produces. The result of both type 1 and type 2 diabetes is that blood sugar levels rise, glucose spills into the urine, and the body can't use its primary energy source.

Type 2 diabetes was originally called "adult onset" diabetes because, prior to the escalation of our consumption of sugar, flour, and other highly refined carbs, this disease affected mostly adults after age forty-five. With the obesity epidemic affecting all ages, children, adolescents, and young adults are part of the type 2 diabetes spectrum.

With high blood glucose levels, diabetes increases the likelihood that a person will suffer from high blood pressure, elevated cholesterol, coronary artery disease, blindness, kidney disease, nerve damage, gum disease, amputation, Alzheimer's disease, cancer, and a shortened life span.

Diabetes is the leading cause of blindness, kidney failure, and amputations of the feet and legs. More than 60 percent of people with diabetes have some nervous system damage, and most non-traumatic limb amputations are performed in people with the disease. The leading cause of death for diabetics is hardening of the arteries, which causes heart disease and stroke.

About one-third of people with diabetes don't even know they have it. Many people don't find out they have diabetes until they are faced with problems such as blurry vision or heart trouble. Before people develop type 2 diabetes, they usually have "prediabetes" a condition in which blood glucose levels are higher than normal, but not yet high enough for a diagnosis of diabetes.

OBESITY

Obesity is a medical condition considered to be a disease, but there is very little empathy from society for those who suffer from it. So many of our eating problems results in serious damage to our bodies, including, most often, weight gain. Fat tissue is an active manufacturer of signals to other parts of the body. The body's fat cell's main job is to store our excess calories as fat. When people grow obese, their fat cells swell with fat and can plump up to three times normal size. As very overweight people get fatter still, they may also layer on many more fat cells.

Here are some of the health consequences of excess weight/fat:

- Moderately obese people live two to five years less than average-size people.

- Severely obese people's life span may be reduced by five to ten years.

- Heart disease—fat cells' chemical flood contributes to heart attacks, heart failure, and cardiac arrest.

- Fat can trigger high blood pressure (hypertension) by making blood vessels narrow.

- Overfilled fat cells affect the body's production and use of insulin, which instructs the muscle to burn energy and the fat cells to store it. Overfilled fat cells blunt the insulin message, thus contributing to insulin resistance. Overfilled fat cells leak fat into the bloodstream, which may infiltrate the heart muscle, contributing to congestive heart failure.

- Misplaced deposits of fat can also ruin the liver and have become the second leading reason for liver transplants after hepatitis B.

- Fat cells produce a variety of proteins that cause inflammation—which cause gunky buildups in the arteries, causing them to burst and triggering heart attacks and strokes; these inflammatory proteins and other fat-driven chemicals may also contribute to cancer.

- Diminished functioning in all areas of one's life especially in social relationships, e.g., family, friends, intimate relationships, education, religious, etc.

- The emotional and spiritual effects of overweight are addressed throughout this book.

GHRELIN AND LEPTIN:
THE HORMONES RESPONSIBLE FOR APPETITE CONTROL

How do we get in trouble with our appetite/eating? Given our understanding of how we get sick as a result of eating sugar/refined carbs, here's the explanation of why our bodies similarly don't respond to our biological mechanisms for appropriate appetite control.

When the stomach runs out of food, our blood sugar levels drop, which triggers the release of the hormone ghrelin from the cells of the stomach. This sends a message to the hypothalamus section of the brain (the part of our brain that regulates the hormone systems in our bodies), which in turn releases neuropeptides, which trigger feelings of hunger, which is really "false starving," telling us it's time to eat. When we have eaten enough, meaning when we're full, our fat tissues release the hormone leptin, telling the hypothalamus to reduce the production of neuropeptides, and it releases another chemical to suppress our appetite. On Mercola.com, Dr. Joseph Mercola states:

> "Metabolism can roughly be defined as the chemistry that turns food into life, and therefore insulin and leptin are both critical to health and disease. Insulin and leptin work together to control the quality of your metabolism, and, to a significant extent, your rate of metabolism."[73]

Again, this is all part of the amazing orchestration of the symphony of our bodies. If leptin is absent, our appetite is uncontrolled and persistent. If leptin is present and the receptors are sensitive, our appetite is inhibited. More body fat means less food is required, and so leptin is secreted to inhibit appetite and the accumulation of excess body fat. Overweight people generally have higher circulating leptin, while leaner people have lower leptin levels, meaning their appetite is stimulated more often. Leptin also responds to short-term energy balance. A severe caloric deficit will result in reduced leptin secretion—this is your body's way of getting you to eat when you need energy. It's the hunger hormone. Overeating temporarily boosts leptin, reducing hunger. Long-term, leptin signals that the body has adequate body fat (energy) stores; short-term, leptin signals that the body has had enough to eat. Both are supposed to result in the reduction in appetite.

If this mechanism is working properly, no one would be overweight.

Understanding Metabolism

171

If it's working correctly, when fat stores are "full," the extra fat will cause a surge in the leptin level, which signals the brain to stop feeling hungry, to stop eating, to stop storing fat, and to start burning some extra fat off. When leptin levels are low, we feel hungry and crave food. It does this by stimulating receptors in our hypothalamus. When leptin binds to receptors in this part of our brains, it stimulates the release of appetite-suppressing chemicals.

But apparently the mechanism is not working because of our out-of-control eating frenzy. People with leptin disorders tend to eat uncontrollably. The belief is that leptin, leptin resistance, and leptin sensitivity are dependent on the dietary environment we provide. Because we have strayed from our evolutionary diets, our metabolisms are unhinged and our leptin pathways are disrupted.

Leptin resistance happens in the same way as insulin resistance—by continuous overexposure to high levels of the hormone. (Leptin receptors in the hypothalamus don't respond to the leptin.) A diet high in sugar (particularly fructose), grains, and processed foods—the same type of diet that will also increase inflammation in the body—as the sugar gets metabolized in the fat cells, the fat releases surges in leptin. Over time, if the body is exposed to too much leptin, it will become resistant, just as the body can become resistant to insulin.

Robert Lustig, M.D., a pediatric endocrinologist, is very vocal about the toxic effects of sugar. He says, "The leptin is being made by the fat cells, the fat cells are trying to tell the brain, 'Hey, I don't need to eat so much,' but the brain can't get the signal. You feel hungrier and the reward doesn't get extinguished. It only gets fostered, and so you eat more and you keep going and it becomes a vicious cycle. If your brain can't see the leptin signal, you're going to get obese."[74]

The only way to reestablish proper leptin (and insulin) signaling is to prevent those surges, and the only known way to do that is through one's diet. Because this process is not instantaneous, those of us who are food addicts overeat because our brain hasn't gotten the message to stop eating; we cannot help but overeat. If we eat too fast, more food than necessary enters the digestive system prior to the suppression of our appetite, which results in overeating.

There is also a relationship between leptin, ghrelin, and sleep. Researchers have found that people who slept less were on average heavier. And people who slept less had lower levels of leptin and higher levels of ghrelin.

A LOOK AT SUCROSE AND FRUCTOSE

Robert Lustig, M.D., a specialist on pediatric hormone disorders and childhood obesity, has most recently brought our attention to some sobering facts about sugar. He stands in the back (or more now, the front—and I stand with him) of the crowd shouting, "The emperor has no clothes—he's really naked!" He says that sugar is a toxic substance that people abuse. He says that it's not about calories but the effect of sugar being a poison and being responsible for the skyrocketing numbers of obese and diabetic Americans and the resultant diseases of Western lifestyles—heart disease, hypertension, and many common cancers.

He uses the word "sugar" to mean both sucrose—beet and cane sugar (white or brown) and high-fructose corn syrup. Refined sugar (sucrose) is made up of a molecule of the carbohydrate glucose, bonded to a molecule of the carbohydrate fructose—a 50-50 mixture of the two. The fructose component of sugar and high-fructose corn syrup (HFCS) is metabolized primarily by the liver, while the glucose from sugar and starches is metabolized by every cell in the body. Consuming sugar (fructose and glucose) means more work for the liver than if you consumed the same number of calories of starch (glucose).

And if you take that sugar in liquid form—soda or fruit juices—the fructose and glucose will hit the liver more quickly than if you ate them in an apple, for example. The speed with which the liver has to do its work will also affect how it metabolizes the fructose and glucose.

If fructose hits the liver in sufficient quantity and with sufficient speed, the liver will convert much of it to fat. This induces the condition we've discussed above, insulin resistance, metabolic syndrome, which is now considered the fundamental problem in obesity, and the underlying defect in heart disease and in type 2 diabetes that is common to obese and overweight individuals.

When a person consumes too much sugar, the liver gets overloaded with fructose and converts some of it into fat. That fat ends up in the bloodstream and generates the bad kind of cholesterol called small dense LDL. These particles are known to lodge in blood vessels, form plaque, in which are associated with heart disease/attacks. This is the source of our population's problems with high cholesterol. We need to stop pointing a finger at eggs and steak.

Also, fructose doesn't affect satiety in the same way as glucose, making you eat more total calories if your fructose intake is high. Nancy Appleton, Ph.D., in her research on sugar has compiled a list of "147 Ways Sugar Ruins Your Health" (it's one of my favorite handouts in my lecture on "Sugar").[75] Fructose is, in many ways, very similar to alcohol in the damage that it can do to your body. Fructose can only be metabolized by your liver, because your liver is the only organ that has the transporter for it.

If you are eating high amounts of fructose (soda, fruit juices, honey, fruit juice sweetened cereals, ketchup, salad dressings, snack foods, fast foods, baked products, dried fruit, breads, pastas, baby foods, almost all packaged foods, etc.), it ends up taxing and damaging your liver in the same way alcohol and other toxins do. Dr. Lustig explains that by "stimulating the 'hedonic [pleasure] pathway' of the brain both directly and indirectly, fructose creates habituation, and possibly dependence [addiction]; also paralleling ethanol [alcohol]."[76]

Fructose and ethanol both have immediate, narcotic effects related to the influence on the brain's production of the neurotransmitter dopamine. In the same way that alcohol can lead to a downward spiral of compulsive overconsumption, fructose tends to generate an insatiable and intense sensation of pleasurable sweetness, often driving us to consume far more than our body can handle; even while it damages multiple organ systems and reduces both the quality and length of our lives, we can't stop consuming it.

There has been so much research on the deleterious effects of sugar and the category it belongs to—refined/processed carbohydrates—that the evidence is overwhelming. It's right before our eyes and in the media. As a reader of this book, you are your own research study (or you're seeing the serious problems of your clients/patients if you are a healthcare professional)—and you are looking for an answer to your eating problems.

Yet, there is so much resistance to seeing what is before our eyes, and our own truth of our helplessness around our eating behavior. We don't want to experience the harmful effects of our eating behavior, but we don't want to let go of what's causing our problems—the sugar and refined/processed carbs.

At Realization Center, Marilyn White has said that everyone who gets off the elevator (we're on the seventh floor) wants the help to feel better but doesn't really want to stop their drinking and/or drugging or change their eating behavior.

Given all of this, for those of us with the extra element of genetic vulnerability, those of us who have struggled with food cravings, weight issues, energy problems, brain function—that is, our functioning in general, have known that sugar, flour, and refined carbs—even though we tried and tried again to control our appetite for them—always beat us up—once we started, we overate them and either sadly accepted the consequence of weight or we found "magic" by purging them. Science is first catching up with what we have known for so long: this is addiction, and we are addicted.

CHAPTER 7
The Culprits and Triggers

All of the conditions discussed in Chapter 6 are a consequence of ingesting the "culprits"—that is, those foods that are too quickly broken down and absorbed by the body (sugar, flour, and all refined carbohydrates). Wheat is included in this category because of its ability to create cravings, which leads to out-of-control eating of these carbs, as I will be discussing. Caffeine also negatively affects blood sugar levels, so it is included in this chapter's discussion. Many of the foods/substances that trigger cravings (i.e., affect brain reward circuits) are also foods that are disruptive to normalized blood sugar levels. In this chapter, I will go into detail about each of these trigger/addictive/culprit foods and substances. Each section concludes with a powerful statement that reinforces our desire to eliminate these culprits and triggers from our food plan. I encourage you to speak these statements aloud.

ALCOHOL AND ALL ADDICTIVE DRUGS

As discussed earlier, normally, when blood sugar begins to drop, the body can respond by making more blood sugar or burning up stored sugar. And when your blood sugar begins to rise, additional insulin is secreted to bring the levels back to a healthy range. Alcohol is considered toxic (a poison) to the body, and all efforts are made to excrete it, including the cessation of maintaining healthy blood glucose levels. Studies have shown that alcohol interferes with all three sources of glucose (foods we eat, breakdown of glucose stored in our muscles [glycogen], and other nutrients in the body) and the hormones needed to maintain healthy blood glucose levels. Heavy drinkers especially deplete their glycogen stores within a few hours when their diet does not provide a sufficient amount of carbohydrates. Over time, excessive alcohol consumption can decrease insulin's effectiveness, resulting in high blood sugar levels.

Research has shown that acute consumption increases insulin

secretion, causing low blood sugar (hypoglycemia) and can also impair the hormonal response that would normally rectify the low blood sugar.

Apart from the powerful biological effects of any and all mind and mood-altering substances, they impair our judgment; they diminish our functioning, and are a total obstacle to the achievement of recovery/discovery.

All alcohol, all drugs, as with all the other culprits, affect brain chemistry and trigger the desire for "more"—and will always prevent the realization of the dream of recovery. To embark on this journey of recovery from food addiction, one must be sober and clean (meaning that you are no longer using alcohol or any drugs). This may be difficult news if you are a smoker. Cigarettes and tobacco in other forms (nicotine) are drugs. Continuing to consume nicotine in any form will always affect the work you do to become abstinent and the work required to live in abstinence.

Therefore, we eliminate all alcoholic drinks and all addictive drugs.

SUGAR

As this book has been discussing and will continue to discuss, sugar is a drug. It's as mood-altering as alcohol or any other category of drug. (Refer back to earlier discussions and the list of studies in Chapter 1: The Disease Concept of Addiction.)

Therefore, we eliminate sugar in all its forms and any food product containing sugar in all its forms.

A NOTE FROM DIANNE

During my lectures, clients sometimes ask, "You mean you *never* eat sugar? What about parties or other special occasions?" and I tell them, "No, I don't. I haven't eaten refined sugar, sugar substitutes, flour, or caffeine, nor have I overeaten in many, many years, and I don't want to. I also don't drink Drano. I have no cravings, *and* I would never go back to the pain and suffering those substances brought me. It's very clear to me, very internalized, that much of my life was lost to the struggle to find relief from my active food addiction. There is no way I would return to that. I can go anywhere, with people who are eating anything, and I have no problem. I don't get triggered, and I don't feel sorry for myself. It's just the opposite—I see the damage others do to their bodies and lives by their behavior with food."

SUGAR SUBSTITUTES AND ARTIFICIAL SWEETENERS

Sugar substitutes and artificial sweeteners affect brain chemistry and keep sugar cravings alive. Studies show that artificial sweeteners may actually cause greater weight gain than sugar by stimulating appetite, increasing carbohydrate cravings, and stimulating fat storage. They may also cause side effects such as headaches, moodiness, lethargy, and dizziness.[77] The substance that fall into this category include honey, aspartame (Equal, NutraSweet, etc.), sucralose (Splenda), saccharin (Sweet'N Low, Sugar Twin), acesulfame K (Sunnet, Sweet One), manitol, stevia, sorbitol, xylitol, and agave. They appear in many products such as diet colas, Crystal Lite, no-sugar added products, sugarless gum/mints, cold cereals, and power/energy bars (which are actually candy bars). Brain chemistry is altered when zero-calorie sweeteners are consumed.

When the sweet taste is not followed by a caloric load, the body craves the calories it was expecting. That's why the use of artificial sweeteners makes us want to eat and drink more—or have more artificially sweetened foods/drinks. They are addictive; we get hooked on them. Artificial sweetness tricks the body so effectively that it still releases insulin into the bloodstream to metabolize the sugar, which is not there. In the absence of sugar for the insulin to act upon, it performs its secondary function, which is to instruct the body to store fat. Note that the first ingredient in artificial sugars is dextrose, which is sugar.

Moreover, these artificial sweeteners have been implicated in numerous health problems and diseases, including multiple sclerosis, lupus, fibromyalgia, tinnitus, vision problems, Parkinson's disease, cancer, headaches, cramps, numbness, memory loss, and mental health problems. Unfortunately, most public health agencies and nutritionists still recommend these toxic substances as an acceptable alternative to sugar. Actually, these sugar alternatives were developed for diabetics, not for weight loss.

In general terms, honey is basically the same as sugar. It is a mixture of sugars and other compounds. With respect to carbohydrates, honey is mainly fructose and glucose. It acts in the body the same as sucrose. Honey gets its sweetness from the monosaccharides fructose and glucose, and has approximately the same relative sweetness as granulated sugar.

Aspartame (Equal, NutraSweet) is metabolized inside the body into wood alcohol (a poison) and formaldehyde (which is a carcinogen used as embalming fluid and is not eliminated from the body through normal waste filtering done by the liver and kidneys). It's been linked to birth defects, cancer, brain tumors, and weight gain. Meanwhile, Splenda came on the market to be a safer alternative to aspartame, the safety of which is being questioned. Splenda (sucralose) is a combination of sugar (sucrose) and chlorine and has been implicated in all of the following (in no particular order):

- Allergic reactions (stuffy nose, runny nose, sneezing, skin redness, itching, blistering, weeping, rash, skin eruptions, hives, red/itchy/swollen/watery eyes)
- Anxiety, dizziness, spaced-out sensation, depression
- Blood sugar increases
- Blurred vision
- Dizziness
- Gastrointestinal problems—bloating, gas, pain nausea, vomiting, diarrhea
- Glycoprotein in the body is affected with crucial health effects
- Headaches, migraines
- Heart palpitations or fluttering
- Intestinal bacteria (the beneficial type) reduced by 50 percent
- Intestinal pH level increased
- Joint pains or aches
- Kidneys, enlarged and calcified
- Leukemia
- Male fertility decreased
- Red blood cells decreased (a sign of anemia)
- Seizures
- Spontaneous abortion in half the population of test animals
- Weight gain
- Wheezing, chest tightness, cough, or shortness of breath

The Culprits and Triggers

179

Sorbitol, a sugar alcohol, is naturally found in apples, peaches, and prunes as well as in food items and beverages made from these sources. It is used as a sugar substitute in a wide range of dietetic foods, such as sugar-free maple syrup, brownies, cookies, pancake/cake mixes, gum, breath mints, licorice, and other candies. It is also used in medicinal products like Milk of Magnesia.

Side effects of food and drinks with sorbitol, especially when consumed in large quantities, could include a range of gastrointestinal problems, including a laxative effect because it is not well absorbed in the small intestine, diarrhea, abdominal pain, abdominal bloating or flatulence (gas), increased or decreased urination, mouth dryness, nausea, vomiting, dizziness, extreme weakness, breathing problems, aggravation of irritable bowel syndrome, swelling of the face and body, seizures, blurred vision, chest pain, confusion and change in heart rate. As will all sugar substitutes, it leads to repeated use, habituation, addiction—triggering our brain mechanism to keep asking for more of that sweet taste.

Contrary to what you might think, agave is not a healthy alternative to sugar. Depending on the source and processing method used, agave syrup can contain as much as 55 percent fructose, the same amount found in high-fructose corn syrup—with the same response in the body as with sugar. Most agave syrup is worse because it is nothing more than a laboratory-generated condensed fructose syrup and has a higher fructose content than any high-fructose corn syrup.

Therefore, we eliminate all sugar substitutes and artificial sweeteners.

A WORD ABOUT DIET SODAS

Caffeine helps alleviate hunger and boost energy; therefore, people with eating issues often consume large quantities of diet soda, which is often high in caffeine and low in calories. But one of the problems with artificially sweetened (diet) sodas is evidenced by soft-drink studies that show they contribute to weight gain by stimulating appetite. Nutrition expert Leslie Bonci, MPH, RD (Director of Sports Nutrition, University of Pittsburgh Medical Center) has stated that people think they can just fool the body.[78] But maybe the body isn't fooled. If you are not giving your body those calories you promised it, your body will retaliate by wanting more calories. That's one of the reasons that you have to keep having "more" soda—to satisfy the body's craving for real food.

FLOUR PRODUCTS

Flour products include bread, pasta, bagels, cakes, cookies, pastries, doughnuts, and pies. Flour converts to glucose too quickly for normal body functioning and rapidly increases blood sugar levels, which requires increase in production of insulin, and "crash" ensues—all this is adverse to the normalization of blood sugar (glucose) levels. Remember, flour is flour, whether it is made from spinach, artichoke, rice, etc. This ground powder regardless of its source is still flour, and it breaks down too quickly for our bodies to manage; they just are not built for it. Stephen Sinatra, M.D., a board-certified cardiologist and certified nutrition specialist, says that bread is the worst thing modern humans introduced into the diet. In *Heart Sense for Women,* he writes:

> "Why is bread (and bagels, and frozen waffles, and crackers) so bad for you? It's mostly processed white flour and sugar. It ferments in the gut, which can cause overgrowth of Candida yeast. These rapidly absorbed, high glycemic carbohydrates trigger your insulin levels to rapidly rise, then fall even more quickly, encouraging insulin resistance and 'rebound hunger.'"[79]

The following is an explanation of the process by which a whole grain becomes the toxic substances, sugar and flour. I am including this information here because the more you understand about the triggers, the more you will be empowered to eliminate them completely.

Anatomy of a Grain

As shown in the illustration at right, the *hull* is the inedible outer portion of any grain. It must be removed before the grain can be eaten (i.e., hulled barley). The *bran* is the layer with all of the grain's fiber, as well as niacin, phosphorus, iron, zinc, and magnesium. Before it is stripped of this layer, the grain is truly a "whole grain." The grain cannot be milled into flour at the "bran" level. Stripped further is the *endosperm*, the next layer with very few vitamins and minerals. The grain cannot be milled into flour at this level. Stripped further is the *germ.* This is the layer at which new plants sprout (think of sprouted bread), full of vitamins and minerals, protein, and a significant amount of fat (think of wheat germ). The grain cannot be milled into flour at this level. What's left is the *starchy center*, the innermost layer that is milled (made into flour). The grain cannot be

The Culprits and Triggers

milled unless it is stripped to this level. When it is stripped to the starchy center, all nutrients have been removed. All the fiber has been removed, and it is anything but a whole grain. The flour is then used for bread, cake, pasta, pretzels, flakes and "O's" for cold cereals, etc.—all then metabolized by the body as sugar. White rice is also found at this level.

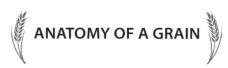

ANATOMY OF A GRAIN

The **HULL**—the inedible outer portion of any grain. It must be removed before the grain can be eaten (i.e., hulled barley).

The **BRAN**—the layer with all the grain's fiber, as well as niacin, phosphorus, iron, zinc and magnesium. Before it is stripped of this layer, the grain is truly a "whole grain." The grain cannot be milled into flour at the "bran" level.

Stripped further:

The **ENDOSPERM**—the next layer with very few vitamins and minerals. The grain cannot be milled into flour at this level.

Stripped further:

The **GERM**—the layer at which new plants sprout (think of sprouted bread), full of vitamins and minerals, protein, and a significant amount of fat (think of wheat germ). The grain cannot be milled into flour at this level.

Stripped further:

The **STARCHY CENTER**—the innermost layer that is milled (made into flour). The grain cannot be milled unless it is stripped to this level. When it is stripped to the starchy center, all nutrients have been removed, all the fiber has been removed, and it is anything but a whole grain. The flour is then used for bread, cake, pasta, pretzels, flakes and "O's" for cold cereals, etc.—all then metabolized as sugar. White rice is also found at this level.

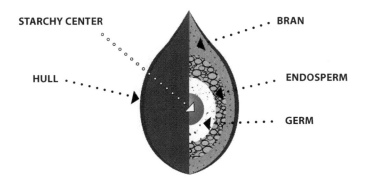

Therefore, we eliminate flour as well as all highly processed/refined carbohydrates.

WHEAT (INCLUDING SPELT AND KAMUT)

When flour is eliminated, then, for the most part, wheat is eliminated, too. (See the comments about wheat in Chapter 11: Realization Center Food Plan for True Recovery from Food Addiction.) Not only does our modern wheat contain a super starch (amylopectin A), which promotes weight gain, and a form of super gluten, which is inflammatory, wheat acts like an opiate in the body, creating the desire/craving to consume it again and again. The way it acts in the body is unique to wheat—not to the other grains. The belief is that when the body digests wheat, it breaks down into polypeptides (short proteins) called exorphins, which attach to opioid receptors in the brain, creating the feelings of "high." As the brain is affected, the phenomenon of craving develops, and you end up wanting more and more. In short, wheat is an addictive appetite stimulant. Research shows that people can be gluten-sensitive without having celiac disease, or gluten antibodies and still have inflammation and many other symptoms, e.g., obesity, allergies, digestive problems, low energy, diabetes, heart disease, cancer, rheumatoid arthritis, and mental illness.

In summary, most people are either allergic to, sensitive to, or intolerant of wheat, which then creates the ensuing craving, causing us to eat more, gain more weight, and the cycle continues. Unfortunately, this is a little-known fact so we don't attribute our "love" for bread and pasta to wheat.

Therefore, we eliminate all wheat.

CORN

Many of us grew up eating corn, believing it was a vegetable. Corn, a whole grain, is in the same category as white rice, a refined/processed grain, in its effect on the body. It is quickly digested, entering the bloodstream rapidly and causing a surge of glucose with the concomitant equalizing amount of insulin to move the glucose into muscles and fat cells. This results in low blood sugar, as described earlier. Theron G. Randolph, M.D., states:

> "Although wheat, yeast, soy and other frequently eaten foods have been described as largely unsuspected causes of chronic reactions [allergy/ addiction] before 1930, corn—the leading cause of food allergy—was not recognized as such until 1944. . . .

The Culprits and Triggers

183

Corn is thus especially important, as many sugars are made from corn, with corn being the leading cause of chronic food addiction in this century. As the food-addicted seek to find a more rapidly occurring and more effective stimulatory effect, this subtle addiction process tends to spread through alcoholic beverages and cigarette smoking. And all cigarettes manufactured in the US since WW I have contained added sugars, commonly corn sugar."[80]

It's not bad enough that corn in its natural cob state is a culprit, converting to glucose too rapidly, canned corn is additionally sweetened with sugar!

High-fructose corn syrup (HFCS) is produced by milling corn to produce cornstarch, then processing that starch to yield corn syrup, which is almost entirely glucose, and then adding enzymes that change some of the glucose into fructose. In the United States, HFCS is among the sweeteners that have primarily replaced sucrose (table sugar) in the food industry. HFCS is significantly cheaper than sugar, and it has become the principal sweetener in breads, cereals, breakfast bars, lunchmeats, yogurts, soft drinks, soups, and condiments.

Therefore, we eliminate all corn.

CAFFEINE

Ahh, caffeine . . . this is also a hard one. We take it as coffee, espresso, soda, chocolate, tea, green tea, and energy drinks). Caffeine is a "thief and a liar"! It's a thief because it robs you of your *natural* stores of energy, and then lies to you, like any good drug (which it is, albeit the most widely used drug in the world), that you have to have it to have your energy.

Caffeine causes increased neuron firing in the brain, which the pituitary gland perceives as an emergency and therefore causes the adrenal glands to release adrenaline—with its concomitant rush of energy (which is what we want and find pleasurable). It also increases dopamine levels, the neurotransmitter that is affected by drugs like amphetamines and heroin.

Caffeine also stimulates the adrenal glands to increase cortisol release. Cortisol then elevates heart rate and blood pressure, readying the body for a fight-or-flight response.

Drinking one or more caffeinated beverages daily results in a short-term energy and long-term fatigue.

Caffeine puts the nervous system into a constant state of "fight or flight," depleting energy reserves. Pushing the adrenal glands to extremes leads to fatigue, anxiety, insomnia, and weight gain. The cortisol triggers the release of glucose from the liver. This freed glucose gives people a sugar high (provoking the release of insulin to bring down spiking levels of glucose), quickly followed by a sugar crash, resulting in tiredness/energy drain and cravings for more caffeine or sugar in the form of simple carbohydrates. These sugar highs and lows add increased stress to the adrenal glands.

MediResource, Inc., provides the following information:

> "Caffeine is one of the two most widely used psychoactive drugs on earth. The other is alcohol. "Psychoactive" means that it has an effect on your mental functioning. Caffeine stimulates the sympathetic nervous system, and triggers stress response. This produces anger, fear, anxiety, increased heart rate and blood pressure, tremor, a jittery feeling, rapid and shallow breathing, change in pain sensitivity, and dozens of other changes. Caffeine is an Addictive Drug. Heavy caffeine users:
>
> —become psychologically [physiologically] dependent
>
> —develop tolerance (requiring more caffeine over time to get the same effects)
>
> —undergo withdrawal syndrome if they don't get it
>
> Withdrawal symptoms include headache, drowsiness, irritability and difficulty concentrating. Many people discover that they are dependent on caffeine when they go for a day or two without coffee and get splitting headaches."[81]

Addiction to caffeine is a serious problem. It can cause problems with stress, anger, and anxiety. Caffeine can aggravate tension headaches, irritable bowel syndrome, chronic pain, and many other physical problems. If you make a decision to eliminate caffeine from your life, don't do it cold turkey. The withdrawal symptoms are too powerful. If your caffeine is in the form of coffee, you should withdraw from it over a month's time, as follows:

- First week—substitute 25% decaf for your regular amount of coffee.

The Culprits and Triggers   185

- Second week—substitute 50% decaf.

- Third week—substitute 75% decaf.

- Fourth week—drink all decaf.

- And then, when you're ready (not more than another month), let go of the decaf.

If your caffeine intake is in the form of soda, reduce the amount you drink over a month's time. A very good substitute for soda is the broad variety of flavored seltzers on the market today—lemon/lime, strawberry, and even coconut and pink grapefruit—they have no sugar and the bubbles are refreshing.

Therefore, we eliminate caffeine in any form.

VOLUME

Although this doesn't fall in to the food category, volume (eating a lot of anything) is one of the reasons many food addicts are in trouble in the first place—we eat too much! And then, we want "more" again and again. It's the phenomenon of craving that gets triggered when we take in more than the body requires. That's why we need to weigh and measure the portions—to take our "will" and "feelings" out of the mix. You know, some days your eyes will say, "Gee, that looks like a lot of food," and on other days, you'll look at a portion and say, "Oh my God, that's so little; it will never fill me up!" The portions set forth in the food plan in Chapter 11 are the appropriate amount of food for your body, recognizing gender differences and assuming about forty-five minutes a day for exercise. If you exercise more than forty-five minutes a day, the food plan needs to be adjusted, as discussed in Chapter 11.

Researchers at Brookhaven National Laboratory wanted to know why some people will still eat a lot even though their stomachs are full. They stated, "We were able to simulate the process that takes place when the stomach is full, and for the first time, we could see the pathway from the stomach to the brain that turns off the brain's desire to continue eating."[82] The overweight subjects had less activation in parts of the brain that signal satiety in normal weight subjects. For all the years of trying to control our weight, losing the battle with those foods that provide brain reward (sugar, flour, fat, and salt), bingeing on them, and then maybe trying to starve, the mechanisms in our bodies that tells us about our hunger and satiety have become deregulated/dysfunctional. See the earlier discussion on leptin and ghrelin on page 170.

The foods we crave, overeat, and try to control are often the scientifically designed processed (junk) foods that don't allow the body to experience fullness and the resultant message to the brain to stop eating—it's enough. We have to allow these functions to return to some state of normalcy by changing our eating behavior. But we won't ever be able to return to them and "play" with them and expect our bodies to react non-addictively.

Therefore, we weigh and measure all food portions.

RESTRICTING/STARVING

This behavior will always backfire and set you up for relapse. Dissatisfaction with weight and body image issues create a decision to eat less and/or exercise more. So periodic diets are the usual tool of the food addict to have control over their appetite and weight problems. The approach becomes "How little can I eat?" And with exercise the approach becomes "How many calories can I burn?" And then it becomes a weight issue. We all know that this thinking and these behaviors don't work—they're temporary Band-Aids to a chronic disease. We go on a diet to lose weight, the diet will, by its very nature, restrict certain types of foods and or quantities, and what happens? We feel deprived, we're hungry, we get angry, we become defiant, and we can't wait to eat our "real" food again. Hunger and cravings take over. We overeat, we binge—and maybe purge if that is in our lexicon of our eating problems. Since we "messed up," we do it again trying harder—more restricting, more feelings of deprivation, and more loss of control.

Maybe it's not a formal diet. Maybe it's attempts to eat better and lose weight by limiting certain foods and/or quantities. The result is the same: overeating/bingeing on those foods the addict is trying to stay away from. The food addict is caught in the cycle and struggle of overeating, restricting/starving, bingeing, maybe purging—it goes on and on, and the food addict is lost in the disease. Sadly, this can go on for years, maybe for a lifetime—albeit, shortened by this disease process.

On the other side of the coin is the food addict who is committed to not eating. The anorexic who is obsessed with food but is able to override

The Culprits and Triggers

her body's need to eat. For the anorexic, the purger, restricting/starving and purging also affect brain chemistry—with triggering the production of endorphins—which are opioid peptides that function as neurotransmitters that allow us to experience pleasure/reward. Again, this creates the set-up for "more" of the same—restricting or starving, overeating with purging.

Therefore, we eliminate restricting/starving.

A WORD FROM DIANNE

Throughout this book, I am attempting to explain that our eating problems are biologically based (with major emotional underpinnings) and expressed in the condition of "food addiction." As I so ardently present the answer to active food addiction as being "recovery," meaning abstinence and a program of support, there is a discussion in Chapter 12: Compliance versus Surrender on why the Food Plan is *not* a diet and is freedom from the bondage of the disease and *not* deprivation. Deprivation is having the disease of food addiction—deprivation does not come from living in the solution; the food plan and involvement in 12 Step food recovery fellowships—that's freedom!

HIGH-FAT, HIGH-SALT, MUNCHY/CRUNCHY FOODS, AND HARD AND SEMI-SOFT CHEESE

Remember Lay's Potato Chips and the challenge to eat only one? They're all fat and salt—the chip itself is just the vehicle! And you really *can't* eat just one. The high-fat and/or high-salt are major triggers for overeating. That's why the food plan presented in Chapter 11 eliminates all of the following:

- **Chips**—potato chips, corn chips, tortilla chips, veggie chips (kale, peas, beans, etc.), and so on. This includes Doritos and Cheetos. In addition, look for sugar in the list of ingredients; it's always there!

- **Popped/puffed grains**—Once a grain is popped or puffed, it becomes a "refined/processed" carb and creates havoc in the body—with the resultant feeling of "wanting more." This includes popcorn, puffed grains (corn, millet, and rice), rice cakes, and corn cakes.

- **Nuts** (and nut butters), which are more a fat than anything else. Nuts are regarded as "snack" foods. They are a hand-to-mouth food, and universally a problem food. Rare is the person who can eat only a few and not want more. The high-fat content creates cravings. Salted nuts are typically a "bar/snack" food to encourage more drinking.

- **Hard, semi-hard, semi-soft, soft cheese** (except cottage cheese and ricotta cheese). This includes Parmesan, cheddar, Colby, Swiss, mozzarella, Velveeta (which is not really cheese), blue cheese, brie, and so on. Another major reason that hard cheese is excluded from the food plan is that it naturally contains a powerful opiate in the morphine family called casomorphins. Eighty percent of a cow's milk protein is casein. As casein breaks down in the stomach, a peptide opiate, casomorphin, is produced. And, yes, it has a druglike, addictive quality. This substance affects brain chemistry that this food plan is designed to normalize and stabilize and eliminate cravings. The casomorphins explain why we like cheese so much and why it's so hard to give it up. Cheese also has high salt content, which is part of the making and aging process. This is not true for low-fat cottage and ricotta cheese—which are acceptable and included in the food plan.

Therefore, we eliminate high-fat, high-salt, munchy/crunchy foods, and most cheeses!

FRUITS WITH A HIGH CONCENTRATION OF SUGAR

While some fruits are recommended and acceptable on the food plan presented in Chapter 11, fruits that are high in sugar are problematic. These include the following:

- Bananas (don't worry—you get more potassium from green leafy veggies than from bananas)
- Cherries
- Dried fruit
- Grapes
- Mangos
- Papayas

Therefore, we eliminate fruits that have a high concentration of sugar.

GUM/MINTS

These bite-sized "foods" are loaded with sugar or sugar substitutes that trigger cravings and hunger. Our bodies are built to stimulate digestion through chewing. When the jaw moves in a chewing motion, a carefully coordinated neurological reflex activates the production of enzymes and acids. Chewing without eating food is harmful. Chewing gum sends the body signals that food is coming. The salivary glands are stimulated. The enzymes and acids that are activated by chewing gum are then released but without food they're intended to digest. This can cause bloating and overproduction of stomach acid, and it can compromise the body's ability to produce sufficient digestive secretions when you actually do eat food. Also, gum chewing causes air to be swallowed, which again causes bloating and gas.

We use gum and mints to stave off hunger and the opposite is the result—it creates hunger. Recent studies showed that while those who chewed gum consumed fewer meals, they ate more at the meals they did consume. And their meals ended up being less nutritious than those eaten by those who do not chew gum.

Results also showed that gum chewers were less likely to eat fruit and instead were more motivated to eat junk food like potato chips and candy. This is likely because the minty flavor in gum makes fruits and vegetables taste bitter.

Sugar-free gum contains artificial sweeteners/sugar substitutes with the negative effects described above. Most sugar-free gum is sweetened with sorbitol, which has been linked to some serious gastrointestinal problems. Sorbitol is used as a laxative, and if taken in sufficient quantities, it can cause abdominal pain, bloating, gas, and diarrhea. Sugar-free gum often contains acidic flavorings and preservatives that may lead to dental erosion, even if it contains cavity-fighting xylitol.

Constant gum chewing can tire our jaws, leading to muscle fatigue, spasms, and pain. It sometimes leads to temporomandibular joint disorder (TMJ), which causes chronic pain in the head and neck, making it painful to open and close the mouth. Studies show the more stressed we are, the harder we chew on our gum—putting more stress on our jaws. It also allows us to chew up or suck down our feelings (particularly anger, unrest, stress, etc.), to be distracted from ourselves. That flies in the face of recovery when we're trying to not run away from ourselves with anything external; even something seemingly so innocuous as a piece of gum or a mint, the focus becomes what's going on in our mouth instead of focusing on our being—our outer and inner life. Some argue that gums and mints help relieve our stress. Our stress is better handled with establishing normalized blood sugar levels by following the food plan in Chapter 11 and the development of healthy coping skills.

Therefore, we eliminate gum and mints!

ENERGY DRINKS

An energy drink is any beverage that contains some form of legal stimulant and/or vitamins, which have been added to give the consumer a short-term boost in energy. Red Bull, Monster, Rock Star, Jolt Cola, Cocaine Energy drink, and many others fall into this category. These drinks tend to contain significant amounts of sugar and the following ingredients:

- **Caffeine**—is a mild stimulant found in cola, tea, coffee, and chocolate. Most energy drinks have 70 to 200 mg of caffeine. Medically, caffeine is useful as a cardiac stimulant and also a mild diuretic (it increases urine production). Caffeine is an addictive drug, and it operates using the same mechanisms that amphetamines and cocaine use to stimulate the brain, though caffeine's effects are milder than amphetamines and cocaine. James D. Lane, professor of medical psychology at Duke University, states that caffeine produces real psychological and physiological dependence. He goes on to say that caffeine's effect at high doses is like having a chronic anxiety condition.[83] It exaggerates the perception of stress and the body's response to it.

- **Guarana** is a climbing plant native to Brazil that contains caffeine. Each fruit contains about one seed, which contains approximately three times more caffeine than coffee beans.

- **Taurine** is an amino acid. One theory is that taurine enhances the effect of caffeine.

- **Ginseng** is actually three different herbs commonly grouped together and called ginseng. There are known adverse effects to the use of excess ginseng, which include headaches, restlessness, and raised blood pressure, especially if it is taken with caffeine and/or alcohol.

- **Inositol** is a member of the vitamin B complex, though it is not considered a vitamin, per se. People who are depressed may have lower

The Culprits and Triggers

191

than normal levels of inositol in their spinal fluid. In addition, inositol participates in the action of serotonin, a neurotransmitter known to be a factor in depression.

- **Choline,** a dietary component of many foods, is part of several major phospholipids, including lecithin, that are critical for normal membrane structure and function. Large oral doses of choline may be associated with hypotension, sweating, salivation, and diarrhea.

- **Sugar** (glucose and fructose), as discussed earlier, is the major carbohydrate used as fuel in our body to supply energy. Glucose is the preferred fuel of brain cells, and also muscle cells in early exercise. Carbohydrates (which sugar is) provide most of the energy needed in our daily lives, both for normal body functions such as heartbeat, breathing, and digestion and for exercise such a cycling, walking, and running. Sugar provides quick energy with the spiking of glucose in our bloodstream and a quick energy drain as blood sugar plummets because the body cannot safely sustain high blood sugar levels.

- **Artificial sweeteners** (if the energy drink is low or no calorie). As discussed, there is a release of gastric hormones when you consume artificial sweeteners. This gives the brain a confusing message: that food is present, but that the food has no "calories." Subsequently, you develop an appetite craving typically thirty to sixty minutes after consuming an artificially sweetened beverage. In addition, these artificially sweetened chemicals, aspartame, sucralose, acesulfame potassium, and sugar alcohols, have been linked to upset stomachs, mood swings, birth defects, cancer, diabetes, emotional disorders, epilepsy, seizures, a variety of neurological disorders and even obesity.

In general, the side effects for energy drinks can include the following:

- Agitation/restlessness
- Chest pain/ischemia
- Dizziness, fainting, irritability, nausea, nervousness, jitters
- Gastrointestinal upset (diarrhea)
- Headache and severe fatigue from withdrawal
- Insomnia
- Palpitations/tachycardia
- Paresthesia (tingling or numbing of the skin)
- Respiratory distress
- Tremors/shaking

All this is to say that these drinks give a whopping energy boost but also an energy drain/crash—prompting the craving for another energy boost: either another drink or caffeine and/or sugar in another form—e.g., candy, soda, coffee, junk food.

Therefore, we eliminate all energy drinks.

THE CARBOHYDRATE "CULPRITS" AT A GLANCE

All addictive substances start out as natural substances that are taken through a refinement process. These addictive substances are quickly absorbed, alter brain chemistry, and change mood. In the follow table, these substances have been "shaded," indicating that they need to be eliminated for **True Recovery**.

TABLE 7.1. THE FOUR BASIC CARBOHYDRATE SUBGROUPS	
UNREFINED/UNPROCESSED CARBOHYDRATES	
Any carbohydrate that hasn't been altered from its natural state. The whole grains listed below have high fiber content and important nutrients—vitamins and minerals. Fiber is important because it slows the absorption of sugar from carbs and helps to stabilize blood sugar levels.	
Complex	**Simple**
Whole Grains— Oats Millet Wheat Quinoa Rye Amaranth Barley Buckwheat (Kasha) Brown rice Corn **Whole Cereals—**Hot **All Vegetables—**carrots, string beans, potatoes, root veggies, sugar beets **Greens** **Legumes** (peas, beans, lentils) **Nuts and seeds**	**All fruit** **Milk, yogurt, buttermilk** **Raw honey** **Sugar cane** **Molasses**

The Culprits and Triggers

REFINED/PROCESSED CARBOHYDRATES	
These products have undergone manufacturing or repackaging processes. Refining removes water, fiber, and nutrients from natural grains, vegetables, and fruits. This helps concentrate taste and improve shelf life. These are not healthy for the body. The sugars in refined foods are concentrated and eating them cause blood sugar levels to spike. This leads to symptoms of increased appetite, irritability, and fatigue—as discussed earlier. Blood sugar fluctuations can also cause the body to store more excess calories as fat. Eating refined carbs can also lead to nutritional deficiencies because they have low nutritional value.	
Complex	**Simple**
Flour—Bread, crackers, pasta, cookies, cakes, pastries, biscuits, pies, donuts, bagels, muffins, pizza, etc. (See Chapter 11 for the complete list)	**Sugar**
	Honey
	Fruit Juice
Cold cereal—all are flour (mostly wheat) pressed into circles or flakes, sweetened with sugar, maltodextrin, fruit juice, honey, artificial sugars (see list of sugars in Chapter 11).	**Sun-dried fruit**
	Agave syrup/nectar
	Maple syrup
Don't be fooled by manufacturers' claims of "Whole grain"—it's a lie! Whole means whole—a grain is no longer whole after it has been ground into flour.	**Pancake Syrup**
	Lactose (powdered skim milk)
	Glucose
Puffed grains (corn, rice, millet) become refined as a result of the "puffing" process	**Fructose**
	Maltose (barley malt)
Popcorn—is "puffed" corn	**High-Fructose Corn Sweetener/Syrup** (made from corn)
White rice	**Brown Rice Syrup**
Corn/potato starch	**With processing/fermentation of grains/ fruit we get: beer, whiskey, scotch, bourbon, sake, vodka, wine, etc.**
Vegetable juice	
	(See Chapter 11, which lists all the names of sugar, including all artificial sweeteners/sugar substitutes.)

Therefore, we eliminate all sugar, flour and refined carbs!

Withdrawal from the culprits—the refined carbohydrates—is a physical phenomenon. The psychological implications, however, are very often ignored or trivialized. There is a grieving process connected with something that was so dear, valuable, and important to us—as if we've lost a lifetime friend. The following "goodbye sugar" letters are some examples of what clients have written as part of the grieving process:

Dearest Beloved Sugar:

I have loved you since our first contact. There was never a moment's doubt about my attraction and fondness for your every feature. I've loved the way you make me feel, the way I see the world through you, your crystalline beauty and your sweet taste.

But Sugar, over the years, I have developed some serious health problems, and they've caused me to learn more about you and your effects on me. I've been surprised and aggrieved to discover that beneath the joy you've brought me, you've been slowly destroying me from the inside-out.

I know our relationship was my choice from the beginning and throughout my acquisition of the little bits of knowledge leading up to my current epiphany. I know that I always had a choice, even before I knew it. You are such an intrinsic part of my culture, my lifestyle, my celebrations, my everydays! I honestly can't imagine even *truly* wanting a life without you.

But here I am. I'm doing my best to remove you from my life. I'm asking God to give me strength, and to replace you in my life with something that's not only less destructive, but that's actually **good** for me. In turn, I am asking you to release your hold on my body, mind, and spirit. Let me go. Don't call me, don't show up and take me by surprise, don't hide amongst others to sneak up on me.

I love you, Sugar, and I appreciate all the years that you've been there for me when no one else was. The times you consoled me. The times you lifted my spirits when nothing else could. The celebrations you made more special. So many empty spaces you've filled in my life. And I thank you with all my heart.

Despite all of that, I know now that you were fake. There was nothing natural about you or your effects on me. Your effect on me comes from a fake, chemical place, and I deserve better than that.

I'm getting to know the real, natural you, and I like what I'm tasting so far. The You that occurs naturally, without being processed or concentrated, or chemically altered will be welcome in my home. The real you is not as intense or dramatic, but the natural you is, and will be, good for me in the long run. I'm no longer willing to let you, in any form, control me, so we won't be as close as we once were once were no matter what happens. For now, I'm cutting you out of my life. You've got plenty of other addicts to keep you busy, and I know that I will miss you dearly, for a while.

But once I've detoxed and remained abstinent for a while, I know the desperate cravings will pass. I'll be happier and healthier, and the space you leave will be filled with something healthy and real.

With heartfelt appreciation,

—CG, a client

The Culprits and Triggers

Sugar Dearest,

Please forgive me for what I'm about to do. I know you deserve more, but in truth, I'm afraid to meet you face to face to say goodbye. I'm too weak to see you in person because I know I'll "eat you up."

I'll always remember our nights together; with you seriously caressing my lit tongue and eager palate. Oh, the bliss! I'll never know what it's like again. How the very taste of you intoxicates me.

Oh, sugar, my beloved. How I will miss our moments together. But life must go on and we must now go our separate ways. I hope it will help you to know that I will think of you every moment and look for you around every corner.

But, my darling, my new life beckons, and I must follow.

His name is brown rice, and while we may never know the same thrilling moments, I will try my best to make him happy. It is with a heavy heart that I leave you. Try to remember me fondly, as I will try to remember you. So, my darling, I will bring a close to our love affair forever, my love. I will always remember you.

—BN, a client

BYE, BYE SUGAR BLUES (Rap Song)

—JZ, a client

Girl, I put you in my coffee
Put you in my tea
'til you run around my brain
and make a mess outta me

I use you in the mornin'
and then again at noon
In the midnight hour
You got me howlin' at the moon

Sugar, urge me on until you're
   all I crave
Teaspoon by teaspoon
you're diggin' my grave
You make a strong man weak
And my hormones moan
As we speak I feel a kidney
   stone growin'

I gotta say good-bye to you
I got the bye-bye sugar blues

Girl, you made me high
You laid me low
You constrict my veins
'til the blood don't flow
You make my eyesight weak
So I can't see
Goddamn the honey bee

So good bye glucose, so long sucrose
Get lost Splenda, I surrender
I'm diggin' myself a 6-foot hole
It's time to lock the sugar bowl
You got my heart now
You want my soul
I'm putting on my walking shoes
And sing the bye-bye sugar blues.

So Haagen-Dazs
Say goodbye, Little Debbie
Please don't cry, Oreo
Please go away

Don't come back another day
It's gonna be hard, letting go,
Dianne Schwartz, tells me so

Candy canes, cakes, and Equal sorry,
there won't be a sequel
I can't live to eat
Gotta eat to live
I took all you had to give
So I say "away with you"
Gonna sing the bye-bye
Don't cry
Don't pine
Don't sigh
Just walk on by
bye-bye-bye Sugar Blues

CHAPTER 8

Denial and Other Defense Mechanisms

Thinking about sense objects
Will attach you to sense objects;
Grow attached, and you become addicted:
Deny your addiction, it turns to anger;
Become angry, and you confuse your mind;
Confuse your mind, the lessons of experience are forgotten
Forget experience, you lose discrimination
Lose discrimination, and you miss life's only purpose.
—BHAGAVAD-GITA, CHAPTER 2 VERSE 62–3

Is food one (or more) of the following to you: Lover? Best friend? Enemy? Isolator? Company? Drug? Soother? Nurturer? Time filler? Distraction? Distancer? Pleasurer?

If food is any one or more of these to you, you automatically and unconsciously stand to defend your relationship with it. Denial is pervasive and persuasive, and it hurts those who suffer from addiction. It allows for the perpetuation of the overeating/undereating or eating/ purging illness. Denial is part and parcel of addiction; it's a major component of the disease. It's the phenomenon that gives us permission to keep overeating, purging, or starving. As a mechanism, denial helps us survive our painful early childhood experiences, but at the same time, as our lives have moved on, it has kept us from being confronted by reality and having to respond and, in most cases, experiencing learning and growth.

Denial allows us to hide from life. It's certainly very damaging to our life process. And it's the major obstacle to recovery. While it's being used, denial eliminates the possibility of change. Denial is a defense mechanism, where the addict is too uncomfortable with the facts of their addiction to face them, rejects them, and instead, insists that it's not true despite the overwhelming evidence.

Denial is multifaceted. The following table categorizes denial.

TABLE 11.1. THE THREE DENIALS—SIMPLE DENIAL, MINIMIZATION, AND PROJECTION (BLAMING)	
The addict may use:	**What the addict tells themselves:**
Simple Denial	**Simple Denial Says:**
Deny the reality of the problem, maintaining there is no problem, and acting as though the problem doesn't exist.	*I have no problem.* *It can't be true.* *This couldn't happen to me.* *No, not me.* *There's nothing wrong with my eating. I just like to eat. I like food.* *I'm big/small because of my genes/body type.* *I'm normal, I can eat like a normal person.* (See page 203.) *If I don't eat, it's like I don't have needs.* *If I keep eating, I can stop the pain.*
Minimization	**Minimization Says:**
Admit to the fact but deny its seriousness or rationalize why there is no need for an intervention. Also, a combination of denial and rationalization—offering alibis, excuses, justification, and other explanation for behavior. The behavior is not denied, but an inaccurate explanation of its cause is given. We take reality and make it smaller. We act as though we don't consider the problem important. We are casual about its existence and its consequences.	*Okay, I have a problem, BUT I can stop anytime.* *Okay, I have a problem, BUT I don't need any help.* *It's no big deal.* *It is not as serious as others think.* *They are overreacting.*
Projection (Blaming)	**Projection Says:**
Admit to both the fact and the seriousness but deny responsibility.	*Okay, I have a problem, BUT I overeat, undereat, and/or purge because of my life's challenges (e.g., spouse, job, boss, kids, living situation).*

Denial and Other Defense Mechanisms

Most often food addiction behaviors—overeating, undereating, and purging—are viewed by professionals as defense mechanisms against underlying emotional issues. It's helpful and valuable to understand that these behaviors had an adaptive function as a response to stress or pain, which allows the food addict to see the behavior(s), not as a problem, but as an attempted solution. For the food addict, however, the solution became the problem. The component that underlies the issue for the food addict is the biology—the mechanism that turns using food as an adaptive function into an addiction. There are those individuals who have suffered childhood stress and pain who do NOT use food to manage their feelings.

OTHER DEFENSE MECHANISMS

The defense mechanisms, other than denial, that a food addict uses to protect her behavior are basically also lies we tell ourselves to evade pain and truth. We carry and use these automatically/unconsciously, so it's valuable to unearth them and bring them to the light. These psychological strategies protect us from anxiety, guilt, and a myriad of uncomfortable feelings. They are not under conscious control. Therefore, they are involuntary. They are:

- **Repression**—tamping down feelings and memories. In a way, all but the most primitive defense mechanisms are forms of repression. Denial can be categorized as repression; we're repressing the awareness of unwelcome truth.

- **Rationalization**—an almost believable but untrue explanation given to justify one's conduct. This is where we have a good excuse. This is the most commonly used defense mechanism. It's something done on an unconscious level. Anorexia is often characterized by the defense mechanisms of denial and rationalization, allowing the person to believe that her judgment and behavior are entirely normal and reasonable. Examples include: "Food is always there for me. It's like the friend I can count on when I'm lonely." Or "I don't want to feel empty and eating helps me to feel full." Or "If I'm heavy, men don't look at me. I feel safer and stronger when I'm big." Or "I need to be thin to feel confident with people."

- **Justification**—offering reasons to prove oneself blameless and without guilt. Examples include: "I'm not hurting anyone because of my eating/purging/starving." Or "I feel strong and confident when I don't eat." Or "I overeat at night while I'm watching TV. I work hard all day, and I guess this is what I do for myself." Or "I get so tired caring for my kids and going from one thing to another. So I have another soda or a candy bar to get through the next hour."

- **Projection**—placing blame for difficulties upon others. Examples include: "My mom doesn't like me being independent, but then when I go to her for help she criticizes me. I hate that! Then I binge and purge.")

- **Intellectualization**—avoiding emotional, personal awareness of eating, purging, or starving, dealing with it on a level of generalization. For example, understanding and explaining behavior from the process of thinking rather than feeling.

- **Diversion**—changing the subject to avoid threatening topics such as diets and body image.

- **Hostility**—becoming angry and irritable when reference is made to one's eating/non-eating behavior.

- **Generalizing**—saying that *everyone* has a problem with food.

- **Joking**—making light of the situation. Examples include: "Hey, I only have a problem with Häagen-Dazs!"

- **Mental avoidance**—We do this in several ways: sleep excessively, become hyperactive, darting from activity to activity, not slowing until we collapse at night (usually after a binge), lose ourselves in earphones, in front of the TV, or in reading materials.

- **Arrogance, entitlement, superiority, and criticism of others**—considered narcissistic defense mechanisms and are often used by those with eating problems. People who are avoiding reality will also go to great lengths to escape situations that confront their denial system.

Another definition for *denial* is: A psychological phenomenon by which reality is not perceived. It's not a matter of deliberate lying or deception. It's a psychological mechanism that operates unconsciously. We use it to shut out our awareness of things that would be too disturbing to know. Or as clients have suggested: Living in the illusion, or, refusal to face reality, unable to be in truth, protection from living in the truth. Not letting yourself know what reality is. Using the "DENIAL" acronym really drives home the meaning:

Denial and Other Defense Mechanisms

Don't

Even

(K)Now

I

Am

Lying

Since we don't know we're lying to ourselves or the world, we call it denial. The illness of food addiction must lie, and it must continue to lie or it cannot exist. The illness cannot live in the light of truth. You can't tell the truth to yourself and continue the addiction. With the truth, you would realize your problem and get some help for it.

HOW DOES YOUR DENIAL SERVE YOU?

So how has denial served you with regard to your food addiction? What comes to mind when you think about it? How do you deny (i.e., protect yourself from knowing) the following realities?

The Seriousness of What You Do With Food?

First of all, what is serious about it?

- Does your eating interfere with or hurt your functioning? Your thinking?

- Do you not feel well because of your over/undereating, and obsessions about your eating? Your body?

- Are you foggy?

- Have you accepted a low level of functioning as your norm?

- Do you go in and out in your head with dissatisfaction with your body/appearance?

- Do you eat foods you know you should not be eating (but can't help it)?

- Are you eating when not hungry and not able to control it?

- Is it the fact that not being able to control your food makes you unhappy? Robs you of the ability to be fully present in your life? To fully focus on your thoughts and be present for your feelings?

- Is it hurting your health, your mood, your energy level, your sleep, your digestion, digestive process, your weight?

- Do you have to starve during the day—knowing you'll be out of control at night—to keep from gaining weight or keep the pretense going that you don't have a problem?

- Do you skip meals and feel a sense of pride? That you can override your need to feed your body?

- Do you tell yourself any of the following:
  - ➤ My habit is pleasurable. Why give it up?
  - ➤ I shouldn't have to change.
  - ➤ I don't overeat; I just make bad choices.
  - ➤ Just this one time.
  - ➤ It's not that bad, that much, or that often (minimization).
  - ➤ Everyone does something with food.
  - ➤ It's hopeless; I'm hopeless.
  - ➤ I've tried over and over but nothing works, so why get my hopes up? I'll just end up feeling frustrated and disappointed again.
  - ➤ I'm in recovery from alcoholism/drug addiction—so it's better than "picking up."
  - ➤ It helps me with my cravings for alcohol/drugs; it helps me stay sober/clean (see Chapter 5: Food Addiction: The Precursor/Gateway to Chemical Dependency).

The Quantities You Eat?

Quantity relates to both overeating and undereating. What do you tell yourself? Here are some examples from clients at Realization Center:

- I'm special. I deserve this doughnut.

- I didn't eat all day, so tonight I can have (fill in the blank).

- I'm only X pounds over a good weight for my body.

- They put it on my plate, so it must be a regular portion.

- I exercised a lot today, a lot of running around, in and out of the car, up and down in the subway, I went to the gym.

Denial and Other Defense Mechanisms

- I worked very hard today, so I'm entitled/deserve to have extra.

- I skipped lunch yesterday (or last month, year) so I can have extra now.

- I didn't eat breakfast, lunch, dinner last night.

- It's the wedding, party, buffet, celebration, dinner party. I can't refuse what's being served.

- I'm naturally a big/small person.

- Everyone else is eating this size serving/taking more. I shouldn't have to feel deprived.

- It wouldn't be polite to refuse the portion, extra, the cake, the cookies, the ice cream, etc.

- It's my favorite.

- It comes with the meal/I paid for it.

- I ate yesterday so I can skip eating today.

- I will eat tomorrow (or later) so I can skip eating today.

- I'd rather eat/starve/purge than face the problems that are bothering me.

- Giving up my habit of over/undereating/purging will be painful and uncomfortable. Ugh! Who wants that?

WHAT IS NORMAL?

NORMAL VERSUS COMMON

Most of us in our society have received our education about nutrition and healthy eating from General Mills, Pepsi, Coca Cola, and others in the food industry via the media—mostly TV. We have come to believe that pizza is a good meal and that a Pop-Tart, McMuffin, the Honey Bee's delivery of a bowl of little "Os," or a shake or smoothie is a good breakfast. Jimmy Dean also gives us a "good way to start the day."

There is a wall of cold cereal in every supermarket represented by delightful characters that children, and we, are connected to: Dora the Explorer, Tony the Tiger, the Keebler Elves . . . The food companies compete with each other to deliver the most seductive meals. Who has the most cheese, bacon, and/or syrup, the biggest bun, and the best sauce?

> And we want it all. It's a war/assault on our senses: sight, hearing, taste, smell, touch.
>
> Certainly those foods deliver pleasure, and we want that pleasure again and again because of our biology—our highjacked brains. We have all become the captive audience for the dealers of our triggers: seductive, addictive foods.
>
> In addition to these erroneous beliefs about food, we are exposed to the reality that "everyone is eating this way" because we have all been led down this path. This destructive way of eating is so ubiquitous in our culture that it's thought of as "normal"! That also gives us the rationale and permission to keep eating in accordance with the dictates of the food industry. BUT IT'S NOT NORMAL! IT'S JUST COMMON!
>
> "Normal" is eating in a way that results in stable blood sugar (glucose) levels. This is the food plan I present in this book. It's basically the only way to eat to have a life that's promised to us.

The Consequences of Overeating/Undereating, Purging, or Starving

I've been discussing the consequences throughout the book, but let's take another look at them:

Physical Health
weight gain/loss, diabetes, heart disease, joint problems, digestive problems (GERD, acid reflux, heartburn, bloating, gastritis, irritable bowel syndrome, colitis, ulcers, diverticulitis, diverticulosis, constipation, hemorrhoids, colorectal cancer), high blood pressure, stroke, cancer, being hyper, episodes of low blood sugar (see below), osteoporosis, teeth deterioration
Brain Function
fogginess, difficulty focusing, poor concentration, memory problems, poor thought processing, poor judgments, poor decision making, poor critical thinking skills, headaches, lightheadedness, "attention deficit disorder" (see Chapter 7: The Culprits and Triggers)
Emotional Health
mood swings, impatience, poor impulse control, depression, anxiety, self-esteem, self-confidence

Denial and Other Defense Mechanisms

Spiritual Health
inability to fully access your creativity, talent, inner spirit, connection to a power greater than yourself, living with serenity, "okayness"
Relationships
poor because of self-esteem issues, lack of confidence, codependency/control issues, people pleasing—the thinking that "relationships are too hard, too much anxiety; the food is easier; I know what to expect, it doesn't threaten to reject me, leave me, abandon me; so let me just stay alone; the food will keep me company."

With regard to the consequence of these behaviors, if you are in fact aware of them, is your self-talk of denial along the lines of any or more of the following:

- It's just this time.

- I can stop any time.

- It's not important.

- It's not so. Couldn't be.

- I don't care.

- I'm too busy or too tired to think about it, much less discuss it.

- I'm not as bad as "Harvey." My situation is not as bad as Harvey's (comparison).

- I don't have these problems, but an awful lot of people around me do (projection).

Loss of Control?

Remember, you're thinking of ways to deny the reality that you've lost control of your eating. People who attempt to control the uncontrollable eating problems often abuse substances such as caffeine, tobacco, alcohol, cocaine, heroin, and over-the-counter medicines such as appetite suppressants, diuretics, laxatives, and emetics. Do you think or say to yourself:

- I'm looking for a silver bullet—in whatever form—and the entire diet industry tries to seduce me. I want to believe what they promise, so I try diet programs, weight-loss programs, exercise programs, magic pills, magic soaps, diet shakes, elixirs, powders, herbs, and some of what's listed below.

- I diet (more successfully in the past than now; now it's harder or impossible). I want to stop my overeating, but it has a life of its own. This is what I try:
  - ➤ skipping meals—especially breakfast (too fattening) or, "I just have coffee (and a cigarette)."
  - ➤ I can skip lunch. I'm able to do than because I'm busy at work, school, appointments, errands.
  - ➤ I purge. It's finding the ultimate magic: I can eat all my disease compels me to and then I can get rid of it by vomiting, using laxatives, enemas, exercising (gym or running), or restricting. I can avoid the consequences of weight. (The lie of this denial is that it doesn't always work to keep weight down and the consequences of purging are dire.)
  - ➤ I try to eat smaller portions.
  - ➤ I try not to eat junk, eat in between, or eat after meals.
  - ➤ I try to not keep sweets or any binge foods in my house.
  - ➤ It's not really loss of control; I just don't have enough willpower.
  - ➤ I use diet pills (from a medical doctor or over the counter).[84]
  - ➤ I use cocaine or crystal meth (now, I have two problems—what did I get myself into? Oh well, it keeps me thin).

ASK YOURSELF

What is my eating problem doing to my life, my relationships, my job, sense of responsibility, my value system, and my peace of mind? Think about this question, and then respond in a notebook or journal.

Need for Help?

Well, first of all, the concept of needing help is really hard. Most likely you're a person who is not used to asking for help. Most likely, you're the person who gives help—a caretaker. So, under those circumstances, asking

Denial and Other Defense Mechanisms

for help is quite foreign. Denying the need for help is like breathing. And if the notion of needing help cuts across the blood brain barrier—there's Weight Watchers, Jenny Craig, Nutrisystem, and asking the doctor for help to get the latest prescription for weight loss. We see ads for quick, cheap, instant, easy weight loss. We get lured by great messages—but this addresses the symptom (weight) not the real issue (addiction).

If the food addict's measure of success is merely weight loss, then any and all of these "work." And another round of the cycle—invariably the weight is back and yet another "failure." However, it isn't us that failed; it's the dieting. Once again, we looked for help in all the wrong places.

There is a new criteria for success—abstinence, addressing the addiction—and healing the mind, body, and spirit. This work is the map and guide for finding that criteria, achieving the goals of healing, having a new experience of yourself, and "living a life beyond your wildest dreams."

EXAMINING DENIAL THROUGH THE STAGES OF GRIEF

As food addiction progresses, the denial system becomes increasingly more pervasive and entrenched. Initially, it is minimal, and with gentle encouragement, the food addict can usually see the problem realistically. In middle stages, as others notice that the problem is getting more serious, stronger defenses appear to shield the food addict from what is really happening to her: more weight gain or loss. In late (advanced) stage, the denial system is usually massive and extremely difficult to penetrate.

A useful way to examine denial is through the view identified by Elizabeth Kübler-Ross, a physician who worked with terminally ill cancer patients, and saw a pattern in patients' psychology as they dealt with grief and tragedy, especially when they were told/learned that they were terminally ill. It's important to understand that coming to terms with having the disease of food addiction and what's necessary to recover creates an experience of loss. You've been in a relationship with food for so many years, and now you're working to change that relationship. That will create the process of grief, which is the normal reaction to loss of any kind. Dr. Kübler-Ross identified five stages, and understanding them helps us understand why we have so much resistance to the recovery. The stages, which can happen in a different order than the order listed, are as follows:

1. Denial

I have no problem! I know what I'm doing. I'm normal—I can eat like a normal person. I throw up my meals as a way to control my weight (what's wrong with that?). Why should I have to live without sugar, flour, caffeine—they work for me (and for everybody else). My weight is because of my meds, my age, my mood, my thyroid, my genes. My mood swings (depression and/or anxiety) or my low self-esteem is because of a brain chemical imbalance, my past trauma, my mother, my kids, my husband, my boss . . .

In facing food addiction, the denial stage is probably the most prevalent and definitely the most deadly. We deny the harsh reality that we have a chronic, terminal illness. We want to believe that what we have is really some minor ailment that we will be able to handle—as soon as we're ready. We deny that the illness is affecting every area of our lives and that its arrest will require major life changes.

"I know I can diet and quit this whenever I want to," we say, "I am going to start tomorrow or next Monday," we promise ourselves. What we are really saying is that we want this to be a simple project that won't require too much effort or too much disruption in our lifestyle. We want to remain self-deluded; we want to believe the whole thing is no big deal and that we can handle it ourselves. We do not see how sadly mistaken we are or how subtly pervasive our denial has become. We do not, or cannot, face the full implication of the First Step of the 12 Step food recovery fellowships—which is to admit we are powerless over food and that our lives have become unmanageable.

Another aspect of denial is the idea, often reinforced by others, "All you need is a little more willpower." Such ideas only serve to feed our guilt and self-loathing. Lack of willpower is not a common characteristic of food addicts. Most of us have exhibited great determination and willpower in laudable professional and personal accomplishments. We often exhibit a great deal of power and strength in our lives. All of this, of course, has nothing to do with our lifelong terminal illness. So, we must fact the fact that willpower has absolutely nothing to do with this illness.

2. Anger

Anger is a natural response to the reality of the loss of something important to us. We become angry that we can't control the food. *What? I have*

Denial and Other Defense Mechanisms

to let go of what? (Sugar, flour, etc.). *Why? Help me moderate—I can be moderate in my eating.* Harm reduction: *That will work! I just stopped drinking, using drugs—and you're asking me to stop eating the way I've eaten all my life? I'm afraid I'll "pick up." I've eaten sugar/flour all my life and now you're telling me they're not good for me, that I have to stop eating sugar/flour . . . that I can't have recovery unless I put down that list of food substances (alcohol, sugar, flour wheat, caffeine, volume, excess fat/salt). This isn't fair! I won't accept this. I can't live without sugar/flour . . . Why me? It's not fair!*

We get angry when we feel threatened. Addicts feel threatened when they are at risk for losing their substance. Of course, underneath the anger is FEAR: fear of the unknown. Food has been the always available companion through all of life's experiences on a moment-by-moment basis: *How could I live without being able to just reach out and get (fill in the blank)?*

3. Bargaining/Negotiating

We want to find a way to not change our eating behavior *and* not experience any of the consequences (weight, lower functioning, fogginess, tiredness, etc.). We want to strike up a deal with the illness so that we can feel some sense of power over it. We want to feel in control of the outcome. We want to change the results without changing what we're doing. No one really wants to hear that, so we search for easier, softer ways, and busy ourselves with half measures. This is exactly what dieting is all about. We want to kid ourselves that this is purely a physical problem. *It's my glands. It's low blood sugar; a high-protein diet will take care of it.*

We bargain with the illness and, in the process, deny the threefold nature of it and how serious it really is. Similarly, we want to bargain with the amount of time and effort required to recover. *I only want to attend meetings once a week. I don't see why I should give up my vacation plans just because they happen to fall smack in the middle of treatment.* In the bargaining stage, we decide to accept the reality that we have a dreadful affliction and that it will not be easy to battle it. But we still want to make some attempts on our own.

- I'll eat less tomorrow.

- Just this one time.

- I can cut down—that would be okay!

We've tried finding the right diet, nutritionist, spa, gym, pills, shots, acupuncture, meditation, hypnosis, protein drinks, health foods, etc. We've read all the recovery books. We know more about food/eating/losing weight than Jenny Craig herself, Weight Watchers founder Jean Nidetch, and Oprah Winfrey, combined. All of these are short-term efforts to pretend we can manage it. Each new plan helps us continue in the delusion that we, like other people, are merely struggling with a few extra pounds. This is not our situation. For us, it is a much more serious problem and requires deeper work to attack the affliction.

Many of us continue bargaining throughout our lives and undergo none of the major changes that could give us a lifelong, stable recovery. The essential nature of bargaining techniques is that we seek to address isolated aspects of our lives. We compartmentalize ourselves, assuming an unrealistic power of mind over the body or vice versa. These approaches (diet clubs, gyms, spas, surgical procedures, nutritional counseling, books, etc.) fail to see the interrelatedness of the mind, body, and spirit. We need to address all aspects of our illness. Also, most of these other methods promote the idea that recovery need not be ongoing, that we can undergo a certain "treatment" and thus achieve a cure. Such a deal has been the lifelong wish of every food addict, and it only serves to keep us in our disease.

4. Sadness/Depression

Wow, this really makes sense—it's something I've known but never wanted or allowed myself to acknowledge. I have to say goodbye to my best friend: sugar/bread/pasta? Oh, that's like losing the closest "being" to me. My life won't be worth living if I can't eat Häagen-Dazs, a bagel, Sara Lee Coffee Cake, M&M's, etc. I'll never feel normal or happy again. Everything is just hopeless.

Despite all the cultural taboos against feeling sorry for ourselves, it is essential that we feel the pain and hopelessness of our condition. The tragedy of our illness must be faced, and we must experience our own mourning and loss. As food addicts, we must give up the delusion that we don't have a problem. We must fact the fact that our life is not a dress rehearsal, but "this is it, and it stinks." It is not going to get better on its own. Recovery won't be easy. In fact, it will be the hardest thing we've ever undertaken. All other life projects will seem easy in comparison.

All of our past was accompanied by the comfort of a lifelong friend and faithful companion—food. We must now experience the loss of this friend, as well as the loss of false hopes. We must look at the wasted teenage years or any other aspects of life that have been damaged by this illness. It is only in facing these things that we can mobilize the energy to confront the difficult and painful process of recovery.

Acknowledging that there are no easy answers results in deep depression and mourning. The mourning is for the loss of a dream. No longer can we hope that the easy, thin life is right around the corner. To recover, we must give up the futile hope of a simple cure.

Most of us have lived our lives as a dress rehearsal, in preparation for the ever-elusive time when we will be thin (without the need to purge if it's the "magic" we use). We avoided the stark fact that this is not a drill—this is it! We must face the reality that, without drastic measures, without a total life reorganization, we are doomed to repeat the same cyclical patterns. Therefore, to accept recovery, we must mourn our old way of life.

"There is no birth of consciousness without pain," wrote noted psychologist Carl Jung. Food addicts who truly enter into and accept recovery must lay old patterns to rest and give birth to change. There is pain, and we need to cry. We need to mourn the loss of our best friend. That relationship, as we knew it, is gone forever. A new relationship with food will take its place. When depression is allowed, it passes. When it is denied, it festers. It is suppressed through the use of food and other drugs, and it serves to help deaden every other feeling.

5. Acceptance (or Surrender)

Surrender is the word used when discussing addiction and the phenomenon of truly letting go. *I give up! I'm waving the white flag. I'm not going to fight anymore. If you tell me to jump, I won't question why—only ask you, "How high?" I'm defeated; I have no more fight left.*

"It is not a resigned and hopeless 'giving up,' a sense of 'what's the use?' or 'I just cannot fight it any longer,' though we hear such statements too," writes Kübler-Ross in *On Death and Dying*. "They also indicate the beginning of the end of the struggle, but the latter are not indications of acceptance. Acceptance should not be mistaken for a happy stage. It is almost void of feelings. It is as if the pain had gone, the struggle is over..."[85]

We are at peace with what is and freely admit out powerlessness over food. God has granted us the serenity to accept that which we could not change. Following acceptance, we grow. This implies we have not merely endured the experience, we have been changed or improved by it. In some way, we consider ourselves enriched. We can accept loss and grow, but the journey is not easy, nor is it particularly comfortable.

In 12 Step food recovery fellowships, we are encouraged. This is the hardest thing you will ever have to do in your life. All your other accomplishments will pale in comparison, because they have all been achieved with food. It is hard, so hard you cannot do it on your own, but we will help you.

When we begin to accept the illness concept, the mind is open to new ideas, and we show a childlike receptivity to following directions. We realize on a very deep level that it has been our own ideas and efforts that got us exactly to this place. We are now ready and willing to accept help from someone else. We are ready to acknowledge we cannot do it on our own, and we are available to hear necessary feedback and direction. We become willing to slow our life down to one day at a time and face our realistic daily projects, rather than the previous goal-oriented fantasies. Recovery can now get underway.

We must let go of our old ideas of what was important and meaningful in life. We must move toward accepting overriding focus on our illness as a central issue for our lives. Once accepting, we are ready to begin work. We will not be interested in anything else but our recovery for a while. We will come to see that if we get the eating in order, all the other aspects of our lives will fall into line. Our attitude becomes one of firm resolve to make our abstinence the most important thing in life, without exception.

I deeply accept that I am different from other people—that I am not "normal" with food and that I must refrain, like the recovering alcoholic, from those food triggers that launch me into my disease. I accept that I must take measures to allow myself to have the support of others and recovering food addicts so that I can work to change my thinking about

Denial and Other Defense Mechanisms
213

myself and learn how to live without "using" food—instead depending on others (and a Higher Power) to help guide my recovery.

Acceptance is not achieved once and for all. If it were, we would not need the lifelong exposure to 12 Step food recovery fellowships and renewed motivation. This is the process by which we achieve that acceptance necessary to the vital Step One of recovery. The road to acceptance is the road to recovery, a road that leads us to admit our powerlessness and unmanageability. Here is ego surrender and acceptance of the need for help. We must come to see that our solo methods were not enough.

There is a difference between admission and acceptance. It's relatively easy to admit something isn't so, but it takes courage to accept it.

The Stages of Grief and You

What do you need to ADMIT to having the problem of food addiction? The answer is simple: your mouth. (We all have big ones!) It's so easy to mouth the words. What do you need to ACCEPT/SURRENDER? Your feet (ACTION). You need to say to yourself, *Feet don't fail me now—get me to a meeting (often)—or to the phone to call a recovery support person (often) or something recovery related, find a food sponsor, ask for help, accept help, use of the tools of the program (food plan, meetings, phone, writing, sponsor, literature, service).* Or another way to see it (as an insightful client put it) to ADMIT you need your head—to ACCEPT you need your heart!

Moving through the stages of grief is not a straight line. Most food addicts go back and forth until they put up the white flag—and truly give up. And, eventually, with a lot of recovery work, conscious, mindful acceptance, and its demonstration (being abstinent) admitting it becomes surrender on an unconscious level. We can think about it as: *I CAN'T eat sugar, flour, drink caffeine—(intellectual understanding) I'm learning what the real problem is with my eating, and I understand I can't have the first one—it's the one that starts me on a binge/purge/starve cycle.*

As the understanding of the nature of the affliction becomes more internalized, the food addict moves to: *I WON'T eat the bagel, the muffin, the cup of coffee.* We are beginning to, as stated by Thom Rutledge, "demonstrate a respect for the responsibility that is ours. I WON'T is an acknowledgement of our personal freedom and our conscious intent to make the best possible use of that freedom."[86]

And, as surrender becomes a part of the food addict's "fiber," the words change to: *No thank you, **I DON'T**—drink coffee, eat sugar, etc.*—(It's been internalized.) The food addict is no longer fighting to get something more/else, no longer looking to an external (food) to fix what doesn't feel right inside.

When you think about your own struggle, where are you? Are you in a form of denial? Or anger? Or sadness or still negotiating? Surrender is a peaceful state of being; it's in your insides where you are no longer go outside the boundaries of your recovery, where you're willing to follow the rules of what will keep you safe from acting out and hurting yourself (i.e., abstinence).

Be careful! Admitting to the having the problem can be a protection in itself. Intellectual (only) admission often leaves the deeper denial in place—intact and poisonous. Ultimately, denial allows you to hide the truth of being out of control and having lost control overeating, eating/purging, or starving.

We do not go through these stages in any particular order, and we do not finish once and for all with each; we sometimes go back and forth. It is a continuous and fluid process. Actually, the analogy to stages traveled in accepting death is not really apart from the process of recovery. In reality, recovery involves laying to rest an old way of life and giving birth to a new personality. The process is often slow, but the timing is accurately paced for each one of us. We needn't worry about getting on with it or pushing too quickly. We have the rest of our lives to travel these stages, to walk the road called recovery.

Remember, denial is insidious—it hangs around—even after recovery begins. It's one of the causes of relapse. It can combine with feeling better, not going to support meetings where your recovery is the priority, getting away from recognizing the commitment to abstinence as number one in your life, and then starting to rationalize you don't need others.

* * *

Denial and Other Defense Mechanisms

WELCOME TO HOLLAND

by Emily Perl Kingsley
Copyright©1987 by Emily Perl Kingsley.
All rights reserved.
Reprinted by permission of the author.

I am often asked to describe the experience of raising a child with a disability —to try to help people who have not shared that unique experience to understand it, to imagine how it would feel. It's like this . . .

When you're going to have a baby, it's like planning a fabulous vacation trip—to Italy. You buy a bunch of guide books and make your wonderful plans. The Coliseum. The Michelangelo *David*. The gondolas in Venice. You may learn some handy phrases in Italian. It's all very exciting.

After months of eager anticipation, the day finally arrives. You pack your bags and off you go. Several hours later, the plane lands. The flight attendant comes in and says, "Welcome to Holland."

"Holland?!?" you say. "What do you mean Holland?? I signed up for Italy! I'm supposed to be in Italy. All my life I've dreamed of going to Italy."

But there's been a change in the flight plan. They've landed in Holland and there you must stay.

The important thing is that they haven't taken you to a horrible, disgusting, filthy place, full of pestilence, famine and disease. It's just a different place.

So you must go out and buy new guide books. And you must learn a whole new language. And you will meet a whole new group of people you would never have met.

It's just a different place. It's slower-paced than Italy, less flashy than Italy. But after you've been there for a while and you catch your breath, you look around . . . and you begin to notice that Holland has windmills . . . and Holland has tulips. Holland even has Rembrandts.

But everyone you know is busy coming and going from Italy... and they're all bragging about what a wonderful time they had there. And for the rest of your life, you will say "Yes, that's where I was supposed to go. That's what I had planned."

And the pain of that will never, ever, ever, ever go away . . . because the loss of that dream is a very very significant loss.

But . . . if you spend your life mourning the fact that you didn't get to Italy, you may never be free to enjoy the very special, the very lovely things . . . about Holland.

PART TWO

The Solution: Abstinence

CHAPTER 9

What Is Abstinence?

*"If you attempt to fill the needs of your soul
through your mouth, you will always fail!"*
—MARCIA BODENSTEIN

The solution to the problem and pain of active food addiction is twofold:

First, eating in a way that *does not cause* an addictive reaction and does not:

- change mood

- trigger the craving to eat more/less

- trigger obsessive thoughts and compulsive eating (which occur when craving is triggered)

- create swings in blood sugar (glucose) levels

Second, participating in a 12 Step food recovery fellowship.

Eating this way and involvement in a structured program of recovery (12 Step food recovery fellowship) is called **"abstinence"** because it allows the addict to abstain from the behaviors of the addiction: overeating, undereating, and/or purging. (This is the same concept as "sobriety," which identifies/describes the alcoholic who is no longer drinking *and* is working a program of recovery.)

Just following the food plan presented in Chapter 11 without involvement in a 12 Step food recovery fellowship is simply being on a diet. It's the same as the alcoholic who stops drinking without participation in AA—they're not "sober"; they're "dry." The term "dry" or "dry drunk" refers to the alcoholic who is abstinent from alcohol but is not working on themselves to change and still exhibits the same personality traits, attitudes, and behaviors as when they were drinking (e.g., anger, grandiosity, being judgmental, intolerance, impulsive, indecisive, mood swings, no emotional spontaneity, no genuine spark, introspection, detachment, self-absorption, evidence of disorganization, easily distracted, complaints of boredom, fantasizing, wishful thinking, etc.).

Abstinence requires the following four components:

1. An effective and realistic food plan[87] that is designed to:

- Meet nutritional needs—to nourish the body and repair damaged cells

- Eliminate refined carbs and all foods to which the food addict is addicted (the "culprits/triggers" that create an addictive reaction; see Chapter 7: The Culprits and Triggers)

- Eliminate cravings to eat more/less, which eliminates obsessive thoughts

- Normalize/stabilize blood sugar levels (by controlling carbs and balancing with appropriate amounts of protein), which results in:
  - ➤ stable and optimized mood
  - ➤ optimized energy
  - ➤ normalized sleep
  - ➤ normalized digestion
  - ➤ optimized brain function
  - ➤ normalization of weight, if it's an issue

- Make meals pleasant

- Not focus on weight

- Be satisfying

- See the discussion of "Diet vs. Food Plan" in Chapter 12: Compliance versus Surrender.

2. A structured program of recovery (*real* participation in a 12 Step food recovery fellowship), which includes:

- Working with a "sponsor" (initially a "food sponsor," who guides/ helps the food addict to follow the food plan on a daily basis, and then a "step sponsor" [maybe the same person], who guides the food addict through the steps)

- Using tools of recovery

What Is Abstinence?

221

- See the further discussion in Chapter 16: 12 Step Food Recovery Fellowships and Relapse Prevention: Tools of Recovery.

3. Behavioral changes, which include:

- Planning meals in advance

- Following rules of the food plan—that is, weighing and measuring, not skipping meals, etc.

- Adhering to rules regarding timing of meals

- Avoiding "HALT" (getting too hungry, angry, lonely, tired)

- Limiting (if not eliminating) weighing oneself (see the discussion in Chapter 16: 12 Step Food Recovery Fellowships and Relapse Prevention: Tools of Recovery)

- Changing associations—"people, places, things" that invite return to the old behavior

- No longer using food for emotional support

4. Consistent movement/physical exercise, which includes walking and participating in sports. Exercise is not to be thought of the way one thinks of a diet (that is, something to start and stop).

Basically, there is *only* one way to eat that normalizes blood sugar levels, which is laid out in the food plan in Chapter 11.

As I explained previously, cravings are triggered when we take in those "foods" that tap into the reward circuit in the brain—which produce a particular chemical (dopamine), which gives us the feeling of joy, pleasure, and euphoria, and then triggers the desire/need for "more." (See the complete discussion in Chapter 1: The Disease Concept of Addiction and Chapter 7: The Culprits and Triggers.) The food plan takes into consideration this concept and excludes those foods that keep us in the cycle of active food addiction. Are you ready to do this? Have you had enough of the pain and suffering caused by your eating/not eating?

Now that you have seen the "list" of the Culprits/Triggers in Chapter 7 and the requirements of abstinence discussed earlier, the question becomes: Are you overwhelmed? Are your eyes rolling back in your head? Is it too much bad news? I would think that you're already aware of the need to let go of sugar and flour (although most people think it's *only* white flour that's a problem). The rest of the items on the list may feel as if they are too much to let go of all at once—that is, unless you're really at "bottom" and willing to go to any length to find relief from the pain and other consequences of your out-of-control eating behavior.

You could start by just eating the food plan breakfast (see Chapter 11)—that's an easy way to begin (instead of trying to change your eating all at once which may set you up for unrealistic expectations, overwhelm you, and may leave you feeling like you've failed). Try that for a week before you venture into the rest of the plan. You will feel better with the first food plan breakfast you have—you'll have more energy for a number of hours and also feel more hopeful.

At some point, however, you do need to "bite the bullet" and really dive in—letting go of the sugar, sugar substitutes, flour (bread and pasta), volume, and the rest of the foods on the list. It will take approximately four and a half days to withdraw from those substances and the volume eating.

WITHDRAWAL SYMPTOMS

Withdrawal symptoms vary from person to person. They can range from no big deal to a very unpleasant experience. The symptoms are listed in Chapter 2 on page 72. Go back and take a moment to review that list now.

Any of these symptoms also appear when blood sugar levels are plummeting—after eating highly refined carbs (including sugary foods), which spike blood sugar levels. As food addicts, we are familiar with them, but we don't connect, make the connection, or attribute these symptoms to our eating, not eating, and/or purging. We think it's the weather, lack of sleep (which may be an issue), our stress level, bad food, our family, our relationships, etc., and we go to food for the fix and other substances such as Red Bull, alcohol, drugs (including cigarettes), or over-the-counter pain relievers (such as Motrin, Tylenol, Aleve, and Excedrin, which contains caffeine), and so on.

Experiencing any of these symptoms feels like living in hell! The food addict in withdrawal, however, is moving toward her best state of health—her body is finally righting itself and moving toward

What Is Abstinence?

homeostasis. The food addict should keep in mind that for years, she has been working against her body—treating it very abusively by eating harmful foods, starving, overeating, purging, overexercising, and extreme diets. Even though it feels awful, the food addict needs to remember that these symptoms are going to pass; they are not forever. She will probably start feeling better on the third day. It's helpful to think about withdrawal being wellness, not sickness; it's a major positive—NOT negative.

The challenge for the food addict to successfully withdraw from the addictive substances/behaviors is the presence of the adversary—CRAVINGS. Cravings for some form of sugar or other refined carb will usually be strongest during the first few days. That's why many food addicts don't go the distance and give in on the second or third day. This is a shame since they've started the detox process and giving in just sends them right back to start.

The food addict who has made a decision to go through this process would be best served to go to 12 Step food recovery fellowship meetings to get support. The decision not to give into the illusory comfort of the food is the decision for success; not having understanding support will make the process even riskier.

Relieving Withdrawal Symptoms

To help in the process of withdrawal, I strongly recommend that you consider taking L-glutamine, which can safely be used to diminish cravings. Glutamine is an amino acid that is quite prevalent in the body naturally and has many functions. L-glutamine has the ability to relieve symptoms of cravings, appearing to act on the brain directly to naturally suppress and relieve them. Research has shown the L-glutamine, in a dose of 500 mg four times daily, decreases craving for alcohol, sugar, and carbohydrates.[88] I recommend taking two 500-mg capsules between breakfast and lunch and two 500-mg capsules between lunch and dinner—separate from food.

Chromium is another supplement to consider. This mineral helps keep blood sugar levels stable, but the amount of chromium found in the body gets used up by a high-carb diet. Putting more back into your body as a supplement restores blood sugar stability and can also help ease the craving for carbs.

Caution: If you are diagnosed with bipolar disorder (manic depression), do not use L-glutamine or chromium without consulting a knowledgeable psychiatrist or psychopharmacologist. These supplements can trigger mania in some people with bipolar disorder. Even if your health-care professional gives you the okay, watch your reactions very carefully.[89]

Here's something else that will also help you during the withdrawal process: the messages you tell yourself. Are you aware of what you tell yourself when you're in discomfort and you look to and pick up food to deal with the discomfort (like you always do)? Most likely you say to yourself, "I can't do this, I can't stand this, I can't tolerate this." When you give yourself this message, you give yourself permission to use food. Changing this message can help you in the process of withdrawal and beyond as you settle into a wonderful life of abstinence. Here's a new message for you to tell yourself:

My New Message
I **can** handle this.

I **can** tolerate this.

I **can** stand this.

I **can** do this.

I don't like it.

I feel or it feels awful.

It stinks/sucks.

It will pass.

I **can** handle this.

I **can** tolerate this.

I **can** stand this.

Repeat it until you believe it—it is the truth!

As those of us who are in recovery and/or treat food addiction know—and is so well verbalized by author and lecturer Kay Sheppard—what is needed to break the binge cycle is to become physically clean and not go looking for substitutes for those addictive foods that create cravings; to accept a way of eating that provides stabilization, i.e., a balance between

What Is Abstinence?

carbs and proteins (as is reflected in the food plan in Chapter 11); and to participate in recovery support groups. In other words, the food addict must:

- Have a complete withdrawal
- Get on the food plan
- Learn about the addictive properties of foods
- Get oriented to a 12 Step food recovery fellowship

Remember, your dignity, self-respect, self-esteem, freedom, hope, and healing will be yours when you do the following:

1. Eliminate foods that promote cravings, obsessional thoughts, compulsive behaviors, mood swings, poor brain function, weight problems, and energy, sleep, and digestive problems and follow a plan of eating that guides you to this end.

2. Develop new behaviors around food, which happens when you commit yourself to the food plan.

3. Become involved in a 12 Step food recovery fellowship.

4. Find new ways to manage your feelings.

5. Resolve unfinished business—especially unresolved family of origin issues that still affect your feelings, beliefs, attitudes and behaviors.

CHAPTER 10

The Basics of Nutrition

When we think of nutrition, we generally think of vitamins, minerals, and other nutrients. However, nutrition is actually about what we put into our bodies and what our bodies do with what we give them. It is important to know and understand nutrition basics and the roles food plays in physical recovery. Optimal physical functioning is a major factor in mental, emotional, and spiritual health. These are compromised by deficiencies in essential nutrients. Along with this, it is essential to become knowledgeable about the sources and how to include them in our daily diets. This chapter will help you on your way.

PROTEINS

The foundation of complete health is formed by the presence of protein and its biochemical activities. Protein is essential to life. Protein sources include:

- Meat (beef, veal, lamb, pork [not bacon] and organ meats)
- Poultry (chicken, turkey, duck)
- Fish
- Eggs
- Dairy
- Beans (legumes)
- Soy products (tofu, tempeh)

Whether you're a mother, a student, an endurance athlete, or a busy professional, your health, stamina, quality of life, and performance depend on protein. Why is protein so important? Here's a list of reasons:

- Essential for normal growth
- Makes up 90 percent of blood dry weight, 80 percent of muscle, and 70 percent of skin
- Provides building blocks for connective tissue
- Acts as a primary constituent of enzymes, hormones, and antibodies

The Basics of Nutrition

227

- Encompasses vital chemicals like immunoglobulins and enzymes.

- Forms the foundation for muscles, skin, bones, hair, heart, teeth, blood, brains, and billions of biochemical activities being performed in our bodies 24/7

What might occur in the case of protein deficiency? Any of the following:

- Chronic fatigue

- Muscle and connective tissue disorders (fibromyalgia, myalgic fibro-myositis, myofascial pain syndromes)

- Deteriorating vision

- Depression

- Slow wound healing

- Decreased resistance to infection

- Grayish complexion

- Hair loss

- Interruption or stoppage of menstruation

- Fragile, splitting, and slow-growing fingernails

- Lack of physical endurance (especially when attempting to exercise)

Proteins are made up of amino acids: the essential amino acids, of which there are nine, are obtained from food sources, and the nonessential amino acids, of which there are eleven, can be made by the body from other amino acids. Although there are more than 100 amino acids found in nature, the human body uses only twenty of them.

Amino acids are used by every cell of the body. They form neurotransmitters and hormones. They are also used for antibody and enzyme production and are responsible for the maintenance of healthy skin, hair, teeth, muscles, nerves, and blood.

All amino acids must be present in adequate amounts for many proteins to be constructed. One by one, specific amino acids are linked together to form a protein. If one amino acid is missing, the amino acid chain falls apart and the protein cannot be made.

The importance of protein to good health cannot be overemphasized. Protein needs must be met at each meal because protein is not stored by the body. When inadequate amounts of protein are consumed, the body cannot manufacture all of the proteins needed to keep the body working at optimum levels. It will begin to break down healthy tissue to meet its needs. This results in muscle weakness, fatigue, irritability, depression, and lowered immune function.

There are incomplete proteins and complete proteins. Here are the characteristics of each:

TABLE 9.1. INCOMPLETE VERSUS COMPLETE PROTEIN	
Incomplete Protein	**Complete Protein**
• Derived from vegetable sources • Low in essential amino acids even when consumed in high amounts • Although vegetable sources contain some protein, they are low in amino acids even when consumed in high amounts. It is not preferable to depend on these for sources of high-quality protein as they alone cannot sustain life. Vegetables are needed for antioxidants, phytonutrients, and fiber, which are also important for good health.	• Derived from animal sources • Contains all essential amino acids • Necessary to sustain health and life

In general, animal-based proteins (meat, fish, poultry, dairy, and eggs) are considered good sources of complete proteins. Complete proteins contain ample amounts of all essential amino acids. Vegetable proteins (grains, legumes, nuts, seeds, and other vegetables) are incomplete proteins because they are missing, or do not have enough of, one or more of the essential amino acids. By combining foods that have complementary nonessential amino acids (as in the table below), you can create a combination that is a complete protein, with all the essential amino acids. Understanding this idea of combining various foods to create complete proteins explains why various cultures can live and survive on rice and beans. Combine any of the grains with any of the legumes in the following table to create a complete protein:

The Basics of Nutrition

TABLE 9.2. MIX AND MATCH GRAINS & LEGUMES

Grains	Legumes
Amaranth	Beans
Barley	Chickpeas
Brown rice	Dried peas
Buckwheat (Kasha)	Lentils
Millet	Soy products (tofu, tempeh)
Oats	
Quinoa	
Rye	

Note: All of these foods are included in the food plan presented in Chapter 11.

Beef

Ideally, beef should be purchased at a butcher shop. Alternatively, if purchasing packaged meat, be aware of the expiration date. Look for red/pink color. If the meat is brown around the edges and/or has a bad odor, it should not be purchased. Meat can be refrigerated one to two days before it is cooked. As with all animal protein, once it is frozen, it should never be refrozen. Wash the cutting board with detergent to avoid salmonella poisoning. To insure the animal was not injected with steroids, growth hormones, and antibiotics, purchase organic meat if possible.

COLD-CUT CAUTIONS

Cold cuts (as opposed to "whole cuts" like roast beef and turkey, which are cooked whole and often flavored with salt and sugar) are sectioned and formed—restructured part, bound with non-meat products. Meat is chopped, seasoned, and formed into symmetrical shapes. Common ingredients in cold cuts include sodium nitrates (color fixative), added solution (meat is cooked in a bag and not drained), "natural juices" (meat is soaked and injected), BHT and BHA (chemicals that retard rancidity), carrageenan (sugar), corn syrup (sugar), hydrolyzed protein (flavor enhancers), emulsifiers (to prevent separation), and gelatin. See the further discussion in Chapter 11.

Poultry

When purchasing poultry, always check the expiration date on packages and choose the furthest date possible. Poultry can be refrigerated for two days prior to cooking.

Commercially raised animals are injected with hormones, growth enhancers, and antibiotics. Their meat contains preservatives, dyes, and chemical additives. The animals are not allowed to run free or see the light of day. Instead, they are kept in cramped, overcrowded cages. Their beaks are removed to prevent them from pecking each other, which also interferes with food and drink intake. Filthy and dehydrated, these animals are highly stressed; their stress hormones also taint their meat.

Free-range poultry is a healthier choice. Some poultry that is not free range is enhanced or "plumped" by being injected with water, salt, and other additives to help it stay juicier and more flavorful. Free-range poultry are allowed to run free in the barnyard. Hormones and antibiotics are not used and their feed is not tainted with chemicals and pesticides. The meat tastes sweeter and is more tender. The cost of free-range poultry has decreased, making it competitive at market as it becomes a more common purchase in many households.

When free-range is unavailable, choose products that state "no additives or preservatives." This helps to avoid additives such as coconut oil, partially hydrogenated oils, and sodium-based phosphates, which are added to increase the juiciness of the bird.

Fish

Fish should never smell "fishy"—not when it's raw, and not when it's cooked. Raw fish should be firm, not hard. The flesh should "spring back" after indenting it with your finger. Avoid overcooking fish and watch out for "smoked" fish because the smoking ingredients usually include sugar.

There are literally dozens of different kinds of fish, each with its own nutritional value—for example, omega-3 fatty acids are found in salmon, albacore tuna, and sardines; vitamin B12 is found in mackerel and bluefin tuna; and iron is found in snapper and sea bass. Most fish is high in selenium and vitamin D. The following is not an exhaustive list of choices; it is just an indication of the most common varieties:

The Basics of Nutrition

231

- Dark and oil-rich: Bluefin tuna, mackerel, salmon, sardines

- White lean and firm: Pollock, catfish, sole, striped bass, swordfish

- Medium-color oil-rich: Coho salmon, mahi mahi, yellowfin tuna, sockeye salmon

- White, lean, and flaky: sea bass, branzino, flounder, snapper, tilapia

- White, firm, oil-rich: albacore tuna, Chilean sea bass, sablefish, sturgeon

> ### COOKING NOTE
>
> Meat, poultry, and fish may be broiled, baked, boiled, roasted, or pan-fried. If grilling, use an electric grill rather than charcoal, since charcoal is a carcinogen. When meat or poultry is potted, the fat is reabsorbed by the flesh, providing excessive fat, so avoid cooking these meats in pots or slow cookers.

Eggs

Eggs provide the highest quality protein on the planet. Egg protein measures a higher "biological value" (the ability to aid growth and repair of body tissues) than any other food source. The protein in the egg is not all in the white. About 3.5 grams is found in the white, and the yolk contains almost 3 grams. Brown and white eggs are the same nutritionally.

Eggs are not a dairy product; they are only kept in the dairy case for refrigeration to ensure freshness. Be sure to check expiration dates and choose eggs from the back of the refrigerator to make sure you are purchasing the coldest eggs possible. Open the carton and check to see that the eggs are intact. Store eggs in the carton in the refrigerator shelf; do not use the egg containers on the door, as this part of the refrigerator does not stay cold enough to prevent bacterial growth.

Eggs have been called the perfect food as they contain complete protein and all vitamins and minerals except vitamin C. Free-range eggs are the best choice. The chickens are allowed to run free in the barnyard. Hormones and antibiotics are not used and their feed is not tainted with chemicals and pesticides. An unhealthy chicken lays unhealthy eggs. Eggs substitutes, dried egg powders, and liquid egg mixtures are poor nutritional alternatives and should be avoided.

Dairy Products

If you choose to consume dairy products, remember that many commercially raised cows are given hormones and antibiotics. They are also exposed to pesticides and other chemicals in their feed. They are under the similar stresses as chickens at the poultry factories. These practices taint our milk supply.

Removing the fat from milk may help lower one's risk of heart diseases, but it also decreases the nutrient value of milk. Fat is important for the absorption of calcium. Removing fat also removes the fat-soluble vitamins A, D, E and K, and only vitamin A and D are returned to milk.

The healthiest advice is to use dairy sparingly. It is possible to obtain adequate calcium without dairy products. Cows make milk on a diet of grass. Avoidance of dairy does not mean you will suffer from osteoporosis; it means that other sources of calcium must be added to your diet daily. Green leafy vegetables and bones added to soup stock and stews can provide needed calcium. Fish eaten whole, such as sardines and herring, or canned salmon with the bones are other good sources. Tofu is also an excellent source of absorbable calcium. When choosing dairy products, use low-fat and organically produced products rather than skim or fat-free versions.

(Most fat-free versions of any food have a lot of sugar added to make up for the taste eliminated by the removal of the fat.) See the further discussion in Chapter 11.

Beans

Beans are incomplete proteins, as they are plant-derived. Combined with any grain listed on page 229, they form a more high-quality protein. Eaten alone they are a good source of fiber and are low in saturated fat.

Soy Products

Soy products, which are made from soybeans, are considered by many to be a low-cost, versatile, overlooked protein. Tofu is the curd made from soybeans that is formed into cakes; it is a good source of protein. It is high in iron, calcium, and magnesium. It is low in the amino acid methionine. Serve with a grain like brown rice, which is high in methionine. Tofu takes on the taste of whatever you prepare it with. Extra firm or firm tofu is best for salads, stir-fry, marinated, baking, broiling, and

The Basics of Nutrition

233

pan-frying. Soft tofu is best for crumbling and preparing like eggs. Silken tofu is best for making sauces and dressings.

Tofu is sold in water. To use it, drain the water and use paper towels to dry as much of the tofu cake as you are going to use, as well as possible. Whatever portion you are not going to use, put back into the refrigerator in fresh water.

Tempeh is also a soy product that is naturally fermented, which binds it. This process retains the whole bean. Tempeh is a great source of protein and fiber. Its flavor becomes more pronounced with age. It stays fresh for a long time, but be aware of the expiration date and honor it. Watch for added wheat. Many varieties also have added grains, making it difficult to weigh properly. A few brands are pure soy. Tempeh may be heated in oven (which makes it crunchy), microwaved, cubed, or sliced. See the further discussion in Chapter 11.

CARBOHYDRATES

Carbohydrates are the first source of energy coming from foods of plant origin. Unlike protein, minerals and fats, carbs are not building blocks for the human body, but rather the fuel that runs the "engine" and is broken down in digestion into glucose, as explained in earlier parts of this book. Everyone needs high-quality, large-molecule carbs like those found in vegetables, beans, whole grains, and brown rice to fuel the body. Here's what you need to know about carbohydrates:

- They are the most common source of food energy.

- Excess of digested/converted carbs (glucose) is stored in liver and muscles. The excess of that becomes fat.

- There is a big difference between complex and simple carbohydrates. See Chapter 6: Understanding Metabolism and the Development of the Disease of Food Addiction for more on this.

- Unrefined or unprocessed (natural) carbs:
  - ➤ Give slow steady energy that lasts over a period of time (especially when combined with protein)
  - ➤ Are rich in vitamins
  - ➤ Are found in whole grains (not flour or wheat; see the illustration on page 181)

> Include vegetables, fruits, potatoes, and beans (which can also be used as a protein)

- <u>Refined or processed carbs,</u> **which must be eliminated:**
  - Give sudden burst of energy (mortgaged energy)
  - Give sudden drop of energy with following symptoms: irritability, nervousness, confusion, suspicion, jumpiness, anxiety, depression, hostility, stress, cravings, hyperactivity, sleeplessness, hallucinations, mood swings, irrational behavior and decisions, inability to focus or concentrate, fogginess
  - Are found in white rice, sugar, corn syrup, high-fructose corn syrup, flour (all bread, all pasta, all cold cereals), potato/corn starch, all vegetable/fruit juices, and alcoholic beverages (liquor, wine, beer)

FAT

Fat has gotten a bad rap. Do you remember when fat was vilified and eliminated from many foods and replaced with sugar? Americans gained more weight and more quickly than ever before. The truth is that fat was never the problem. Actually, we need fat. Here's what you need to know about fat:

- Contain heat and energy for the body
- Slowest burning in the body—long lasting
- Body needs more with physical activity
- Body needs less (but still needs some) with little/limited activity
- Includes all liquid oils, butter, avocado, and mayonnaise (no sugar)

As fat was never the problem, the distinction is not between healthy and unhealthy, but between saturated (stable, hard at room temperature—i.e., butter) and unsaturated (unstable, liquid at room temperature, i.e., vegetable oil). Hydrogenation is a process in which liquid unsaturated fat is turned into a solid fat by adding hydrogen. This processing results in a type of fat called trans fat. Eating trans fats increases risks for heart disease, stroke, and diabetes. For example, margarine is still being thought of as healthier than butter even though it contains trans fats.

The Basics of Nutrition

VITAMINS AND MINERALS

Why do we need vitamins and minerals? What are their functions? They are considered essential nutrients. Acting together, they perform hundreds of roles in the body. They maintain bone health, heal wounds, and bolster the immune system. They also convert food into energy and repair cellular damage. The body uses vitamins and minerals to regulate metabolic processes. They direct the body how to use ingested proteins, carbohydrates, and fats.

WATER

Water is one of the most vital of all nutrients. In fact, the water you drink is as important as the food you eat. You can survive long periods of time without food, but several days without water can be fatal. More than half of the body (40 to 50 quarts) is water. Eight to ten cups of water are lost daily through perspiration, urine, breath, and through the intestinal tract and must be replaced.

Water is necessary for every function of the body. Drinking 8 to 10 (8-ounce) glasses of water throughout the day is necessary for good health. (Water can be in the form of water, seltzer, and club soda.)

Here are eleven reasons to get your 8 to 10 glasses of water a day:

1. Keeps your mind sharp by hydrating the brain.

2. Carries nutrients to cells and transports wastes to kidneys and lungs for excretion.

3. Carries hormones and disease-fighting cells through the bloodstream.

4. Necessary for many chemical reactions of digestion and metabolism.

5. Assists in temperature regulation; cools through sweat.

6. Protects and cushions tissues; lubricates joints, thereby decreasing muscle cramps.

7. Prevents headaches by keeping the brain hydrated.

8. Provides satiety, gives a full feeling.

9. Moisturizes skin—no need for expensive chemical-laden skin moisturizers.

10. Critical to food digestion and absorption.

11. Assists with constipation relief.

This chapter was just the tip of the iceberg when it comes to nutrition-related information, but it is a good foundation to get you started. The food plan discussed in the next chapter ensures that you get sufficient amounts of all the nutrients your body needs to keep you healthy and in recovery from food addiction. You also now have a better understanding of the reasons behind the food plan choices, and knowing the reasons can help keep you focused on the food plan.

CHAPTER 11

Realization Center
Food Plan for True Recovery
from Food Addiction

As you have learned throughout this book, food addiction is a chronic, progressive biochemical illness. Processed and refined foods are the drugs of choice for food addicts and are usually combinations of sugar, flour, wheat, caffeine, and fat. To provide relief from emotional distress and physical craving, the addict self-medicates and perpetuates the cycle of binge eating/guilt/craving.

The purpose of the plan is to stabilize your blood sugar and at the same time address issues of the addiction (which resides in the brain [just as with an alcoholic]). When we talk about the brain and addiction, what we're really talking about is **CRAVING!** And craving takes place in the brain.

If you are committed to not having to put up a fight, that is, fighting the cravings, then the **triggers** (just like the alcohol for the alcoholic) must be eliminated.

I guarantee that once they are gone from your realm (not by giving them up but by relinquishing them (an issue of your decision, your choice), you will no longer experience cravings (which are a physiological phenomenon).

It takes about 4 to 5 days to detox from sugar, sugar substitutes, wheat, flour, etc. Caffeine should be eliminated over a month's time—using decaf

---

Disclaimer: Before starting the food plan, it is important to consult with your healthcare professionals for approval. When you present them with the REALIZATION CENTER FOOD PLAN FOR TRUE RECOVERY FROM FOOD ADDICTION, we are certain they will be as enthusiastic and supportive as we are as you return to better health and vitality. (In addition, we would be pleased to speak to your health care professional upon your request).

(25% for the first week, 50% for the second week, 75% for the third week, then 100% for the fourth week, and then eliminate the decaf).

Withdrawal symptoms vary from person to person. They may include cravings, sleep disturbances, digestive disturbances, headaches, and/or irritability.

Once the cravings are gone—ahhhh—then you get to experience the urges.

As you learned earlier, I make a distinction between cravings and urges: in my definitions, **cravings** are a physiological/biological phenomenon produced in the reward/pleasure circuit in the brain; **urges**, on the other hand, are experienced only when cravings are no longer triggered and result from feelings that are uncomfortable and have been historically medicated/numbed by eating/not eating or eating and purging.

Urges don't come from the brain—because you're no longer taking in the substance that create the craving! Urges are about your heart, your feelings—e.g., when you get angry, or you feel vulnerable or less than and you want to bury your face in an Entenmann's cake.

Urges are not being driven by your biology—they're being driven by uncomfortable feelings, and your emotional memory is such that you know what can make you FEEL better. But using food to manage your feelings is a deception. You'll feel better for a very short time and then feel the shame and remorse and then you hurt yourself again.

Please do not modify this food plan; its principles will afford you the most comfortable detox from addictive substances, elimination of cravings, the greatest satiety, an increase in energy, stability of mood, sleep, digestion, brain function (clarity of thinking, concentration, memory, perception, and more), normalization of weight (if it's an issue), improvement in overall health, and the ability to pursue your recovery and your life.

These benefits are attained because the food plan will immediately normalize/stabilize your blood sugar levels—and you will then experience yourself so much better/healthier than you have been in the past. You will become a star in your own movie. I promise!

This food plan, along with your food recovery support system, will allow you to be **ABSTINENT**—to no longer overeat, undereat, or purge. **ABSTINENCE** is the goal, and it is the solution to breaking out of the bondage of the disease of food addiction.

Realization Center Food Plan for True Recovery from Food Addiction

You deserve to be and feel the absolute best you can—and it all starts with what you put in your mouth. The food is everything!

PRINCIPLES OF THE FOOD PLAN

1. **Weighing & Measuring:** All foods must be weighed and measured according to specifications. As volume is a trigger for relapse, this is an important principle. Weighing and measuring take the emotion out of meal portions. Portions may appear large when you don't want to eat and may appear small when food urges hit. Correct portions for your body have been determined. Individual modifications can be made if necessary.

   A digital or mechanical kitchen or postal scale, measuring cups, and measuring spoons are necessary tools for your recovery. "Eyeballing" always results in too much or not enough and leaves room for obsession—e.g., "I ate too much," "I did not eat enough," "I need more . . ."

   In a larger sense, weighing and measuring is a very spiritual act.

2. **Do not leave out any of the portions or skip any meals.** Remember, as food addicts, we are the best accountants—always keeping track of what we didn't eat—and then when we may be feeling inadequate, angry, scared, etc., we give ourselves permission to add an extra "whatever" that we didn't eat a while ago—and then we're in trouble— maybe off to the races.

   This is a very tricky, cunning, baffling, and powerful illness. We have to stop trying to be in control—it always backfires!

   Skipping meals is NOT the secret to recovery, weight loss, or better health. Your body needs a consistent source of fuel throughout the day to maintain your energy level and to keep your brain alert and alive.

   When you regularly skip meals, you're not "saving" calories; you're just scaring your body into thinking that it might not get any more fuel. When you tease your body in that way, it tries to store up all of the energy it can—so your metabolism slows down, which can actually lead to future weight gain!

   Also, do not combine meals (e.g., "brunch," instead of breakfast and lunch) as it does not allow a timely flow of meals and plays havoc with blood sugar.

3. **Personal Trigger Foods:** Refrain from your personal trigger foods—even if they appear on the food plan, they may stimulate a desire to overeat.

4. **Meal Timing:**

- **Breakfast** must be eaten within 1 hour after arising.

- **Lunch** must be eaten no more than 4 to 5 hours after breakfast.

- **Dinner** must be eaten no more than 5 hours after lunch.

- **Metabolic adjustment (MA)** must be eaten approximately 4 hours after dinner (before bedtime).

The MA can also be eaten between breakfast and lunch OR lunch and dinner if the time between those meals is going to be longer than 5 hours.

Please do not think of the MA as a "snack." Its purpose, as the name suggests, is to regulate your metabolism to insure that there is no sudden drop in blood sugar, leading to crash, and then leading to overeating/using.

5. **Protein at Every Meal:** Protein produces the secretion of the hormone glucagon, which helps to maintain blood sugar stability.

6. **Sugar, Flour, Wheat:** We refrain from all forms of sugar, artificial sweeteners, flour, and wheat. It is especially important to check all labels when grocery shopping—and to do it each time, as manufacturers often change ingredients without notification. ANY FORM OF SUGAR, FLOUR, or WHEAT in any amount can be a trigger. Please refer to "Names of Sugar" on page 252 and "Names of Wheat" on page 255. Become familiar with those sugars most frequently used in products, including but not limited to refined sugars, high-fructose corn syrup, evaporated cane juice, fructose, lactose, maltose, modified food starch, molasses, inulin, sorbitol, Splenda (Sucralose), aspartame (NutraSweet), and honey.

Note: "Low-Calorie" or "Lite" on a label does not mean that the product is sugar free. You must read the list of ingredients on any product you might purchase.

Realization Center Food Plan for True Recovery from Food Addiction

241

7. **Sweeteners:** Diet products feed the obsession to restrict and diet. Research on artificial sweeteners has shown that they have little or no effect on weight loss. The body may use aspartame (NutraSweet, Equal, Splenda) in the same fashion that it does sugar, i.e., raising blood sugar levels with the resulting crash. Studies show they also trigger cravings for real sugar. They may also cause side effects such as headaches, moodiness, lethargy, and dizziness. This also includes stevia and agave. See the list of artificial sweeteners on page 253.

---

8. Typical/Common Foods That Must Be Excluded:

Sugar—all forms*; fructose, sucrose, corn sweeteners, dextrose, honey, glucose, barley malt, maltodextrin, polydextrose

Alcohol—all forms

Artificial Sweeteners—all forms**

Bananas

Bouillon cubes

Caffeine-containing foods— coffee, tea, sodas, beverages

Cakes, Pies

Chocolate

Cocoa

Cold cereals—all

Cooked, processed meat dishes

Cooked sausage, bologna, liverwurst, wieners

Cookies

Corn and cornstarch

Crackers

Cream Cheese

Dates

Doughnuts

Dried fruits

Exotic fruits

Figs

Flour—all forms; spaghetti, macaroni, all pastas, breads, pizza, crackers, spinach/ artichoke/all noodles, bagels, pita

Wheat—all forms*; durum, bulgur, kamut, semolina, spelt

Fried foods

Gravies

Griddle/pancakes

Hard cheese

Ice cream and cones

Malt products, foods containing malt

Nuts/seeds—all (except using seeds as an oil)

Puddings

Puffed grains***—rice, rice cakes, millet, corn, popcorn

Raisins

Salty snack foods

Soy sauce****

Sugar-free Candies

Vitamin water

* See "Names of Sugar" on page 252.

** This includes Equal, Splenda, Stevia, Truvia, Agave, Xylitol, Saccharin, Sugar Twin—any and all of them.

*** Once a grain is puffed, it becomes a refined carbohydrate, which is too rapidly converted to glucose and acts in the body the same way sugar does.

**** Soy sauce contains wheat. A better alternative is wheat-free tamari, or, still better "Braggs Liquid Aminos," which tastes like soy sauce.

9. **Caffeine:** We avoid all forms of caffeine—coffee, tea, chocolate, and caffeinated sodas as they are potent appetite stimulants and serve to lower blood sugar levels. Limit decaffeinated beverages, as they, too, contain some caffeine. Caffeine-free teas are accepted alternatives.

10. **Eating Out:** When dining out or eating foods that you have not personally prepared, ask for the list of ingredients in the dish. Sugar in its many forms is often added to foods we would not expect to find it in, such as sauces, salad dressings, yogurts, vitamins, and/or soups.

    Even when eating out, please follow principle 1 listed earlier: Weigh and measure your restaurant meal—don't put your "life" in the hands of others; they really don't understand and compromising for the sake of "appearances" is never worth the ensuing consequences.

11. **Planning:** Plan menus carefully, write them down, and include sufficient variety to avoid boredom and possible triggering. It will also help with food shopping. You cannot afford to be spontaneous or chaotic in your eating.

12. **Shopping:** Fresh fruit and vegetables should always be the first choice. Frozen is next, making sure there is no added sugar to frozen fruit or, if canned, that it's packed in water or its own juice, making sure to drain the liquid before eating. Rinse canned vegetables and fruits under cold water, as they are usually packed with large amount of salt.

13. **Water/Beverages:** It is important to drink 8 to 10 cups of water daily. The body needs water for every function—digestion, circulation, elimination, blood flow, and respiration; even the fat-burning process requires water.

Realization Center Food Plan for True Recovery from Food Addiction

Bottled water and seltzer are acceptable provided they have no sugar or sugary flavorings of any kind. (A very good substitute for soda is the broad variety of flavored seltzers on the market today – lemon/lime, strawberry, and even coconut and pink grapefruit—they have no sugar and the bubbles are refreshing.)

As juice is basically 100% sugar; *all* fruit and vegetable juices are avoided. Also the "designer" waters, such as Vitamin Water, Gatorade, Glaceau, etc., have added sugar (or artificial sweetener), so we exclude them from our program. Plain water or seltzer is the answer to hydration and better health.

14. **Gum & Mints:** There is no chewing gum or mints/candy permitted. They are mostly sugar or sugar substitutes. These stimulate the salivary glands and create a feeling of hunger/craving. Also, chewing gum or sucking on mints allows you to chew away your feelings, which is in conflict with a major purpose of this process—to discover who you are, what you feel, and what you really want.

15. **Be Prepared!** Call ahead to restaurants, conferences, and friends to make sure that food on your plan will be available. Explaining your nutritional needs in advance helps to avoid conflict later. Many abstainers choose to bring their own meals in uncertain situations (airplanes, meetings, conferences). This is the ultimate act of self-respect/self-love.

16. **Food Preparation:** Food may be baked, broiled, oven-roasted, or grilled. Use nonstick pans and nonstick sprays. When dining out, avoid ordering sautéed or fried foods, as they contain much more fat than is abstinent (healthy).

17. **When in Doubt . . .** If you are unsure about anything, leave it alone. If something listed in this food plan becomes unclear to you, avoid it. When in doubt, leave it out.

18. **Turning Over Your Food:** Every day, write down your meal plan and discuss it with your sponsor *before* you eat anything. Include foods you intend to eat and the amounts. Do not make any changes without consulting your sponsor.

19. **If this plan seems overwhelming to you, start simply**—start with the "Food Plan Breakfast."

As you become comfortable with making changes to how you eat, you will be eager to continue.

21. **Breakfast:** As you were likely told by your mother, breakfast is the most important meal of the day.

- It gently raises your blood sugar, which has dropped during the night.

- It prevents drops in blood sugar levels, which lead to poor food choices later in the day.

- It helps start the day feeling like you're taking care of yourself, setting a positive tone for the day.

- Improves productivity, learning, and focus.

There are no rules about which proteins are proper for breakfast. Meat, fish, and poultry as well as eggs and dairy are acceptable. It is essential to eat breakfast even if you do not feel hungry or "don't feel" like it. Avoid the temptation to make up for the mistakes of yesterday. This thinking only serves to perpetuate the cycle of chaotic eating.

22. **Eat Consciously:** Sit down for meals. Remain seated for meals. Eat gently and slowly. Chew your food! Chewing is the first step in proper digestion. Food needs to be ground and mixed with saliva for the proper absorption and digestion of nutrients. This helps to avoid issues such as gas, bloating, esophageal reflux, nausea, stomachaches, heartburn, and belching.

Do not engage in "distracted eating" (watching TV, reading, or talking on the telephone). Focus on the meal. Try to give THANKS for your food before and after each meal.

23. **Weighing Yourself:** Never weigh yourself more than once per month, if at all. I personally believe you should throw away your scale. Unless required by your physician, you don't need to know what you weigh!

Your clothes will tell you about your weight loss or gain. I think weighing yourself is most often a setup to eat or to restrict—the number will often be more or less than you expected, and disappointment or excitement about your weight is a trigger. The idea of weighing yourself also keeps the focus/emphasis on the physical aspect of recovery. If you remain abstinent, following the food plan, your body will find its proper, healthy weight. Your body is very smart and will appreciate your treating it with the care and respect it requires and will return the "favor" umpteen fold by becoming highly functional and healthy! **Trust the process!**

24. **Exercise:** Getting regular exercise is very important and, in moderation, is part of the recovery equation. It is not a weight-loss/control tool; rather, it is an integral part of a healthy lifestyle. In moderation, it enhances feelings of well-being, increases your energy, and stabilizes mood.

    Overexercising negates the benefits of this recovery process and is or becomes yet another element of food addiction. It can actually be harmful and counterproductive to health and recovery.

    This food plan supports 45 minutes per day of exercise, including warm-up and cooldown. We are built to move—no matter how old we are. Mild walking, stretching, yoga, aerobics, and strength training with the advice and consent of a physician and ideally under the tutelage of a professional is often the best way to go.

25. **If You Are Pregnant:** Again, be sure to speak with your doctor before adopting the food plan. When you receive the go-ahead from your doctor, you will follow the food plan for the first trimester, and then, at the beginning of the second trimester, you should make additions to your meals.

    You must gain weight in a pregnancy. If you are following the food plan, you can rest assured that the weight gain is baby/pregnancy weight and not "fat" weight. During this time, it is essential to follow a plan of healthy eating. Your physician will probably prescribe prenatal vitamins, so be sure to take them. Morning sickness is a sign of a healthy pregnancy and may not be limited to the morning. Mint, chamomile, non-caffeinated, and non-sugared herbal teas may be helpful and soothing.

Add the following to the food plan during the second and third trimester:

- 1 more metabolic adjustment (with a dairy as the protein)
- 1 additional ounce of protein at each meal
- 1 additional starchy vegetable/grain selection at lunch
- 1 additional tablespoon of oil per day

26. **Vitamins and Supplements**: A good-quality multivitamin is important to take daily as are other basic supplements. Consult with your physician. Suggestions include:

- Multivitamin (Solgar M75 is a good choice)
- Blue Bonnet B-complex 100 (one with breakfast and one with lunch)
- Fish oils
- Vitamin C (Ester C is preferred) 500 mg, three times per day
- Vitamin E—Maxi-Gamma Tocopherols
- Calcium
- L-Glutamine
- Vitamin D

Realization Center Food Plan for True Recovery from Food Addiction

247

— FOOD PLAN FOR WOMEN —

(See "Food Plan Selections" on page 248.)

Breakfast (within 1 hr. of arising)	Lunch (4–5 hrs. after breakfast)	Dinner (4–5 hrs. after lunch)	MA* (Metabolic Adjustment) (3–4 hrs. after dinner)
1 protein	1 protein	1 protein	1 dairy or ½ protein
1 fruit or 6 oz vegetables	2 servings vegetables** Combination of cooked and raw	2 servings vegetables** Combination of cooked and raw	1 Fruit
1 grain or 1 starchy vegetable	Option***	2 grains or starchy vegetable ***	
	Oil/fat ****	Oil/fat****	

* **Metabolic Adjustment**—This is not a "snack" as we typically think of "snacks." It is a "mini-meal" with the purpose of keeping blood sugar levels stable. It is also a "moveable" meal; if there is going to be a period longer than 5 hours between lunch and dinner, then it may be eaten between those meals—**3 to 4 HOURS AFTER LUNCH.**

** **Vegetables**—a combination of cooked and raw (both lunch and dinner). Option: Add up to 6 oz of vegetables per day—3 oz at lunch and 3 oz at dinner.

*** **Lunch Option**: You may move ½ of Dinner grain/starch selection to Lunch.

**** **Oils/Fats**—2 tablespoons (6 teaspoons) of oils/fats must be used daily and may be divided anyway you choose provided that the selections are used at a meals.

All weights are AFTER cooking.

FOOD PLAN SELECTIONS*

Proteins (all weights are after cooking)		Dairy		Fruits	
Beans	1 cup	Buttermilk	1 cup	Apple	6 oz
Beef	4 oz	Low-fat cottage cheese	½ cup	Apricot	6 oz
Chicken	4 oz			Berries (all varieties)	6 oz
Duck	4 oz	1% milk	1 cup		6 oz
Edamame	¾ cup	Non-fat or low-fat yogurt	1 cup	Clementines	6 oz
Eggs	2			Grapefruit	6 oz
Egg substitute	¾ cup	Ricotta cheese—part skim	½ cup	Kiwi	8 oz
Egg whites	6			Melon	6 oz
Fish	4 oz			Nectarines	6 oz
Lamb	4 oz			Orange	6 oz
Low-fat cottage cheese	½ cup			Peach	6 oz
Low-fat or non-fat yogurt	1 cup			Pear	6 oz
Pork	4 oz			Pineapple	6 oz
Ricotta Cheese Part Skim	½ cup			Plums	6 oz
Shellfish	4 oz			Tangerine	
Soybeans	¾ cup				
Soy milk—unsweetened	1 cup				
Tempeh (no grains) (Soyboy or Litelife soy only)	6 oz				
Tofu	8 oz				
Turkey	4 oz				
Veal	4 oz				

The items within each category can be combined to equal the indicated portion, e.g., steak and eggs, cottage cheese and yogurt, fruit salad.

Realization Center Food Plan for True Recovery from Food Addiction

Vegetables (6 oz)		Grains/Starchy Vegetables ½ cup after cooking (unless otherwise noted)	Oils/Fats 2 tablespoons per day
Alfalfa sprouts	Mushrooms	* Grains (typically ¼ raw):	Avocado (¼)
Artichoke hearts (canned)	Okra	Amaranth	Butter
Asparagus	Onions	Barley	Canola oil
Bamboo shoots	Pickles	Brown basmati rice	Corn oil
Beans—all beans	Peppers	Brown rice	Flax seeds or flax seed oil
Beets (3 oz or ½ Cup)	Pimientos	Buckwheat (Kasha)	Mayonnaise (no sugar)
Bok choy	Radishes	Cream of Rye	
Broccoli	Rhubarb	Millet	Nut oils
Brussels sprouts	Rutabaga	Oat Bran	Olive oil
Cabbage	Sauerkraut	Oatmeal (not instant)	Safflower oil
Carrots	Scallions	Quinoa	Salad dressing (no sugar)
Cauliflower	Sea vegetables (hijiki, nori, arame, dulse, wakame, etc.)	Rye	Vegetable oil
Celery		**Starchy Vegetables:**	
Chicory	Shallots	Beans—lima, navy, all dried beans	
Cucumber	Snow pea pods		
Daikon radish	Spinach	Parsnips	
Eggplant	Spaghetti squash	Peas—green	
Endive	Sprouts (Not wheat grass)	Potatoes—all including sweet (6 oz)	
Escarole			
Greens—beet, collard, dandelion, kale, all lettuces, mustard, turnip, etc.	Swiss chard	Sun chokes or Jerusalem artichokes	
	Tomatoes		
	Turnips	Winter squash—acorn, butternut, Hubbard, kabocha, pumpkin	
Hearts of palm	Watercress		
Jicama	Water chestnuts		
Kohlrabi	Yellow squash (summer squash)	Yam	
Leeks	Zucchini		

Condiments:

The following condiments may be used provided they contain <u>no sugar</u>:

- herbs, spices, and vinegars (except balsamic)
- ½ cup tomato sauce, ketchup
- ½ cup salsa, mustard (check for sugar), lemon juice, lime juice

We exclude soy sauce from this category because it contains wheat. A good substitute is Braggs Liquid Aminos (available in most health food stores and some supermarkets) or tamari.

— FOOD PLAN FOR MEN —

(See "Food Plan Selections" on page 251.)

Breakfast (within 1 hr. of arising)	Lunch (4–5 hrs. after breakfast)	Dinner (4–5 hrs. after lunch)	MA* (Metabolic Adjustment) (3–4 hrs. after dinner)
1 protein	1 protein	1 protein	1 dairy or ½ protein
1 fruit or 6 oz vegetables	2 servings vegetables** Combination of cooked and raw	2 servings vegetables** Combination of cooked and raw	1 fruit
1 grain or 1 starchy vegetable	2 grains or 1 starchy vegetable or 1 fruit	2 grains or 1 starchy vegetable	
	Oil/fat ***	Oil/fat***	

* **Metabolic Adjustment**—This is not a "snack" as we typically think of "snacks." It is a "mini-meal" with the purpose of keeping blood sugar levels stable. It is also a "moveable" meal; if there is going to be a period longer than 5 hours between lunch and dinner, then it may be eaten between those meals—**3 to 4 HOURS AFTER LUNCH.**

** **Vegetables**—a combination of cooked and raw (both lunch and dinner). Option: Add up to 6 oz of vegetables per day—3 oz at lunch and 3 oz at dinner.

*** **Oils/Fats**—2 tablespoons (6 teaspoons) of oils/fats must be used daily and may be divided anyway you choose provided that the selections are used at a meals.

All weights are AFTER cooking.

Condiments:

The following condiments may be used provided they contain <u>no sugar</u>:

- herbs, spices, and vinegars (except balsamic)
- ½ cup tomato sauce, ketchup
- ½ cup salsa, mustard (check for sugar), lemon juice, lime juice.

We exclude soy sauce from this category because it contains wheat. A good substitute is Braggs Liquid Aminos (available in most health food stores and some supermarkets) or tamari.

Realization Center Food Plan for True Recovery from Food Addiction 251

FOOD PLAN SELECTIONS*

Proteins (all weights are after cooking)		Dairy		Fruits	
Beans	1 cup	Buttermilk	1 cup	Apple	6 oz
Beef	5 oz	Low-fat cottage cheese	¾ cup	Apricot	6 oz
Chicken	6 oz			Berries (all varieties)	6 oz
Duck	5 oz	1% milk	1 cup		6 oz
Edamame	¾ cup	Non-fat or low-fat yogurt	1 cup	Clementines	6 oz
Eggs	3			Grapefruit	6 oz
Egg Substitute	¾ cup	Ricotta cheese— part skim	¾ cup	Kiwi	8 oz
Egg Whites	6			Melon	6 oz
Fish	6 oz			Nectarines	6 oz
Lamb	5 oz			Orange	6 oz
Low Fat Cottage Cheese	¾ cup			Peach	6 oz
Low Fat or Non-Fat Yogurt	1 cup			Pear	6 oz
Pork	5 oz			Pineapple	6 oz
Ricotta Cheese Part Skim	¾ cup			Plums	6 oz
Shellfish	5 oz			Tangerine	
Soybeans	¾ cup				
Soy Milk—unsweetened	1 cup				
Tempeh (no grains)	6 oz				
(Soyboy or Litelife soy only)					
Tofu	8 oz				
Turkey	6 oz				
Veal	5 oz				

The items within each category can be combined to equal the indicated portion, e.g., steak and eggs, cottage cheese and yogurt, fruit salad, etc.

Vegetables (6 oz)		Grains/Starchy Vegetables ½ cup after cooking (unless otherwise noted)	Oils/Fats 2 tablespoons per day
Alfalfa sprouts	Mushrooms	* **Grains** (typically ¼ cup raw)**:**	Avocado (¼)
Artichoke hearts (canned)	Okra	Amaranth	Butter
Asparagus	Onions	Barley	Canola oil
Bamboo shoots	Pickles	Brown Basmati Rice	Corn oil
Beans—yellow or green	Peppers	Brown Rice	Flax seeds or flax seed oil
Beets (3 oz or ½ cup)	Pimientos	Buckwheat (Kasha)	Mayonnaise (no sugar)
Bok choy	Radishes	Cream of Rye	Nut oils
Broccoli	Rhubarb	Millet	Olive oil
Brussels sprouts	Rutabaga	Oat Bran	Safflower oil
Cabbage	Sauerkraut	Oatmeal (not instant)	Salad dressing (no sugar)
Carrots	Scallions	Quinoa	Vegetable oil
Cauliflower	Sea vegetables— hijiki, nori, arame, dulse, wakame	Rye	
Celery	Shallots	**Starchy Vegetables:**	
Chicory	Snow pea pods	Beans—lima, navy, all dried beans	
Cucumber	Spinach	Parsnips	
Daikon radish	Spaghetti squash	Peas—green	
Eggplant	Sprouts (not wheat grass)	Potatoes—all including sweet (6 oz)	
Endive	Swiss chard		
Escarole	Tomatoes	Sun chokes or Jerusalem artichokes	
Greens—beet, collard, dandelion, kale, all lettuces, mustard, turnip	Turnips	Winter Squash—acorn, butternut, Hubbard, kabocha, pumpkin, Yam	
	Watercress		
	Water chestnuts		
Hearts of palm	Yellow squash (summer squash)		
Jicama	Zucchini		
Kohlrabi			
Leeks			

NAMES OF SUGAR

Ace-K

Acesulfame-K (Sunette, Sweet & Safe, Sweet One)

Aguamiel

Alcohol/Alcoholic Drinks

Alitame

Amasake

ARTIFICIAL SWEETENERS (see end of list)

Artificial Flavors

Barley Malt, Syrup

Beer

Blackstrap Molasses

Caramel Color (used in diet or regular colas

Chewing Gum

Clarified Grape Juice

Realization Center Food Plan for True Recovery from Food Addiction

Concentrated fruit juices (i.e., pear, grape, pineapple, orange)

Corn Sweetener

Cyclamates

Date Paste

Dextrin

Dextrose

Dried/Dehydrated Fruit/Vegs: apricots, bananas, dates, figs, pears, kale, veg chips, etc.,

Evaporated Cane Juice

Extracts

Fat Substitutes (made from concentrated fruit paste)

Fructooligosacchrides (FOS)

Fructose

Fruit Juice Concentrate

Glucosamine

Glycerin

Heavy Syrup

Honey—any type or form

Jaggery

-ides, any additive with this suffix: Monosodium, Glycerides, Olyglycerides, Saccharides (any), Trisaccharides, Diglycerides, Glycerides (any), Mono- Glycerides, Onosaccharides, Polysaccharides, etc.

Licorice Root Powder

"Light"/"Lite" or "Low" Sugar

Malted Barley

Maltodextrins/dextrose

Malto-anything

Mannitol

Molasses, Blackstrap Molasses

Monosaccharides

"Natural" Flavors/Sweeteners

Nectars (All)

Neotame

-ol—any additive with this suffix: Carbitol, Glucitol, Glycerol, Glycol, Hexitol, Inversol, Maltitol, Mannitol, Sorbitol, Xyltol, etc.

-ose—any additive with this suffix: Colorose, Dextrose, Fructose, Galactose, Glucose, Lactose, Levulose, Maltodextrose, Maltose, Mannose, Polydextrose, Polytose, Ribose, Sucralose, Sucrose, Tagatose, Zylose

Raisins—Juice, Paste, Syrup

Rice—Malt, Sugar, Syrup, Sweeteners

Sorghum Molasses, Syrup

Succanat (evaporated Cane Juice)

Sucraryl

Sucrose (cane or beet)

Sugar –All Forms: Apple, Barbados, Bark (Zylose), Beet, Brown (any color), Cane Sugar/Juice, Caramel Sugars, Confectioners, Date, Fruit Sugar/ Sweetener, Granulated, Grape, Invert Light or Lite Sugar, Lo or Low, Maple, Milled, "Natural" Sugar, Powered, Raw, Turbinado, Unrefined

Sunette/Sweet-One

Syrups –any type: Agave, Barley, Brown Rice, Corn, Date, Fig, High Fructose Corn, Hydrogenated Glucose, Invert, "Light" or "Lite", Malt, Maple

Table Salt (dextrose is added)

Vanillin

Whey (71% Lactose)

Xanthan Gums

ARTIFICIAL SWEETENERS (all artificial sweeteners are considered sugar!!): 100% Natural Sweetener, All-Natural Sweeteners, Pure Natural Sweeteners, Naturally Sweetened, Saccharine in Packets, Liquid Saccharine, Aspartame (Equal), Sweet N Low, Splenda (Sucralose), Stevia, Truvia, Sugar Twin in Packs or bulk, Low-Calorie Sweeteners of all kinds, Lite/Light Sweeteners of all kinds

Flour: Sugar's Twin

Flour is sugar's twin. Flour is absorbed almost as quickly as sugar is, and it raises/spikes your blood sugar followed by a severe drop and then affects brain chemistry to create all the adverse effects that sugar has—triggering cravings and altering mood.

Once a grain, vegetable, nut, or bean is ground into flour, it becomes a refined carbohydrate, which is an addictive substance to the food addict. Whole-grain flour is still flour. And once a grain is ground into flour, it's not whole anymore.

The Prevalence of Wheat

In the book *Intelligent Medicine* (Simon & Schuster, 1997), Dr. Ronald Hoffman states, "Wheat is one of the most common causes of food allergy or intolerance. Some individuals experience a profound sensitivity to all wheat products. In their system, improperly digested wheat fragments appear to mimic powerful neurotransmitters that are similar to opium. This results in symptoms of fatigue, feeling 'stoned' or 'high' because of the opiate-like compound, intestinal bloating, and possibly constipation. These individuals [food addicts] may develop food cravings for their offending substance that can lead to binge eating."

We therefore eliminate all wheat. However, wheat is prevalent in many foods. Be aware that it is found in all of the following:

BEVERAGES: Beer, cocomalt gin (any drink containing grain neutral spirits), whiskey, malted milk, ovaltine and postum. Remember, the food plan excludes ALL alcoholic beverages.

BREADS: All breads are excluded from the food plan. These include bagels, biscuits, crackers, muffins, popovers, pretzels, rolls and breads, including those sold as corn bread, graham bread, pumpernickel, rye bread, etc. They may contain a portion of wheat flour as well as other grains.

CEREALS: These include cooked cereals such as cream of wheat and malt-o-meal. ALL cold cereals contain wheat and/or sugar.

FLOURS: White flour (bleached or unbleached), all-purpose flour, whole wheat flour, graham flour packaged baking mixes, semolina flour and durum flour (found in pastas and bread).

Realization Center Food Plan for True Recovery from Food Addiction

MISCELLANEOUS: Bouillon cubes, cooked processed meat dishes, fried food rolled or dipped in flour mixtures, gravies, griddle cakes, pancakes, ice cream cones, malt products or food containing malt, cooked sausages (bologna, liverwurst, wieners), thickening in ice cream or bottled condiments, soy sauce. A better option is Braggs Liquid Amino (tastes like soy sauce—even better) or tamari (make sure the label says "wheat free").

PASTRIES AND DESSERTS: Cakes, cookies, doughnuts, pies, puddings, candy.

PASTAS/FLOUR: We avoid ALL forms of flour. All pastas/noodles are made from flour—This includes pastas/noodles labeled: spinach pasta, artichoke pasta/flour, rice noodles. (Most pasta including spaghetti, macaroni, noodles, etc. is made of wheat flour—so they are excluded on two counts—one because they are made from flour and also because of the wheat.)

WHEAT-FREE PRODUCTS: Read the labels. Check the ingredients list to make sure it is wheat and flour free. **Spelt and Kamut** are in the wheat family, so we avoid them.

NAMES OF WHEAT

Abyssinian Hard (Wheat Triticum durum)	Filler	Malt Extract, Flavoring, Syrup, Vinegar
Bleached Flour	Food Starch	Matzo Semolina
Bran	Fu (dried wheat gluten)	Miso
Bread Flour	Germ	Modified Starch, Food Starch
Brown Flour	Graham Flour	MSG
Bulgur (Bulgur Wheat/Nuts)	Granary Flour	Natural Flavoring
Calcium Caseinate (Contains MSG)	Gravy Cubes	Pasta
Cereal Binding	Groats (barley, wheat)	Red Winter
Couscous	Hard Wheat	Seitan
Durum (Duram) Wheat Tritium	Hydrolyzed Plant Protein (HPP)	Semolina
Edible Starch	Hydrolyzed Vegetable Protein (HVP)	Semolina Triticum
Einkorn Wheat	Kamut	Shoyu (soy sauce)
	Malt	Soba Noodles
		Spelt

Sodium Caseinate (Contains MSG)

Soy Sauce

Spelt (Triticum Spelta)– cousin to wheat

Sprouted Wheat

Starch

Stock Cubes

Strong Flour

Suet in Packets

Tabbouleh

Tamari with wheat

Teriyaki Sauce

Textured Vegetable Protein—TVP

Triticale X triticosecale

Udon (wheat noodles)

Vegetable Starch

Vital Gluten

Wheat Any Kind:
Abyssinian, Bran, Berries, Bulgur, Durum, Germ, Germ Oil, Nuts, Sprouted, Starch, Triticum aestivum, Triticum Mononoccum

Wheat Grass (can contain seeds)

White Flour

Whole-Meal Flour

PART THREE

Dealing with Food Addiction

CHAPTER 12

Compliance versus Surrender

"If eating is out of control, the addict will have a marginal life."
—MARCIA BODENSTEIN

It is virtually impossible to be fully awake, alive, aware, and present for life and all of its layers and nuances if one is drunk (yes, drunk) on sugar. At the forefront of the obsessed mind is "Why did I do this?" and "When can I get more?" and "How can I ever stop?" and "God, I feel awful." Thinking is cloudy and fuzzy, decisions are not thought out, the quality of relationships suffers, and the addict circles around the rim of life rather than in the center of living.

As Marilyn J. White, founder of Realization Center, has said, "We lower our standards to meet the needs of the disease." Values are compromised as far as truthfulness with others, hiding food, sneak eating, lying about what and how much, and generally behaving in ways that the food addict would not if she were not affected in a major way by what was eaten. When abstinence is achieved, these compromises fully come to light and the disparity is often astounding.

Recovery is a process—not an event. It takes time (often too much) to get to the place of raising the white flag. The problem for most addicts and food addicts especially is that we have a high tolerance for pain and suffering. The denial is powerful, the food is powerful—and the cravings are in charge; they're "driving the bus." So what is it going to take? What has to happen to make a shift?

Previous chapters have discussed and examined the nature of addiction, cravings, denial, *and* the key component of the solution—detoxing (withdrawing from sugar, sugar substitutes, flour, caffeine) and using the food plan, becoming abstinent (sober with food). But let's drill down a little further. All action (recovery from addiction) requires a first step: making a **DECISION** to do something (in this instance, change). You're reading this book because you made a decision to change.

259

When behavior becomes unacceptable and intolerable, and the pain of continuing the behavior is worse than the fear of changing it, we are moved to make a decision to change. Each of my addictions required its own individual DECISION, the process of which I share with you in the following inset.

DECISIONS, DECISIONS

I started smoking when I was fifteen years old. I became an inveterate smoker, and it progressed to four packs a day—for many years. I loved to smoke. I was soooo addicted to it. I was always smoking—even in the middle of the night, waking up to get my fix of nicotine. My brother, who had his own struggle with stopping smoking, and his family were on my case to do the same. I wanted none of it. I had no intention or desire to stop.

One day, when I was thirty-eight years old, I remember waking up, sitting on the side of the bed, and trying, unsuccessfully, to take a deep breath. I was gasping for air. At that moment, I said to myself ('cause I knew), "I have to stop smoking." I didn't stop smoking at that moment, but I had at that moment made a DECISION to stop, and I immediately sought help. I went to SMOKENDERS (see smokenders.com) and went through the program—successfully. I have (gratefully) not had a cigarette since my cut-off day of June 9, 1979.

My decision to recover from my food addiction was not so clear cut (unfortunately)—as my understanding of the recovery did not form until years after I wanted to stop my overeating. The decision I did make, however, was that my eating was out of control, and it was affecting every area of my life. The sign of an intelligent person, I was told, isn't having all the answers, it's knowing where to go for them. The same way I went to SMOKENDERS for smoking cessation, I was leveled enough by my eating that I had to find out where to go for help. So, with that decision in place, I found my own 12 Step food recovery program, and by continuing the process, my abstinence has evolved over time.

Let's examine the options for this decision to change—to become abstinent.

Compliance versus Surrender

DECISION BALANCE SHEET

To Not Change—To Continue Your Current Behavior With Food

Costs of Not Changing

Health issues:

- Malnutrition
- Diabetes
- Low blood sugar episodes (hypoglycemia) i.e., "Crashes"
- Heart disease/damage (high blood pressure, high cholesterol, stroke, heart attack)
- Low blood pressure
- Electrolyte imbalance (potassium and other electrolyte loss may eventually lead to muscle cramping and even fatal heart rhythm disturbances)
- Irritation in the mouth, esophagus, and stomach from constant exposure to stomach acid
- Tears in the stomach and esophagus
- Ruptured esophagus
- Swollen glands
- Digestive problems (heartburn, gastroesophageal reflux disease [GERD], constipation, diarrhea, stomach pain, gas, diverticulitis/diverticulosis[90], colorectal cancer[91]
- Joint problems (arthritis, stiffness)
- Osteoporosis
- Dental problems—erosion of tooth enamel, cavities, receding gums
- Weight problems (abnormal weight)

In bondage/enslavement to the addiction

Cravings (which MUST be satisfied—always on quest for a fix from an external substance or behavior)

Low or no sex drive (libido)

Headaches

Dizziness/lightheadedness

Dehydration

Inability to withstand surgery

Remain out of control

Sleep problems (waking up tired [we're supposed to wake up refreshed and energized], restlessness, poor "REM" sleep cycle)

Low energy, fatigue, extreme tiredness (lethargy)

Weakness

Low motivation (for everything) (dreams, goals, ambitions not realized)

Low enthusiasm for living

Poor brain function (focus, concentration, thought processing, memory, distorted perception of the world, decision making, poor critical judgment skills, fogginess)

Reinforces low Self-esteem, Self-respect (not feeling good enough, codependency)

Guilt, shame

Work issues

Undermines opportunity

Undermines respect

High relapse risk (for recovering alcoholics and recovering drug addicts)

Mood issues (mood swings, depression, anxiety, irritability, anger, grumpiness)

Poor access to one's creativity, talent, spirit

Spirituality issues

Relationship problems (with self-esteem issues, mood swings, irritability, health problems, one is not good relationship material—you don't even want to be in a relationship with you—and it makes it near impossible for anyone else to be in a relationship with you—even if they love you)

Tolerate the intolerable	Lack of authenticity (generated by the belief that you're not good enough)
Need to continually escape life	
Takes up time	Poor (distorted) self-image
Isolation/need to hide from one's self and others	Years off one's normal life span and sickness during one's life, especially as the food addict ages

Benefits of Not Changing

No effort/work necessary	Relieves the stress to use the food, anxiety
Familiar	Avoid problems
Instant gratification/comfort/quick fix	Forces relaxation
To get high	To feel normal
Easy	Sense of power
Not scary	Provides a feeling of control
Comfort always available	Prevents success/failure conflict
Provides security	Keeps the peace
Keeps you company	Puts off responsibility
Never leaves you	Alleviates Guilt
Remain arrogant (that nothing needs to change)	Masks unhappiness
	Provides an excuse to eat
Continue to experience the numbing of feelings/of life's challenges, repress feelings	Fit in with the crowd
	Takes up time
Continue behaviors to cope	

Remember, IF NOTHING CHANGES, NOTHING CHANGES! Let's now look at the other side of the Decision Balance Sheet.

TO CHANGE—TO BECOME ABSTINENT

Costs of Changing

Experience withdrawal symptoms from sugar, sugar substitutes and flour, volume (four a half days), and caffeine (over a month's time)	Feelings start to surface including vulnerability
	Expense (with planning, can be done on a tight budget)
Work/effort	Feelings of loss of sugar, flour, caffeine, i.e., best friend, lover, companion, energizer, boredom fixer, medication
Time (planning, shopping, preparing—more time in beginning, i.e., learning curve)	
Having to ask for help (anathema to most food addicts)	Requires discipline
	Be more responsible

Compliance versus Surrender

Being honest

Deal with problems

Giving up old beliefs, thinking & behaviors

Face reality of your past

Having to make amends

Being responsible for your own future

Reconstruct your own life

Benefits of Changing*

No cravings! Guaranteed!

Awareness of one's self, discover one's self

Realize feelings and deal with them

Quiet time enjoyed without fear of being alone

New hobbies, interesting activities

Improved health

Normalization of blood sugar levels which creates:

Increase in energy—consistent throughout day

Stable mood—even emotional keel

Improved brain function—clarity, focus, concentration, Memory, thought processing, decision making, judgment, perceptions more clear

Elimination of "crashes" during the day

Motivation increases

Weight Loss (if it was an issue)

Guilt-free eating/stable weight

Feel good

Become happy

Increased enthusiasm for living

Regain self-esteem

Self-confidence

Develop new confidence

Trust in yourself and others

Like yourself

Establish your own self-identity

Broaden horizon

Proper handling of stress

Less self-imposed pressure and procrastination, more accomplished

Learn that anxiety passes

Ability to speak up for your rights

Enjoyable and effective ways to relax

Able to celebrate life

Acceptance into the adult world

Actions not motivated by guilt

Regain respect of friends, family

Save money, health, life, marriage

Develop new friends

Available for new romances (not in the first year!)

Caring about self

Spirituality

Improved self-image

Hope returns

Lower risk for relapse (if recovering from alcohol/drugs)

Increased sex drive

Improved relationships

Open potential for new activities (achieve goals)

Enjoy the holidays

Become authentic, be one's true self; the belief about the need to be other than oneself dissipates.

Basically, all the opposites of the Costs of Not Changing.

Examining the pluses and minuses of becoming abstinent, you still have options:

1. A decision not to change (we call it "doing more research").

2. Compliance to "your rules"—*A diet, but, what the heck, I need to lose weight.*

3. True surrender.

THE MIND OF AN ADDICT

In the late 1940s and early 1950s, psychiatrist Harry Tiebout, MD, wrote three articles exploring the thoughts, behaviors, and psyche of the alcoholic.[92] His understanding and discussions give us particular insight into the mind of the addict in general and the food addict in particular. He asserts that surrender precedes acceptance. In applying Tiebout's insight to the food addict, we can see that a major characteristic of the food addict's personality is "defiant individuality" (obstinate and rebellious). The food addict who "hits bottom" because her eating behavior and failed attempts to find a solution aren't enough to stop the behavior, the food addict then makes a decision to "do something." If that "something" is recovery related—i.e., treatment, 12 Step meetings, a recovery support system (12 Step meetings, sponsorship), learning that the triggers (see list of Culprits/Triggers on page 46) are what fuels the addiction and that they have to be eliminated—the food addict can take one of two paths. She may make what appears to be complete surrender but, in truth, she is only a half-heartedly relinquishing control. In other words:

> "[S]He accepts as a practical fact that [s]he cannot at that moment conquer reality, but lurking in his [her] unconscious is the feeling 'There'll come a day'—which implies no real acceptance and demonstrates conclusively that the struggle is still on."

What the food addict at this point is experiencing is submission (superficial yielding), half-hearted acceptance, concession, resignation. According to Tiebout:

> "With each of these words there is a feeling of reservation, a tug in the direction of nonacceptance."

Compliance versus Surrender

It should be noted that no one can force themselves into acceptance. Again, according to Tiebout:

"One must have a feeling—conviction—otherwise the acceptance is not wholehearted but halfhearted with a large element of lip service."

I often see clients who, fairly early in treatment, express and demonstrate a surrender to the recovery process by accepting the food plan as the key to their recovery. They become abstinent. At that point, no one knows if the food addict is surrendering with reservations—still maintaining her "infantile ego." That state is a very young one that involves a belief in one's omnipotence. Take the case of Margaret:

Margaret came into treatment feeling defeated and powerless over her eating behavior. She was seeing a therapist and going to 12 Step meetings for codependency. She agreed to stop drinking at the beginning of treatment to address her alcohol abuse/dependence and started to be educated about the nature of her food addiction. She participated in early recovery groups for the alcohol and the food. In the beginning, she struggled to let go of the sugar/sugar substitutes and flour and in time began to follow the food plan.

Her adherence to the food plan continued for thirty-two days—she stated that she felt more energetic, slept better, had no cravings, experienced more stable mood, and noticed that she felt more confident about setting boundaries, especially with her sister (with whom she had a difficult relationship).

Margaret was attending OA meetings (which was required to be in treatment for her food addiction). One evening, she had a difficult exchange with her sister and decided to get relief the way she was accustomed to getting it in order to cope with her feelings—cake. She had not been able to regain her abstinence.

Margaret would eventually experience a true surrender—conscious and unconscious—white flag up the flag pole! She finally realized that her customary coping tool (the food) was not going to change her relationship with her sister (except probably to make it worse), and ultimately, she would be the one to suffer—like taking poison and expecting the other person to die.

When the food addict makes the transition from old eating behavior to accepting and following the food plan, a pink cloud often ensues. She feels invincible and powerful. When the inevitable emotional upheaval appears combined with an unwillingness to sit with the discomfort, the food addict reverts back to old coping behavior—using the food for comfort and relief. It is not unusual after each such episode to find it more difficult to resume following the food plan. Fortunately, recovery teaches healthier skills and coping mechanisms.

Early surrender is the sure knowledge of "I am going to be abstinent no matter what." A goal of true surrender is that when trigger situations arise, there is no thought of food to fix the problem. According to Tiebout:

"Acceptance appears to be a state of mind in which the individual accepts rather than rejects or resists....to go along with, to cooperate, to be receptive. [S]He is not argumentative, quarrelsome, irritable or contentious."

The food addict learns and accepts that the food plan is the solution to her addiction (as the alcoholic learns and accepts the alcohol plays a part in her alcoholism). The addict begins to follow the food plan and, after the four and a half days of detox/withdrawal, she experiences relief. She is "taking the First Step" *(We admitted that we were powerless over food [sugar and the sugar substitutes, flour, wheat, caffeine, volume, hard/soft cheese, high fat, high salt, and personal triggers] that our lives have become unmanageable).* At this point, the food addict is accepting that they are unable to control their eating behavior and are willing to follow a plan of eating as a solution. Likewise, the alcoholic must accept without reservation that she cannot take the first drink, that it's the first drink that gets her into trouble (wanting "more"), and then it's "off to the races." The food addict must surrender to the fact—accept—that the following are the culprits that cause her to want "more" (see Chapter 7 for the complete list):

- Alcohol/drugs (marijuana, cocaine, crack, amphetamines, crystal meth, heroin, pills, nicotine etc.)

- Sugar/sugar substitutes (which also includes gum and mints)

- Flour (bread and pasta)—*all* flour

Compliance versus Surrender

- Highly processed and refined carbohydrates
- Wheat, corn
- Caffeine
- Hard/soft cheese
- Nuts

- Volume/overeating
- Restricting/starving/purging
- High-fat, high-salt
- Skipping meals—not eating on a schedule

It's important to try to understand this part of our psyche because it's integral to whether or not we have True Recovery or relapse over and over again.

WHAT IS COMPLIANCE?

When you were growing up, were you a good kid? Did you go along with what you were asked or told to do? Most likely, you started out being "good"—that is, compliant. One definition of *compliance* is "action of obedience; yielding to the wishes of others." So when we're compliant, we're really agreeing to something we really don't want to agree to. *I agree to what you want—not what I want, and it is definitely not okay with me. (I'm telling you yes, but inside I am screaming NO!).* When we're compliant, we experience a lot of the following:

- **Pressure**—You're told, made to believe, or tell yourself that there are unwanted consequences of not cooperating, not changing your ways. You're pressured by the people and circumstances (punishment in one form or another). *(My weight—my body is larger than I want it to be—what a pain in "butt" that is! Damn, I can't eat the way I want without weighing more than I want or gaining more.)*

- **Stress**—Created by the "shoulds" and "have to's"—the eternal conflict/inconsistency between making someone else pleased (with you) and that of honoring your own wants and needs. *(I know I should go on this diet and lose weight. My blood pressure is high, my blood sugar is at a dangerous level, my knees hurt, I can't breathe, but all I really want to do is to be left alone, lie on my couch, and eat and eat . . .)*

- **Anger**—*I really don't want to do this (do what you say). I'm being made to do this. I'm being forced to go along with what you want—and*

I'm pissed—or they're pissed for having to make the effort to manipulate me or cajole me or convince me to do what they want/(I really don't want to eat differently [i.e., stop eating sugar, bread, pasta]—I'm angry that my body is making me do this because it's not the size that I want—I want to scream!)

- **Guilt**—The yes on the outside and the no on the inside make the addict feel like a fraud, a two-faced liar, a sham. This creates a conflict with one's truth—and the feelings of shame and guilt ensues. *(I'll go on this "diet" [even though you keep telling me it's not a diet, it's a food plan and the focus is recovery].)*

- **Low self-esteem**—The addict experiences an inability to stand up for herself. Compliance (going along with the program), not having a voice to say no, becomes routine and cements the belief that one is unable to speak one's truth and therefore feels "less than"—not worthwhile. *(I know I'm not going to stick with this. I've failed so many times before with diets and attempts at recovery, and I tell myself this time I'll do it and I tell others the same. I feel that I'm different—like there's something's wrong with me. Other people can do it—other people "get it.")*

- **Empty promises**—Think back to your early life: Were you promised something if you complied, and then when you did what was asked of you, you didn't get what was promised? (Food promises everything [to soothe, comfort, etc.] and delivers nothing.) *"The peanut butter calls me. It's in the cabinet saying my name in a seductive musical come-hither voice. Its smell and feel are already invading my senses. It's promising me comfort, love, friendship, activity, conversation, physical attachment—everything I need. And, as I open the lid, inhale deeply, sink my tablespoon into its smoothness, bring it to my lips, swallow it, and it SMACKS ME IN THE FACE! It's a liar, a faker and will never deliver what it promises. What emptiness, what despair . . ."*

After a while, what happens? Being compliant leaves YOU out of the mixture. *"I'm not doing this for me; I'm doing this for you and your approval."*

Defiance Follows Compliance

Then you become defiant. *Defiance* is defined as "bold opposition and resistance"—a challenge to meet in combat—"The hell with this!"—then rebellion, retaliation ensues. Defiance shows up in being closed, not being teachable, giving lip service (yeah, yeah, yeah)—not following directions, not being honest with both oneself and others.

If you are attending 12 Step food recovery fellowships (see Chapter 16: 12 Step Food Recovery Fellowships and Relapse Prevention), the following is a list of behaviors that evidence defiance/resistance. If you plan to attend (I hope that you do sooner than later), be aware of these. Remember that our behavior says more about us than any of our words.

- Not being honest about your abstinence.

- Arguing each point.

- Coming late to meetings.

- Picking people apart and what they say or don't say in a meeting.

- Not giving out your phone number.

- Not getting any recovery literature.

- Not allowing anyone to know what you are doing.

- Focusing *only* on people who are *not* making it—being judgmental/critical.

- Giving lip service.

- Not saying what you feel or think.

- Setting yourself apart—being different from *those* people. You probably do this unconsciously by comparing yourself to others. When we do this, we lose! Because when we compare, we are either better than or less than others. This separates us (and makes us miserable). The healthier mindset is to try to relate to or identify with others—this allows us to connect—to be a part of instead of being apart from. There's a wonderful slogan in the 12 Step meetings: **Compare and Despair!**

And since a diet is about compliance, did you become resentful—angry, and if you experienced weight loss, complacent? Compliance is really a short-term Band-Aid for a long-term problem. So what is the answer? What is the needed internal position for all this battle to stop? It's SURRENDER.

SURRENDER IS THE ANSWER

To give up—to put up the white flag—to say that "my way doesn't work"—just tell me what to do. To give over entirely.

Surrender is for myself, not for you. Compliance is for the outside; surrender is for the inside. It comes from me and even though it is hard, it is okay with me. It's my decision. My disease tells me to be angry at giving up my substances and wants to find a way for me to become defiant. My surrender allows me to tell someone when these feelings begin because it is me who voluntarily wants be abstinent. When you give up, it is for you—your decision.

Even though you may still want to eat sugar, sweeteners, flour, caffeine, excess food, etc., or starve or purge, it has become okay with you that you don't. When you're not eating those trigger foods, and you're in compliance/not surrendered—that's "white knuckle" abstinence (in other words, you're sitting on your hands and clenching your teeth!).

Abstinence is number one when you really believe you are powerless.

- The struggle (the decision) is over.

- You experience release from the conflict.

- Your attitudes toward what you need to do to stay abstinent change.

- Your willingness will change and you will allow help.

Surrender is a very personal experience. It's a shift in one's being. It's the addict saying, "I've had enough—I'm done—I will go to any length to be free—I will do whatever I have to do." The experience is one of a real "psychic change."

You will begin to experience the beginning of freedom from bondage. It will be okay with you to use whatever tools are necessary to follow the food plan, or not purge or starve because it is now okay with you if they work.

FOOD PLAN (ABSTINENCE) VERSUS DIET (COMPLIANCE)

Upon first view of the food plan, one can unarguably say it is a diet. True, it looks like a diet (with permitted foods, specific portions, rules, written on a piece of paper, etc.) in the typical sense we're used to understanding the meaning of "diet", i.e., for weight loss (dictionary: n. a regulated selection of foods, as for medical reasons or cosmetic weight loss; adj. of or relating to a food regimen designed to promote weight loss). Diets, though, are a perfect example of compliance. *I'm going on a diet to lose weight for:*

- Fitting in; to look like others
- The beach (bathing suit or summer clothes in general)
- The wedding, party, celebration, conference, big dinner
- The vacation/trip
- My job/career
- My family—spouse, children

- My diabetes
- My liver, heart
- My legs, my knees
- My doctor
- My therapist, treatment program
- To get a date, relationship

But *not voluntarily* for myself.

In compliance, what you are really saying is, "I'm going along with you, but I have conditions and reservations, and I have a silent contract that you don't know about. If I am doing this (staying away from my substance) for my family, job, boss, etc., and they disappoint me or I get mad at them, I no longer have a reason to go back. I had reservations in the first place. I was just complying." When you are doing it only for compliance, you are also thinking that when you lose the weight, you can eat as you want. Or, after a time on the diet, either you begin to lose weight and think, *That's enough* or *Ugh! This is too hard, uncomfortable, takes too much work.* Or you're not able to get past the first four and a half days of the detox/withdrawal process.

You need to ask yourself: *Why do I want to stop the out-of-control eating?*

Intention, purpose, desire, pain (from the overeating, overeating/purging), hopelessness, defiance, resistance, and grandiosity—they all figure into this process of compliance, surrender, acceptance.

Okay, so why are you reading this book? If you're not reading it for professional purposes or to help out a family member, I would think you're reading this book to find an answer to your inability to control your eating, your inability to will yourself into eating the way you want. You've probably read other books on diets and weight loss and have been told to "stop the insanity (of crazy eating)," listen to your body, stop when you're full, lose weight forever, recover from "eating disorders," etc. My assumption is that you're in a lot of pain (or call it frustration, despair, shame, or hopelessness). You haven't been able to stop your eating behavior, even though you now want to, maybe more than anything else. You feel you're at the end; you're ready to do anything. So, you are offered this solution (idea of addiction, food plan, and need for recovery), it makes sense to you and you buy into it (as a start). You want to try this. You're committed. Let's look at two scenarios:

Scenario 1

You say to yourself, *Let me try this "food plan"—I'm willing to try to let go of sugar/sugar substitutes, flour (bread and pasta) as is described (I'll deal with the coffee later). I don't need any help with this. I've been on other diets and have been successful (in the short term). I've lost weight before—so I know how to do this.*

So what happens? Let's say you're able to push through the withdrawal stage—those four and a half days—and you make it through the first week. The food plan is working: you begin to feel fewer cravings, more energy, and clearer thinking, and your clothes feel looser in the second week. The food plan becomes more workable—a little easier. You start to feel hopeful (and powerful).

Scenario 2

Let's say you start the process (i.e., you begin the food plan, maybe you look up FAA or OA meetings, and maybe you begin to go). You start to feel inspired, hopeful. All that's promised is starting to happen. In a week's time, you start to feel better, more energy, cravings are gone (after the first four and a half days), and maybe in another week clothes feel a little looser. The food plan is becoming more familiar, a little less scary. Another week or so passes. You start feeling proud of yourself. Let's say you do go to an FAA or OA meeting—and you hear and identify with

Compliance versus Surrender

273

others who share their stories and struggles, and maybe you begin to share. You feel that you've found the answer. And the clothes get even looser. And the scale (you can't resist staying off the scale) shows lower numbers. *Hey, this way of eating is okay—it's working.* And you say to yourself, *I can do this. I don't think I need these meetings. I just can follow this plan.*

In both scenarios, you may also begin thinking, *I don't have to be so "strict"—I can have some of those foods they say have to be eliminated. I can have a cookie, a piece of cake, a candy bar, one slice of toast, croutons on my salad, an extra piece of fruit, a second helping, etc.* Bingo! This is the disease starting to assert itself, the creeping in of the addict's "defiant individuality and grandiosity," which Harry Tiebout says may very well explain why the addict is typically resistant to the point of being unreasonable and stubborn about seeking help or being able to accept help even when she seeks it. Defiance and grandiosity operate on the unconscious level, and they are powerful influences against surrender.

What happens with the food addict who initially appears to have surrendered but, in fact, is just going along with the food plan (as a diet), being "compliant" with the rules. As the food addict begins to feel better—maybe some weight loss, the food addict starts to become annoyed and resentful—*This is too hard, it takes too much time, why do I have to do this, I can change the "rules" and do it my way.* Defiance says, "It's not true that I can't manage my eating, and grandiosity says there is nothing I cannot master and control" (even though the whole history of the food addict has proven again and again her inability to control and manage her eating behavior). So slowly and gradually, after a time of the food addict looking as if she has let go and settled into recovery, as stated by Harry Tiebout:

> "The memory of his/her own acute period of anxiety and pain and hopelessness is swallowed up by the defiance and grandiosity. Thus, the addict loses the effectiveness of the anxiety as a stimulus to create suffering and a desire for change. This cycle will go on repeating itself as long as the defiance and the grandiosity continue to function with unimpaired vigor."[93]

As long as the food addict uses the food plan as a diet, she is in compliance. In other words, say Tiebout:

"Accepts reality consciously, but not unconsciously. He or she accepts as a practical fact that he or she cannot at that moment lick reality, but lurking in the unconscious is the feeling, there'll come a day (when I can eat as I want), which implies no real acceptance and demonstrates conclusively that the struggle is still on. With compliance, which at best is a superficial yielding, tension continues."[94]

According to Tiebout, surrender precedes acceptance. Unless food addicts accept that they have an illness (a disease over which they truly have no power), that they *can't handle* their eating (which has been proven and demonstrated too many times to count), and that they must settle into a way of eating that does not trigger their overeating/undereating behavior, they will never find True Recovery: peace and freedom.

The first step of all 12 Step programs states this idea—that addicts admit their powerlessness over their behavior. I would like to believe that implicit in the word "admit" is this idea that surrender leads to acceptance. Maybe when the founders of AA developed the first step, a better word choice would have been "We *surrendered* to our powerlessness over . . . or *accepted* that we are powerless over . . ." As Tiebout states:

"Many an AA meeting has been devoted to quibbling about the difference between admit and accept. Time and again slips are explained on the basis that the one who slips has not truly accepted his alcoholism."[95]

This first step is seen as the one that lays the foundation for recovery. It is the one that requires the (food) addict to stop the behavior—to put down the substances (i.e., sugar, sweeteners, flour, wheat, caffeine, volume, hard/soft cheese, nuts, excess fat/salt for the food addict; alcohol for the alcoholic; drugs for the drug addict). It's the only step that must be done perfectly. Whenever the 12 Step literature mentions the concept "progress, not perfection," it is referring to Steps Two through Twelve— never Step One. As Tiebout states:

"When an individual surrenders, the ability to accept reality functions on the unconscious level, and there is no residual battle; relaxation with freedom from strain and conflict ensues. In fact, it is perfectly possible

Compliance versus Surrender

275

to ascertain how much acceptance of reality is on the unconscious level by the degree of relaxation that develops. The greater the relaxation, the greater the inner acceptance of reality."[96]

For the food addict, that means following the "directions" that will achieve abstinence. Those directions involve attending 12 Step meetings (FAA, OA, CEA-HOW armed with this food plan), finding someone to be a food sponsor, and "turning over" her food daily to the sponsor.

As a rule, food addicts tend to shift into "diet mentality" using the food plan as a diet, rather than turning over their food and honoring their commitment in terms of what foods they committed to, the amounts, and the times (all of which are critical to live in abstinence—a day at a time). Evidence of "diet mentality" is seen when the food addict is not eating everything committed to and minimizing this "because I won't be gaining weight." Or eating too much and thinking it's okay because it's "abstinent food." Equally as dangerous, however, is to get preoccupied with abstinence and forget about working the steps. According to Tiebout:

"Surrender can be viewed as a moment when the unconscious forces of defiance and grandiosity actually cease to function effectively. When this happens, the food addict is wide open to reality; he or she can listen and learn without conflict and fighting back. He or she is receptive to life, not antagonistic. The food addict senses a feeling of relatedness and at-oneness that becomes the source of an inner peace and serenity, the possession of which frees the individual from fighting the food plan. In other words, the act of surrender is an occasion wherein the individual no longer fights life, but accepts it."

Moving from understanding an "act of surrender" to examining the emotional "state of surrender"—which can be defined as a state in which there is a persisting capacity to accept reality—Tiebout further says:

"There is no sense of 'must'; nor is there any sense of fatalism. With true unconscious surrender, the acceptance of reality means the individual can work in it and with it. The state of surrender is really positive and creative."[97]

So, the final question is: *Do I have a disease (food addiction) or a weight problem?*

If you focus on the weight, you will lose the recovery. If you focus on the recovery, you will lose the weight!

Let's assume you're beginning to make changes: maybe beginning with "the breakfast" set forth in the food plan in Chapter 11, or maybe you've taken on the entire mission. Let's look at how you're doing this—is it as a diet or have you embraced it as a plan of eating for your life? Review "Diet versus Realization Center True Recovery Food Plan" on page 279.

If you follow the food plan without following a food recovery program and creating a food recovery support system for yourself, you will have made the food plan into a diet—with the resultant consequences—and it will eventually go the way of all diets: failure.

An article in an old edition of the *Grapevine* magazine (published by Overeaters Anonymous) (date unknown) titled "What's the Difference between Dieting and Abstinence" states the following:

"Dieting is going through a day obsessed with eating as little as possible without actually losing consciousness (dizziness is OK). Abstinence is eating 3 nourishing meals a day [and a Metabolic Adjustment], with life in between."

"Dieting is having a goal weight, a goal day, clenched fists and gritted teeth. Abstinence is accepting powerlessness over food, relaxing and giving up the fight."

"Dieting is scaring myself so I'll look good at my high school reunion. Abstinence is accepting and liking myself just as I am today, and realizing that my worth does not hinge on the size of my body."

"Dieting is life-threatening. Abstinence is life-giving."

"A diet is something you start on Monday and go off on Thursday. Abstinence is an ongoing daily reprieve from the disease of compulsive overeating."

"Dieting is placing all the emphasis on food, which must be controlled in order to solve the problem, which is believed to be fat. Abstinence is knowing that fat is not the problem but only a symptom of an illness called compulsive overeating [food addiction], and that the solution lies not in trying to control the food but in practicing the twelve steps."

"Dieting is rigidly adhering to 700 calories a day because my boyfriend said he would marry me at 115 pounds. Abstaining is knowing that the jerk should be so lucky to marry me at 315 pounds, and telling him so!"

Compliance versus Surrender

"Dieting is being obsessed with calories, carbohydrates and charts, always jumping on the scale to monitor my weight. Abstinence is letting go and letting God, just following a simple food plan one day at a time and trusting the results to my higher power."

The diet industry is an industry that is dependent on the failure of its products/services. It's the only industry that thrives on failure of its customers. How ironic is that? And it's dependent on the support of the medical establishment and the media proclaiming and focusing on the symptom (overweight) and not the cause (food addiction)! Weight Watchers, Jenny Craig, NutriSlim, Optifast, SlimFast, the shakes promoted on TV and in magazines, and all the diet pills and pill pushers are the manifestation of the collective denial about the truth of the problem—that it's not the weight but rather what's causing the overweight: food addiction.

The following story "I Am Not a Duck" is a clever analogy about. . . . no, let's see if you can guess what it's about.

I AM NOT A DUCK
BY JOHN FOSTER

I may look like a duck and walk like a duck and quack like a duck and drink like a duck . . .

But I am not a duck. I'm an eagle in disguise.

If you could prove to me that it's respectable to be a duck, I might consider being one. But don't waste your time—my mind is made up.

I think it's shameful to be a duck. I won't be a duck.

It's so lonely here among all these ducks. I'm so out of place here.

But for some reason, none of the other eagles will have anything to do with me.

Why are eagles so cruel?

Some of the ducks are quite nice. It's too bad I'm an eagle.

No, it isn't! I'm glad I'm an eagle.

Even if I WERE a duck, I wouldn't stay a duck. I'd become an eagle.

I can be anything I want to be and I owe it to myself to be an eagle.

Ducks are terrible. I HATE ducks.

I keep trying to swoop down and grab a rabbit in my claws. But I can't do it.

I have webbed feet.

> It's all GOD's fault. Why would he make an eagle with webbed feet?
>
> If I starve to death, God will have only himself to blame.
>
> I do my part—why doesn't he do his?
>
> The ducks all want to help me. But how can they? What does a duck know about an eagle's problems?
>
> Why can't they mind their own business?
>
> Why don't the eagles offer to help? Someday I'll get even with those eagles. I HATE them!
>
> I'm beginning to like ducks better than I do eagles.
>
> Being an eagle is killing me.
>
> >Not being a duck is killing me.
>
> I don't know what's killing me.
>
> I just know I'm dying.
>
> >Help me, God.
>
> >God, help me.
>
> Guess what, God!
>
> >I am a duck…whether I like it or not…I'm a duck.
>
> Why didn't you tell me?
>
> I've forgotten how to act.
>
> >Show me, God, how to be a duck.
>
> >Help me.
>
> Help me be a good duck.
>
> Ducks are the best people in the world.
>
> >I love ducks.
>
> >I'm grateful to be a duck.

What does this story mean to you? It's an interesting and clever metaphor about the process of acceptance. Where are you with regard to food? Are you still trying to be an eagle ("normal" with food; see page 203), or do you accept that you're a "duck" (i.e., food addict)?

In *Healing the Shame That Binds You*, John Bradshaw says:

"For the most part diets are the greatest hoax ever perpetrated on a suffering group of people. Ninety-five percent of the people who diet gain the weight back within five years. Diets underscore one of the most paradoxical aspects of toxic shame [Ed. note: see discussion on self-esteem in Chapter 14: Self-Esteem and Family Systems]. In dieting and losing weight, one has the sense of controlling and fixing the problem....Control is one of the major strategies of cover-up for shame. All the layers of cover-up are attempts to control the outside so that the inside will not be exposed."[98]

Control, though, is an illusion; it's white-knuckling. Eventually, that illusion is shattered and old behavior surfaces and then the search is on for the next diet, and the next, and the next . . . This perpetuates the belief that "I am defective, I am deficient, something's wrong with me," when the real issue is that a "diet" is never the solution. This "diet failure" continues the core of shame.

What is the distinction between a diet and a food plan? Let's look at the differences:

TABLE 12.1. DIET VERSUS REALIZATION CENTER TRUE RECOVERY FOOD PLAN		
	Diet	**Food Plan**
Purpose	Weight loss	Normalize blood sugar levels Eliminate cravings, develop healthy eating patterns for life Although the normalization of weight is one of the benefits of this food plan, it is not the entire focus; it is integrated into a larger scope, i.e., True Recovery.
Basis	That weight is the problem.	The food addiction is the problem.
Concept	Restrictive in nature—often neglects long-term nutritional needs/problems Calorie counting, calorie restriction, "points," "exchanges"	Healthy way of eating—nutritionally sound (once started can last a lifetime)
Term	Short term (not meant to last—when weight loss is accomplished, okay to return to old way of eating—understood to be a short-term answer to a long-term problem, i.e., food addiction)	Lifetime—one day at a time

| Focus | Symptom centered on weight and weight loss* Does not take into consideration those foods an individual is addicted to or triggered by Many diets permit periods where one can use the addictive substances and use "free foods" or reward with snacks of the very foods one is addicted to. Not for the food addict who has a progressive disease. Is not integrated in any kind of social or psychological aspects of the individual's life. Does not address trigger situations Limited kind of enterprise

In actuality, when a person is eating in a way that normalizes their blood sugar (the food plan), the body finds its true weight. The body is very smart and wants to be at the appropriate weight. We have become the obstacle to that by our distorted beliefs about what we should look like and weigh. | Eliminates those foods the food addict is both addicted to and triggered by (alcohol, sugar/sugar subs, flour, wheat, caffeine, volume, hard/soft cheese, excess fat/salt, personal trigger foods); recognizes the relationship between specific foods and the addictive process and requires the person to remain abstinent from these foods. (These foods are not necessary for maintenance and they are not healthy foods.) There are **no negative health consequences** by adhering to the food plan set forth in Chapter 11. Will integrate into the overall life of the individual. It addresses more than just a short-term problem with a limited perspective. It helps the individual eat differently and eventually takes the focus off the food—(initially, however, the focus is on the food—learning selections, portion sizes, etc.) Centered on the disease—integral part of one's overall recovery process. Recognizes that any major change, including symptom change—of weight loss—is going to take a long period of time and any excessive claims for progress will promote disappointment and failure. Becomes integrative and addresses specific issues in the individual's recovery Will lower cost of expenditures for doctors and hospital visits/insurance rates. Even though we speak of recovery on a "one day at a time" basis, it also takes place within the context of the intention to stay in recovery forever.[99] |
|---|---|---|
| Claim | Instant results or instant gratification; promise to be easy—e.g., eat all you want and lose 20 pounds in two weeks; It's magic! (does not look at long-term necessity for hard work; promise results that they cannot deliver); tends to be gimmicky | Eliminates (not just satisfies) cravings (after the first four and a half days that it takes the body to cycle out the addictive foods). By normalizing blood sugar levels, the food plan allows the individual to experience stabilization of mood, optimization of energy, brain function (focus, concentration, thought processing, memory, perception of the world, decision making, judgment), normalization of sleep, digestion, weight, allows the addict to experience all the promises of True Recovery—in full measure. |

Compliance versus Surrender

Consequences	Most often the temporary weight loss experienced from restriction and dieting very predictably does not last. (See "Weight Cycling" on page 281.)	None

WEIGHT CYCLING

Study after study has confirmed that 95 percent of people who follow organized weight-loss programs subsequently gain back almost all of the weight they lose and oftentimes more. The person is likely then to ricochet out of the restriction phase and begin binge eating. This bingeing can lead to weight gain over time. The "serial dieter" repeatedly goes from restriction to bingeing, and overtime may gain more and more weight. This cycle is called weight cycling and can lead to very serious medical, physical, and emotional consequences.

Effects of weight cycling include:

- Increased inflammation

- Damage to heart and cardiovascular system

- Reduces muscle mass and increases risk of hip fractures

- Increases risk of gallstones

- May cause DNA damage or abnormal cell changes in breast tissue

- May increase risk of hysterectomy

- Causes physical weakness

- May alter tryptophan levels and effect serotonin function, and ironically, increase impulsivity and depression

Comments: Going on a diet is like the alcoholic going on the wagon—they attempt to quit, slow down, or control their intake over a brief period of time. There is a big difference between going on the wagon and getting into recovery.

You may know the yo-yo pattern that many overweight women follow as they make the rounds of Weight Watchers, Optifast and Nutrisystem: they lose weight, remain in craving, fight their hunger, become irritable and socially isolated, snap at their children or other family members, become even more sedentary and "fall off the wagon" and gain weight (even more than when they started) again.

"Dieting" is a euphemism for starvation. The consequences of food deprivation are always the same, whether the deprivation is voluntary or not. Among the most common of these consequences are depression, obsession with food, and chronically, overeating and weight gain.

Many of these symptoms, particularly depression and preoccupation with food, are misinterpreted as psychological rather than metabolic by physicians, psychotherapists, and the dieting victims themselves. The real problem—the malnutrition—goes untreated.

Most dieters alternate overeating and starving. All chronically skip meals, particularly breakfast, and undereat whenever possible. Rebound cravings and overeating escalate along with weight gain. Slow metabolism, a classic feature of malnutrition, leads to further weight gain. "Diet foods," typically containing large doses of caffeine and NutraSweet, are now known to increase bloating, carbohydrate craving, depression, and weight gain while further depleting vital nutrients.

CHAPTER 13

The Language of Feelings and Food Addiction

"We use food to say what is not being said in words and wanting what can only be provided by another person."
—MARCIA BODENSTEIN

Those of us who use food to deal with feelings lose the ability to regulate how we feel and our ability to maintain healthy ways of resolving problems. Overeating, restricting, and eating and purging often lead to feelings of shame, guilt, and hopelessness. To reduce the impact of these feelings, people often eat, restrict, and purge more, thus creating a never-ending cycle of distress. In this chapter, I'll discuss feelings and the language of feelings, but first, let's take a look at why the food addict "uses" food by overeating, overeating and purging, or starving.

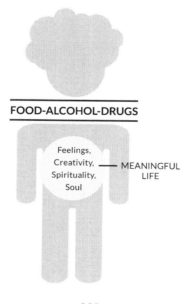

REASONS FOR "USING" FOOD

When I talk about using food, I mean "using" in the sense of using an addictive substance. What would be *your* reasons for "using" food? Stop for a moment, before you read further, and think about what drives you to eat when you're not hungry and/or what drives you to purge the food you've eaten. What drives you to not eat, to postpone meals maybe indefinitely? Perhaps you're not aware of the reason because it is in response to a physical craving that's been triggered by a "culprit" or, as your blood sugar may be crashing, the craving shows up and takes charge of your behavior. Remember, once you're in craving, obsession takes over, then compulsion, and then you have lost control and act out on your compulsion—in other words, all bets are off!

Here, however, I want to examine the emotional aspect of our addictive eating behavior. Eating behaviors (overeating, undereating, and purging) are an easy go-to to deal with emotional issues, but what has happened to many of us is that what was the "solution" of the food became the "problem," if we bring to it our vulnerable biology, i.e., our genetic vulnerability.

As discussed in Chapter 3 and discussed later in Chapters 14 and 15, most food addicts don't have a firm foundation established for the development of healthy coping mechanisms. Whether consciously or not, when people cannot cope in a healthy way, they most often develop adaptive measures, the purpose of which is to make them feel whole, safe, secure, and in control. Those of us who use food (e.g., bingeing, purging, restricting, weight loss, eating rituals) to cope with other problems and to either avoid or meet emotional needs lose the opportunity to discover ourselves and grow and mature.

The following list of reasons for "using" food has been developed over many years of lecturing with clients who offered their reasons. Many of these can be seen in terms of "needs."

- For comfort or soothing
- For relief; to release tension
- For distraction; to create drama or excitement
- To feel powerful or express autonomy
- To feel in control
- To get rid of feelings; to avoid, annihilate, obliterate, regulate, numb, stuff, anesthetize,

The Language of Feelings and Food Addiction

extinguish, suppress, paralyze, bury, deaden, kill, sedate, medicate, or push down feelings of boredom, loneliness, anxiety, depression, hurt, disappointment, guilt, deprivation, fear, anger, loss, etc.

➤ As a safeguard against anxiety

➤ To sleep, which is an effective anesthesia

- To connect; for company

- To disconnect, dissociate

- To feel safe, to insulate, or to reduce anxiety, including:

  ➤ To dissociate from intrusive thoughts, feelings, and images

  ➤ To attempt to "disappear" (as with anorexia)

  ➤ To create a large body for protection

  ➤ To create small body for protection

- For nurturing

- To hide

- To isolate

- To fill the void, the emptiness; to feel complete, whole

- To get high

- To take revenge or to punish

- To celebrate

- To reward, relax

- To protect against unmourned losses and issues

- As an expression of or discharge of feelings, i.e. anger, rage, pain, guilt, shame, rebellion

- To avoid or encourage feelings of deprivation

- To avoid intimacy

- To avoid risk-taking

- For fear of failure or success, confrontation, or responsibility

- As a replacement for relationships

- Behaviors and resulting consequences are evidence for self-blame ("I am bad") instead of the blaming of abusers

I'm sure you can add your own reasons and descriptions to this list. The following sections examine some of these in more depth.

For Comfort and Relief, and to Release Tension

This one works well at the end of the day (and it most likely is not a conscious decision or rationalization/justification): *Oh, what a day this was! I was so stressed! I need/I have to have/I deserve (fill in the blank).* From a very young age, we are given food to ease a discomfort. If we fell down or got hurt, we got a cookie, candy, or a meal, which told us that it's okay to use the food to get soothing. And, of course, the food works to soothe us. As a child, we went to the doctor for an injection and what did he give us? A lollypop! And forty years later, we're sitting in front of him and he's telling us to lose weight, that we have heart disease, cholesterol issues, insulin resistance—what a sad joke! How ironic. At many turns in our early years, we got the connection: food for comfort, relief! One client stated, "If I don't purge, I'm anxious and distracted. After I purge, I can calm down and get things done."

In a letter on Twitter commenting on the premature death of jazz singer Amy Winehouse, her friend Russell Brand wrote:

> All addicts, regardless of the substance or their social status, share a consistent and obvious symptom; they're not quite present when you talk to them. They communicate to you through a barely discernible but unignorable evil.
> .... They have about them the air of elsewhere, that they're looking through you to somewhere else they'd rather be. And of course they are. The priority of any addict is to anaesthetize the pain of living to ease the passage of the day with some purchased relief.

As a Distraction

The food addict says (consciously or unconsciously): *I'm too uncomfortable with being with myself, being aware of myself, my thoughts, my sadness, my guilt, nervousness, fear, my need to focus and concentrate. Let me eat something or, if not, think about eating something.*

So, back in the doctor's office, he may have told us if we were good and brave and not cry, we would *get* a lollypop to distract us from feeling the fear or pain of the shot. As so clearly stated by Rebecca Cooper in *Recovery Today,* "We focused on getting the lollypop instead of feeling the fear or pain of the needle. We effectively blocked the pain and focused on the reward, the sugar. Is it any wonder that later in life when we

The Language of Feelings and Food Addiction

experience pain, emotional or physical, that we think of a candy bar to make us feel better?"[100]

For Power or Control

Did you ever skip lunch? You felt hungry, but you told yourself, *No I'm not going to give into my hunger. I'm too busy. I'm on a roll (with whatever project or focus), and I don't want to stop. I'm too angry, I'm too (fill in the blank).* Do you remember how you felt? Powerful? In control? It is a powerful feeling to override your need to eat, and maybe you can override your other needs, too?

As for purging (i.e., vomiting, laxatives, enemas, restricting, over-exercising), that feeling of being clean and empty can be very euphoric and gives rise to feeling amazingly powerful and feeling as if you could erase, by magic, the consequences of the loss of control (i.e., overeating/bingeing).

Unfortunately, in all of the hard work and effort to be in control, food addicts are always on the verge of feeling out of control. The "out-of-control" monster is always breathing down their necks and will, without the protection of the addiction, get them.

Food addicts believe they have to constantly exert more effort to be in control, follow more rigid rules to keep the control, and put up more rigid walls and defenses to protect themselves from potential experiences that will make them feel vulnerable, stupid, or powerless. Unfortunately, the consequence of this kind of pursuit is a deep sense of loneliness, which leads to more self-contempt, which indirectly feeds the addiction.

To Get Rid of Feelings

Since food (eating, not eating, eating and purging) is a mood changer—that's what's being accomplished: the changing or stuffing or medicating or anesthetizing or sedating or deadening feelings. So if you were furious at your friend, family, an abuser (or anyone), a dish of ice cream or a doughnut or chips will succeed in pushing away (actually pushing down) the anger.

From a very early age, most of us experience getting food (most often candy, cake, ice cream, etc.) to ameliorate a hurt or to quell a strong feeling, the message being, "You shouldn't feel that feeling! Here's something

The Big Book of True Recovery from Food Addiction and Beyond

to eat. Get rid of or stuff that feeling with food." We learned early on that food can deaden our feelings. Our parents or caregiver "used" the food for the same purpose, so they passed on the "use" (the addictive behavior) of the substance to us.

What about that very early feeling of disappointment? Restricting can be an expression of and defense against early childhood needs and feelings like, *It's too scary to need anything, I try not to even need food.* According to writer and columnist Caroline Knapp, who struggled with addiction:

> "Starving becomes a solution to a wide variety of conflicts and fears, or at least it starts out resembling a solution: Something feels perversely good, or right, or gratifying about it, some key seems to slide into place, some distress assuaged, and the benefits of this are strong enough to outweigh whatever negative or painful feelings are aroused, such as shame, confusion, or physical hunger."[101]

In her book *Appetites,* Knapp goes on to describe bingeing, wherein the endlessly, daunting business of defining oneself—naming one's needs, speaking up for oneself, tolerating pain and frustration and disappoint-ment—simply grinding to a halt in the narcotizing stupor of a binge, all anxiety focused on the procuring of food, then eased, briefly, but power-fully in its consumption.

Think for a moment; what do you recall regarding the "use" of food in your childhood home to relieve feelings? Did your mother or grand-mother give you something to eat to make you *feel* better, *feel* different, or *not feel*? That's the goal: to obliterate any feeling and replace it with the "pleasure" of food.

To Connect

A major need for all of us is to connect with another person—to have a heart connection. Whether or not we deny it, we need to feel that we are known, heard, and understood and that we belong—you know, heart to heart. Since most of us (that is, "food people") have trust issues as a result of our trust having been broken way back, we look to the food for that fulfillment of the need of connection. And the food works.

To Disconnect and Dissociate

On the other hand, there are those times we need to "pull the plug." Life is too much, people are too much, work, the world, my caretaking—too, too much! So, going to bed with "Ben and Jerry" or "Little Debbie" becomes a perfectly reasonable solution.

The idea of "dissociation" is an extreme form of disconnection. We often think of dissociation as the response of a sexually abused child who, in defense against the horrendous act, emotionally splits off from himself or herself and mentally separates from his or her body. We also can use eating behaviors as a powerful tool to create and maintain separation from interpersonal issues and as a means for a person to dissociate from intrapsychic (occurring within the mind) conflicts.

What about the times that you have gone to the movies? After buying your ticket, you stop by the candy counter and buy the industrial-size popcorn and soda. The excitement and anticipation is building. You go into the theater and make your way down the aisle to a row with an empty seat, moving over people and being *very* careful not to spill the popcorn or soda because they are valuable treasures. You settle into the seat and carefully arrange yourself again, being very careful not to spill the precious treasures. The lights get dim and then go out, and the trailers or movie begins. And you start the hand-to-mouth movement from the box and the cup. You're eating and drinking—and it taste oh so good! And you are not alone; you are surrounded by a group of people, albeit strangers, laughing together, fearful together, sharing the same feelings. You are not alone. Now you're in a trance and disconnected from yourself. Or do you accomplish the same sate just staying home, lying on your couch with food for company and watching TV?

To Feel Safe or Insulated

Eating to feel safe or insulated include the following reasons:

- To dissociate from intrusive thoughts, feelings, and images
- To attempt to "disappear" (as with anorexia)
- To create large body for protection
- To create small body for protection

How often have you looked to eat something when you were frightened? It's probably automatic and you probably don't even know you feel unsafe. The overriding "feeling" is, "I'm hungry," and eating or not eating to feel safe works for the moment.

When there is sexual abuse, frequently the body, sexuality, and gender (masculinity and femininity) become the enemy. The survivor may think, *I was abused because of my femaleness, my attractiveness, my genitals, my breasts* . . . Similarly, a distorted survival strategy is to make the body unattractive to keep abuse away. Intrusive trauma memories can be displaced by food and/or weight obsession and provide an internal structure of dissociative states or aspects of the self.

In his 2002 book *The Heart of Addiction*, Lance Dodes, a Harvard trained psychiatrist, offered the idea that addiction is displacement, i.e., that the addictive act is a substitute response to unacceptable feelings of powerlessness and shame that arise in situations that have personal meaning for the addict. The addict perceives that directly facing the cause of these intolerable feelings is not permissible, and she resorts to the addictive act to repair the feeling of powerlessness and restore her sense of having control over her life.

To Nurture

We think of nurturing as feeling soothed, supported, cared about. The dictionary definition of "nurture" is: 1) To feed and protect; to nurture one's offspring, 2) to support and encourage as during the period of training or development, and 3) to bring up; train; educate. Even though the definition includes "feeding," I think the implication is more about feeling loved and cared about, not about "using" food. We have lost the distinction between "nurture" and "nourish"—they do not have the same meaning.

Often, when I'm going to a diner for dinner, as I'm led to my seat, I always look to see what everyone is eating (a hazard of my profession). When I see a man alone, what do you think he's eating? Often I see meatloaf, mashed potatoes, gravy, peas (maybe)—a comforting, nurturing "mommy meal."

Eating is a ritual that some families frequently use to signify, "We are loving and caring parents because we provide for our children and we sit at the table as a family." This nourishing with food can easily be

The Language of Feelings and Food Addiction

pointed to as proof to the unloved child or the parent that the family is a loving one. Thus, food comes to represent a substitute for affection: "I know I have love if I'm fed." Such parents can also use food to mask an incapacity for genuine affection. This dynamic also creates the obstacle to food addiction recovery because it requires the food addict to "leave home." (See the further discussion in Chapter 16: 12 Step Food Recovery Fellowships and Relapse Prevention.)

To Hide or Isolate

Food can serve as company when the food addict wants to retreat from the world. Since trust is an issue, isolation becomes the safe state to live within (see to the fortress illustration in Chapter 3: Little Food Addict in Training on page 138). Isolation is a major problem for most food addicts. The food makes the loneliness that isolation brings not just tolerable, but enjoyable, so loneliness is not really experienced. But think about it: without the food, the isolation is potentially a big, black cavernous hole.

To Fill the Void, the Emptiness

Food addicts typically experience a big empty space inside. (I often ask clients to describe it: How big? What shape? What color?) It starts very early when those developmental dependency needs are partially met or not met at all—again, back to those most important needs of being listened to, heard, understood, and taken seriously. If they were mostly ignored, then the emptiness started and grew. How many times have you tried to fill this hole with food? When do you do it? At night when there's less distractions? Does it ever fill the hole? Do you ever feel whole or complete? Definitely not. But we go back again and again to try. It's automatic.

To Get High

Overeating or undereating, eating and purging, or not eating are all mood changers. All that sugar and sugar substitutes, flour, soft/hard cheese, volume, and caffeine affect brain chemistry in the same way that alcohol does.

Have you ever "passed out" from overeating? Maybe you don't think of it as passing out, but rather as being so exhausted from all the sugar, etc., or being so stuffed that you just went to sleep. That's passing out.

Restricting or starving and purging also affect brain chemistry by triggering the production of endorphins, which are opioid peptides that function as neurotransmitters (brain chemicals) that allow us to experience pleasure or reward.

How about those energy drinks? All that sugar or sugar substitute and caffeine, and then the rush, with explosive energy, laser focus, raciness, the rush—wow! (I loved this feeling.) And then the crash—the exhaustion, irritability, crankiness, lightheadedness, headache, nervousness, maybe an anxiety attack with heart palpitations, a fogginess, lack of focus, inability to concentrate, loss of memory, and nausea—*Oh well, guess I better get another one.*

For Revenge or to Punish

Eating for revenge or to punish is not even a conscious thought—it's just a knee-jerk reaction. Because of her history, the addict is unwilling or unable to confront another person directly with her difficult feelings, such as anger, disappointment, and hurt so she turn these on herself: *I'm so angry, I want to tear their ears off their head! I'm so angry because someone is controlling, is yelling at me, and I can't get a word in! I've lost my power. I'm not being heard. What can I eat? I have to have something! Let it begin.* If the addict is a bulimic, she might also think, *I'll then vomit my guts out (symbolically, my anger) out,* or, *I'm so angry, I won't eat.* This makes perfect sense to a food addict.

To Celebrate or Reward

Most likely, food was used in your family—by everyone—as a reward. And it was so intertwined with the holidays, which laid the foundation for patterns that continue into adult years. Also, sharing a meal equated to family love.

When food is a main focal point during the holidays, children learn to connect their intimacy with food. They may experience their parents eating many times throughout the day, overeating and expressing how stuffed they are. The mid-afternoon turkey dinner has escalated into a second and third helping, a turkey sandwich a couple of hours later, and a late-night snack and more the next day.

Most of us have learned as families to socialize around food. Certainly, the holidays are a time of "eat, drink, and be merry." Parents and grandparents alike reward their children with cookies or a special treat. Food has been reinforced as a reward instead of as fuel for their bodies.

So when do you use food to celebrate or reward yourself? The obvious times are parties, holidays (including Thanksgiving, the national food celebration eating day; Christmas, the entire season, with cookies and cakes and candy; Easter with chocolate bunnies, candy, etc.; and Valentine's Day, with go-to-hell chocolate candy fest), the weekend of the Super Bowl, birthdays, anniversaries, and the list goes on. Then there are the personal celebrations such as, "I passed the test," "Something went well at my job," "I got the deal," "I got the apartment, house, car, bike, coat, grade, certificate, telephone call, second interview, audition, etc.," "I lost weight," I gained weight," etc. How about just surviving the day? That's reason enough.

To Protect Against Unmourned Losses and Issues

This is a scenario in which everyone has ostensibly "moved on" and made the "best of it" through compulsive working, eating, drinking, or taking care of others. We have so much grief and loss that we medicate with the food. As I mentioned in Chapter 3: Little Food Addict in Training, we are so sad about and have grief over what we didn't get from our caretakers (for example, understanding, consistent kindness, affection) that we should have gotten and what we did get—abuse and trauma—that we should not have gotten. We have lost so much of our lives because of the messages that we're not good enough. And from an early age, the food serves to protect us from these potentially overwhelming feelings. Food, though, has no arms, so it can't hold us—but we pretend that it does.

As an Expression of or Discharge of Feelings

In some families who have sit-down meals, there may be such verbal abuse and uproar that eating itself is associated with terror and fear. In homes where children are not permitted to express emotions, are treated unfairly, and are then prohibited from the expression of natural frustrations and anger related to daily injustice, rage begins to develop. Because the natural responses are suppressed, strong emotions must seek release in indirect and surreptitious ways. Strong emotion can be suppressed and sated by eating behavior. Thus, "I'm frustrated and overwhelmed" equals "I'm hungry"; "I am out of control" equals control of food intake; and "I am lonely and afraid" equals "I am hungry." Let's discuss this more now.

Such expressions of feelings include rebelliousness, avoiding intimacy, and using food as a replacement for relationships. Using the food can have calming effects, with the food addict thinking, *If I don't eat, I don't feel,* or *I'll eat so I won't feel.*

Purging accomplishes the release of painful and negative emotions and has a physiological calming effect over mood. The physical feelings created by the act of purging or hunger can be a substitute for psychologically experiencing emotions. Symptoms also serve to regulate emotions, in that the person projects feelings and conflicts onto the symptom (e.g., feeling guilt or shame because of purging rather than thinking about what in the person's life causes feelings of guilt or shame).

Using food also can also be viewed as a metaphor. The behaviors represent symbols that individuals are unable to express and experience emotionally, verbally, and relationally. For example, rejection of food can symbolize the rejection of other appetites in life, such as joy, sex, emotional connectedness, relationships, and work fulfillment. Food can be a replacement for what is unfulfilling in life. The taking in and purging out of food can be a statement of ambivalence about intimacy. Not eating can signify a need to control or an act of separation or individuation—rebellion—i.e., "You cannot control my eating."

To Avoid or Encourage Feelings of Deprivation

For most, if not all, food addicts, there is a core of shame—feelings of *I'm less than, I don't matter.* Those feelings exist in a space of emptiness, a void—a sense of deprivation. For example, *I overeat to make up for everything I felt deprived of!* or *I starve because I feel or believe deprivation is what I deserve.*

For Evidence of Self-Blame

This was listed earlier as "behaviors and resulting consequences are evidence for self-blame ('I am bad') instead of the blaming of abusers." As long as a victim of abuse believes she is defective and deserving of the abuse, she can avoid acknowledging that she was helpless and that her parents were abusive or neglectful. Believing that "I am to blame" is much more tolerable than, "I am helpless and there is no one to protect me."

Keep in mind that all of the interpretations discussed exist with addiction as the underlying problem. These behaviors, however they started, have taken on a life of their own. All the reasons discussed can be boiled down to these specific purposes:

- Power
- Control
- Connection
- Safety
- Nurturing
- Revenge or Punishment

All of these purposes can be place under the category of "to get rid of feelings." Using food for any of these reasons is an illusion, a deception! There is no power or control or connection or safety or revenge in food. And just like there's no crying in baseball, there's no nurturing in food. Nurturing comes from other people. When we look to food for nurturing, it only leaves us lonelier and more isolated and empty and bereft. It's only when we recognize that we need people—that nurturing comes from people—that recovery can begin. When we deal with our feelings openly and honestly in the presence of others, healing begins. That's why it's imperative to attend and participate in 12 Step meetings for food recovery—but more about that later.

THE LANGUAGE OF FEELINGS

Language is the communication of thoughts and feelings between human beings by means of speech and hearing (and expression). The term "feelings" means to be emotionally affected,[102] or a physical reaction to a thought process that creates energy somewhere within the body, which we then act on or react to. This is illustrated in the basic action chain:

Stimulus > Thought > Feeling > Action

Please stop reading this book for a moment and think of some feelings words. On a piece of paper, write down all the words you can think of. Note that *hungry, tired, sleepy, nauseous,* and similar types of words are physical feelings, not emotional feelings; the words you choose must have an emotional connection. Are you stuck? The list of feelings words is very long.

Did you ever say to yourself or to someone else, "I can't talk about my feelings! I CAN'T talk about my feelings!" Not knowing how to express feelings is very common. Many people were simply never taught how. Think about how you learned language; It was modeled for you. You heard it, absorbed it, copied it—all those thousands of words. When you were very young, did you hear any of the words you listed on your piece of paper? Did you hear, "I'm hurt, I'm sad, I'm furious . . . disappointed, excited, scared, frustrated, confused, jealous, envious, angry, inadequate, overwhelmed, useless"? Maybe you saw them acted out, but mostly, you didn't hear the words. Ergo, one of the reasons you say and believe that you can't talk about your feelings is because you never learned the words to express them. And maybe, even though you spent years in therapy, you still have a short list!

Especially in alcoholic, chemically dependent, food-addicted families, people learn more about how to conceal their true identities than how to reveal them. So we continue to accept and play our roles, rather than risking being real and genuine. Another reason for not being able to talk about your feelings is that you were shut down by your parents or caregivers from an early age. Maybe the messages to not have your feelings were subtle, or maybe they were outright threatening: "Why are you crying? What are YOU crying about? I'll give you something to cry about!" The message here is, "You have no reason to cry, to feel pain, so you'd better stop and get rid of the feelings!"

Maybe you heard, "Boys don't cry! Don't be a sissy!" or "Better wipe that smile off your face, missy!" Or maybe you heard such statements aimed at another person or perhaps you overheard something like "I don't know why she's like that" in response to your outward show of fear, sadness, or any other emotion.

All these messages are very rejecting and shaming—shaming because they say that something is wrong with the child for having a feeling. When a child is exhibiting a strong feeling, the loving, healthy response in the parent or caregiver should be acknowledgment, caring, and kindness. "Sweetheart, what's wrong? I see how upset you are. Please tell me what happened," and, once they've explored the situation, "Let me give you a big, long hug."

I'm not talking about a tantrum, where little Sarah is not getting what she wants; there are different approaches to dealing with tantrums. Ignoring the child or saying, "I can't hear you right now. I will wait until you can use your words," tells the child that this behavior is not the means to get her what she wants but never as a means to shame or reject. "I love you, but I don't like your behavior" should be the message. The comment, "When you calm down, I will be happy to talk with you," tells the child that she is important but her behavior is unacceptable.

Feelings are never right or wrong, good or bad, in a moral sense. They just are! They can be based on inaccurate information, but they are still valid. If someone feels angry at a presumed injustice, that anger is still the "right" feeling; the anger may and should dissipate when the person learns the truth (i.e., no injustice or harm was meant). Experiencing certain feelings may be comfortable or uncomfortable, pleasant or unpleasant. But the feelings themselves are neither right nor wrong. It's what we do with our feelings that's important. Think about the following statement:

What I think and how I feel are the fingerprints of who I am.

As a human being, you have thoughts, feelings, and a body to house it all in (that's true for animals, too). That's it! That's what makes you who you are—and, of course, how you express those thoughts and feelings. But without the thoughts and feelings, there's nothing.

Okay, so what's my point?

Now, the truth is that apart from using food for our fuel—having nice meals, eating something because we are really hungry—we have used it as a mood changer, to get rid of feeling feelings we are uncomfortable with, feelings we don't want to feel. And, certainly, the food works! We give a lot of power to food and have a lot of expectations from it, and it never delivers!

When we understand that, in large measure, who we are is defined by our feelings, we have accomplished getting rid of ourselves—and how sad that is. Most of us have abandonment issues, and we succeed in perpetuating the experience of abandonment by doing it to ourselves—leaving ourselves—by trying to obliterate our feelings.

Your feelings are perhaps your most personal possessions, and when they are not well managed, they can be devastating. You must be able to identify your feelings, accept them as an integral part of yourself, and manage each one as it comes, avoiding suppression when possible.

Becoming aware of our feelings and constructively dealing with them is crucial to the process of healing.

Growing up in troubled or dysfunctional families, our needs weren't met. That is a painful experience. We feel the painful feelings. Because our families did not function in a way that provided us with nurturing, support, acceptance, respect, and a listening ear, and most had the rule of "don't have feelings," there was no one with whom we could share our feelings. We used food to defend ourselves, to shut the feelings out, away from our awareness. Doing so allows us to survive, although at a high price. We become progressively numb, out of touch, false, and codependent. For the food addict, every feeling translates into feeling hungry—"I'm hungry. I want something to eat." But the hunger is never for food.

When we are thus not our real, authentic selves, we do not grow mentally, emotionally, and spiritually. We begin to experience life as victims because we feel stifled, unalive, and often frustrated and confused. We are unaware of our total self, and we feel as though others, "the system," and the world are "doing it to us," i.e., we are their victims, at their mercy.

When we begin to identify and experience our feelings, we make our way out of our position as victim and its suffering. Certainly talking about our feelings with safe and supportive people is the way to know and experience them. That's where 12 Step meetings are essential in this process, as well as therapy, if possible.

We can make our feelings our friends. Appropriately handled, they will not betray us; we will not lose control or be overwhelmed or engulfed, as we fear.

Our feelings are the way we perceive ourselves. They are our reaction to the world around us, the way we sense being alive. Without awareness of our feelings, we have no real awareness of life. They summarize our experience and tell us if it feels good or bad. Feelings are our most helpful link in our relationship with ourselves, others, and the world around us.

As explained by Charles Whitfield, M.D., in *Healing the Child Within*, our feelings both warn us and assure us. They act as indicators or gauges of how we are doing in the moment and over a stretch of time. They give us a sense of mastery and aliveness. Our real self feels both joy and pain, and it expresses and shares them with appropriate others.

However, our false or codependent self tends to push us to feel mostly painful feelings and to withhold and not share them.

Our feelings exist on a spectrum, starting with the most joyous, going through the most painful, and ending with confusion and numbness, as follows:

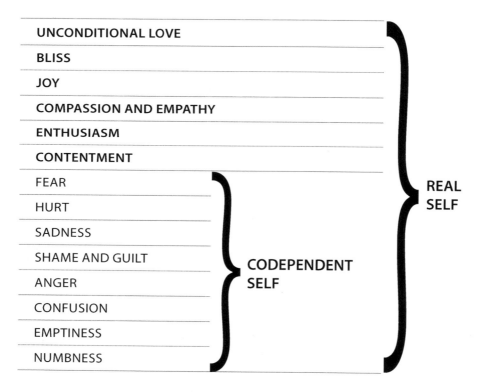

According to Charles Whitfield, in viewing our feelings in this way, we see that our Real and True Self—our child within—is empowered with a wider range of possibilities than we might have believed. The maintenance and growth of our Child Within is associated with what psychotherapists and counselors call a "strong ego," i.e., a flexible and creative ego that can "roll with the punches" of life. In contrast, the codependent self tends to be more limited, responding to mostly painful feelings—or no feelings at all, i.e., numbness. To cover up the pain, we use relatively unhealthy ego defenses, food being a major one, which give us fewer possibilities and choices in our lives. In the course "Eat to Kill," Dr. Matthew Anderson states:

"Instead of eating to kill these feelings, [with the use of the food plan] we can learn to identify, experience and work them through. As we learn to manage our feelings [and with the guidance of the food plan] we change our relationship to food and to ourselves. We increase our self-esteem, self-acceptance and self-empowerment."[103]

As you begin to make changes toward settling into the food plan, moving away from "using" food for your feelings, feelings will begin to surface, so it's important to begin to develop a vocabulary of feelings and to exercise their use. **Remember: Your feelings will not kill you, your addictions will!**

If you can substitute "I think" for "I feel," it's not a feeling. For example, "I feel that this is an uplifting experience" is a judgment, not a feeling. If you can substitute "I am" for "I feel," it is a feeling. For example, "I feel lonely" or "I am lonely." That is "you" at that time.

Feelings can be about:

1. Situations, actions, and/or things (e.g., embarrassment, nervousness, relaxation)

2. Other people (e.g., annoyance, anger, love, sympathy)

3. Self (e.g., loneliness, confidence, inadequacy, lovability)

Feelings are here and now. All of us have feelings—here and now. We are interacting with each other constantly on the feeling level. Therefore, we have a common ground for relating and communicating, regardless of our differences in age, education, socioeconomic status, political and moral values, intellectual opinions and prejudices, and physical abilities or disabilities. The words in Table 13.1 can help you be more exacting when identifying your feelings. We are always feeling, and when the strength of your feelings overpowers what you are thinking, then it's time to pay attention to what you're feeling.

You can photocopy this spreadsheet. Keep it with you at all times or on your beside table for four weeks. During the day or at the end of the day, check off the feelings you experience(d). This practice helps you identify your emotions. According to the well-respected addictions expert Pia Mellody, there are eight basic emotions: anger, fear, pain, joy, passion, love, shame, and guilt. Table 13.2 offers a closer look at these eight emotions.[104]

The Language of Feelings and Food Addiction

TABLE 13.1. VOCABULARY OF FEELINGS

Pleasant Feelings

Open	Happy	Alive	Good	Love	Interested	Positive	Strong
Understanding	Great	Playful	Calm	Loving	Concerned	Eager	Impulsive
Confident	Gay	Courageous	Peaceful	Warmth toward	Affected	Keen	Free
Reliable	Joyous	Energetic	Tranquil	Considerate	Fascinated	Earnest	Sure
Easy	Jolly	Excited	At ease	Affection for	Intrigued	Intent	Certain
Amazed	Lucky	Liberated	Comfortable	Sensitive	Absorbed	Inspired	Rebellious
Free	Fortunate	Optimistic	Sheltered	Tenderness toward	Engrossed	Determined	Unique
Sympathetic	Delighted	Provocative	Pleased	Gentle	Inquisitive	Excited	Dynamic
Interested	Overjoyed	Impulsive	Encouraged	Devoted	Nosy	Enthusiastic	Tenacious
Satisfied	Gleeful	Free	Clever	Caring	Snoopy	Bold	Hardy
Receptive	Thankful	Carefree	Surprised	Attracted by	Curious	Brave	Secure
Accepting	Important	Frisky	Content	Infatuated	Congenial	Daring	Strong
Kind	Festive	Spry	Quiet	Passionate	Cordial	Challenged	Arrogant
Accountable	Ecstatic	Lively	Certain	Admiration		Optimistic	Bold
Appeased	Satisfied	Animated	Relaxed	Touched		Reinforced	Capable
Noticed	Glad	Sparkling	Serene	Sympathy		Confident	Competent
Wanted	Cheerful	Spirited	Free and easy	Close		Hopeful	Determined
	Sunny	Thrilled	Bright	Loved		Composed	Invigorated
	Merry	Stimulated	Blessed	Comforted		Dignified	Powerful
	Elated	Wonderful	Reassured	Drawn toward		Helpful	Robust
	Jubilant	Activated	Healthy	Benevolent		Pleasant	Vigorous
	Amused	Active	Honorable	Charitable		Important	Virile
	Blissful	Involved	Honored	Generous		Qualified	Vital
	Contented	Lucky	Proud	Sentimental		Successful	Possessive
	Delighted	Vivacious	Loyal	Protective		Relief	Need for
	Pleased	Accepted	Modest	Nurturing			Independent
		Needed	Rested	Concern for			
			Restored				
			United				
			Wanted				
			Justified				

Difficult/Unpleasant Feelings

Angry	Depressed	Confused	Helpless	Indifferent	Afraid	Hurt	Sad
Mad	Lousy	Upset	Incapable	Insensitive	Scared	Crushed	Tearful
Irritated	Disappointed	Doubtful	Alone	Dull	Fearful	Tormented	Sorrowful
Grouchy	Discouraged	Self-doubt	Isolated	Nonchalant	Frightened	Deprived	Pained
Moody	Ashamed	Uncertain	Paralyzed	Neutral	Terrified	Pained	Grief
Enraged	Powerless	Unsure	Fatigued	Reserved	Terrorized	Tortured	Anguish
Hostile	Diminished	Indecisive	Useless	Weary	Suspicious	Dejected	Desolate
Frustrated	Guilty	Perplexed	Inferior	Bored	Anxious	Rejected	Desperate
Aggravated	Dissatisfied	Exasperated	Limited	Preoccupied	Alarmed	Discarded	Discontented
Insulting	Miserable	Hesitant	Limp	Cold	Panic	Ignored	Drained
Sore	Detestable	Shocked	Vulnerable	Disinterested	Nervous	Neglected	Exhausted
Annoyed	Repugnant	Stupefied	Empty	Lifeless	Worried	Deceived	Fatigued
Upset	Despicable	Disillusioned	Forced	Accommodating	Vulnerable	Misunderstood	Pessimistic
Hateful	Disgusting	Unbelieving	Hesitant	Distant	Timid	Injured	Hopeless
Unpleasant	Abominable	Skeptical	Flustered	Docile	Shy	Offended	Unhappy
Offensive	Terrible	Distrustful	Despair	Placid	Insecure	Embarrassed	Lonely
Overbearing	In Despair	Misgiving	Frustrated	Idle	Overwhelmed	Afflicted	Solemn
Bitter	Sulky	Ignorant	Hindered	Inactive	Shaky	Aching	Melancholy
Disgusted	Bad	Lost	Dependent	Inhospitable	Restless	Victimized	Forlorn
Aggressive	A sense of loss	Unsure	Imprisoned		Doubtful	Harassed	Grief
Resentful	Defeated	Vague	Distressed		Troubled	Heartbroken	Mournful
Inflamed	Empty	Uneasy	Woeful		Threatened	Agonized	Dismayed
Provoked		Pessimistic	Inadequate		Menaced	Appalled	Alone
Incensed		Tense	Pathetic		Trapped	Humiliated	Forsaken
Infuriated		Bewildered	Tragic		Cowardly	Shamed	Withdrawn
Cross		Disturbed	In a stew		Quaking	Wronged	Miserable
Worked Up		Jumbled	Dominated		Wary	Alienated	Blue
Boiling		Restless	Censured		Apprehensive	Abandoned	Gloomy
Fuming			Confined		Bashful	Absurd	Heavy-hearted
Indignant			Destitute		Cautious	Abused	Regret
Agitated			Frail			Betrayed	Selfish
Closed			Weak			Denied	Sulky
Cranky			Weary			Deserted	Bored
Wicked			Overworked			Despised	
Malicious			Pressured			Disgraced	
Mean			Defensive			Mortified	
						Plagued	
						Ridiculous	
						Scorned	
						Unwelcome	
						Blamed	

TABLE 13.2. THE EIGHT BASIC EMOTIONS: THEIR GIFTS AND LOCATIONS

Eight Basic Emotions	Their Gifts	Where Felt
ANGER Resentment Irritation Frustration	Assertiveness Strength Energy	All Over Body Power Energy
FEAR Apprehension Overwhelmed Threatened	Preservation Wisdom Protection	Stomach Upper Chest Suffocation
PAIN Hurt Pity Sad Lonely	Healing Growth Awareness	Lower Chest and Heart Hurting
JOY Happy Elated Hopeful	Abundance Happiness Gratitude	All Over Body Lightness
PASSION Enthusiasm Desire Zest Affection	Appetite Energy Excitement	All Over Body Energized Recharged Spontaneous
LOVE Tenderness Compassion Warmth	Connection Life Spirituality	Heart Swelling Warmth
SHAME Embarrassment Humble	Humility Containment Humanity	Face, Neck and/or Upper Chest Warm Hot Red
GUILT Regretful Contrite Remorseful	Values Amends Containment	Gut Gnawing sensation

"I" MESSAGES

To express yourself, it is important to begin developing healthy communication techniques. Another exercise to practice is to use "I" messages. The "I" message is a tool that enables us to get in touch with what we feel and to communicate this feeling in a clear and nonjudgmental way. It is a declaration of our own feeling stemming from *our* perception. Here are some examples of the feeling part of an "I" message:

- *I feel overwhelmed.*
- *I feel rejected.*
- *I feel sad.*
- *I feel afraid.*
- *I feel let down.*
- *I feel anxious.*

A complete "I" message contains three parts. The first part describes the behavior that is unacceptable, the second part conveys the feeling, and the third part tells the effect of the behavior on you. The format of the three part "I" message is:

- *When* (describe behavior)
- *I feel* (your feeling)
- *Because* (effect of the behavior)

An optional fourth part could be:

- *I would like* . . . (describe the change you'd like)

Here are two examples:

- *When I see clothes left on the couch, I feel resentful because I have to pick them up.*
- *When you were late, I was frightened because I thought something had happened to you.*

We often avoid vulnerability by changing the feeling into a thought or an opinion and use phrases such as: *You're driving me to an early grave, you're selfish, you make me mad* . . . These are called "you" messages. "You" messages are criticisms and judgments. They moralize, command, threaten, distract, reassure, question, ridicule, lecture, advise, and give solutions. They are roadblocks to communication.

The Language of Feelings and Food Addiction

305

Here's another way of seeing the formula for communication:

When you said/did (fill in the blank), **I felt/feel** (fill in the blank), **because** (fill in the blank).
  or
I felt/feel (fill in the blank), **when you said/did** (fill in the blank), **because** (fill in the blank).

I suggest that you first practice this with friends or your recovery support system, not your family. When you communicate from an "I feel" place, you are not being accusatory, critical, or judgmental (as in "You made me so angry"), you are stating your feelings. The "You made me so (fill in the blank)" statement requires the person to whom this statement is directed to become defensive and fight, to argue back.

Here's an example:

You: "**When you** didn't call me back, **I felt** rejected/ignored/abandoned/hurt, **because** I didn't feel important enough for you to call me back."

Friend: "Oh, you shouldn't feel that way (we've heard that all our lives). I was so busy/away/I forgot/lost your number/erased the message/etc."

You: "I'm just telling you how I feel/felt."

You *are* just stating your feelings; you're not asking them to fix you or extracting a promise or an apology, although that's what most people will want to do. This is a very honest way to communicate and leaves you empowered, *and* you don't have to take care of your friend, if they have feelings.

Here's another example:

You: "**When you** walked out of the meeting with some people (and didn't say anything to me) and left me, **I felt** lost/abandoned/ignored/like I didn't matter/jealous, **because** I hadn't made plans with anyone else. I went home alone."

Friend: "You shouldn't feel that way. I saw you talking with someone/I totally got wrapped up with so and so and became oblivious (or _____)."

You: "I'm just telling you how I felt."

For practice (and fun), try this on checkout line in the deli or supermarket or when you're trying to be served in an appetizing section or at a deli counter:

You: "**When you** waited on that lady before me, **I felt** rejected/ignored/invisible/hurt/not important **because** I was on line before her and I will be late for an appointment if I have to wait any longer."

The cashier or helper might think you're crazy, but it doesn't matter—you're practicing being you! I do this whenever I have the chance to exercise my "voice"! Remember, the more you are able to identify and communicate your feelings, the less the need to use the food to get rid of them. The formula is:

Stress/Pain/Problem > Powerless/
Uncontrolled Craving + Medication (food) =
Relief (for 2 minutes), Shame, Remorse, Guilt, Self-hatred
or
Stress/Pain/Problem + Communication
(Sharing the Feelings With a Safe Person[s]) = Real Relief

This is one of the major reasons that the food addict needs a 12 Step food recovery program. Those who suffer from food addiction started early to deny their feelings as a result of having them shamed, dismissed, discouraged, ignored, etc., and used food as medication, comfort, solace. Therefore, feelings became laundered through a filter of "I'm hungry" as *the* feeling. One does not know one is feeling sad or mad or anxious; the experience is "I'm hungry. I want something to eat."

To have food in its rightful place in our lives, it's critical to work on feeling your feelings. Of course, the food recovery needs to be first—with the use of the food plan. But soon, the feelings will start to surface, and it's necessary to understand what is happening and to have a vocabulary and structure to deal with them.

7 FACTS ABOUT FEELINGS

1. **Feelings follow change:** Feelings often come about when changes are taking place. When you rethink, redo, reorganize, or rearrange, feelings just happen.

2. **Feelings and other people:** Feelings come in relationships with other people, including your parents, your spouse or partner, your boss, your children, you neighbors, your friends—anyone with whom you communicate.

3. **Feelings don't just disappear:** If feelings are ignored, they don't just go away. Feelings stick around and take other shapes and forms. Often, they do damage to your physical or mental health.

4. **Feelings can be sneaky:** Often your feelings come in disguises. You can mislabel your emotions. For example, you can feel you are angry when you are really afraid, or you can feel you are sad or confused when you are really angry.

5. **Feelings can lead to relapse:** If you do not learn to accept and express your feelings honestly and appropriately, you may be tempted to use the temporary, ineffective, and damaging alternative of food.

6. **Feelings just are:** Feelings by themselves are not right or wrong. They are just part of you.

7. **Feelings can change:** No matter how strong or how quiet they may be at first, feelings can change.

I Feel the Feeling

by Hugh Prather

I am beginning to think that there are no destructive feelings, only destructive acts, and that my actions become destructive only when I condemn and reject my feelings. If I say that I don't want to feel a certain way, I disregard the fact that I do feel that way and that the feeling is me. Feeling a certain way is one feeling; not wanting to feel that way is another feeling, and it does not cause the first feeling to stop. I can change my response to a feeling, I can no more get rid of it than I can get rid of myself. When I disown a feeling, I do not destroy it; I only forfeit my capacity to act it out as I wish. By condemning it, I stop believing it to be me and so it seems to take on a life of its own and force me to respond to it in a habitual way. But if I see that I feel the feeling, then I retain my ability to act on it in the way I choose rather than the way I fear.

Tonight a little boy fell in my lap and looked up at me for affection. I felt tight and awkward. I was battling so hard about how I "should" feel that I didn't pause long enough to see how I *did* feel. Maybe the fear that I didn't feel the love I thought I should was groundless and would have been there if I had not been afraid to look at myself.[105]

CHAPTER 14

Self-Esteem
and the Family System

There is a vast disparity between the image the active food addict tries to project to the outside world and her inner world of shame and negative self-talk. In this chapter, we will take a look at the inner world of the food addict and, again, at how family dynamics played a part in the development of the addiction.

"For as long as I can remember, I have been a food addict. I started my first diet when I was nine and spent the next 25 years attempting to lose weight and eat normally. . . . I always failed. I felt worthless as a human being. As I progressed through my life, I became more and more hopeless. . . . .

As a child, I was a champion swimmer, I played two instruments and did well in school, but nothing I ever accomplished was strong enough to counteract the negative feelings I held for myself, because I couldn't control my eating or my weight. Depriving myself of foods that everyone else got to eat made me feel even worse.

I have learned since coming to OA and being abstinent and working the 12 Steps . . . that no amount of "outside" accomplishments could have given me what I found inside of myself when I stopped using food to numb my feelings and stuff down my pain. Abstaining from compulsive eating and living the 12 Steps each day is all I need to do to feel worthwhile.

I have also learned that I wasn't deprived because I couldn't eat sweets or three times as much food as my body needed. The true deprivation in my life was the punishment I endured at the hands of my disease. By overeating all these years, I deprived myself of self-esteem, good health, peace of mind, and an attractive appearance."

—Anonymous

UNDERSTANDING DYSFUNCTIONAL FAMILY SYSTEMS

In the article "Understanding Addictions," Ann Crumpler, LCSW, wrote:

> "Addicts struggle to control their behavior, and experience despair over failure to manage urges [cravings]. This lack of competency creates a perpetual loss of self-esteem, fueling the need to escape further into the addictive behavior."[106]

This quote speaks to the shame that results from being in active addiction (any addiction, not just food). When we're in our addiction, we feel "less than" because we know we are behaving in self-destructive ways—even though we say, *Hey, I'm only hurting myself, and no one else,* which is against our higher self and better instincts—and at the same time we are lying, stealing, cheating, acting crazy, hiding, hurting others, and keeping a big, ugly, shameful secret. What we must consider, however, is the underlying shame we carry from early childhood. And that brings us to an examination of some family dynamics.

Do you come from a dysfunctional family? Your answer is probably "Yes, who doesn't?" I think the term "dysfunctional family" is redundant; by virtue of putting people together who have different personalities, genders, perspectives, and ages with children who have different needs and parents who have troubled histories and expecting them to function well, just because of blood connections, is basically unreasonable, ergo "dysfunctional."

In the book *Forgiving Our Parents, Forgiving Ourselves: Healing Adult Children of Dysfunctional Families,* authors David Stoop and James Masteller explain:

> "A dysfunctional family is one in which conflict, misbehavior, and often abuse on the part of individual members occurs continually and regularly, leading other members to accommodate such actions (both in behavior and in molding themselves to enable it). Children sometimes grow up in such families with the understanding that such an arrangement is normal. Dysfunctional families are primarily a result of codependent adults and may also be affected by addictions (alcohol, drugs, food, etc.). Other origins include mental illness and the parent emulating or over-correcting their own dysfunctional parents. In some cases, a 'childlike' parent will allow the dominant parent to abuse their children."[107]

Four different kinds of dysfunctional family systems have been identified. They are:

1. The alcoholic and/or chemically dependent (including food addicted) family system.

2. The emotionally or psychologically disturbed family system.

3. The physically abusive or sexually abusive family system.

4. The religious fundamentalist or rigidly dogmatic family system.

Many of our families fit into more than just one of these categories. All these types of family systems have rigid rules. The members of these families usually have poor communication patterns, low self-image, and loss of identity. They very often behave in self-destructive ways.

When dysfunction exists in the home, the focus is usually centered on the dysfunctional parent or parents. The needs of the children are often neglected. When the emphasis in the home is on the dysfunction, there are sacrifices that have to be made. The primary sacrifice is most often in the area of healthy family interactions. Those who must make the most sacrifices or who usually feel the most negative effects of such sacrifices are the children.

An understanding of family systems is important to see that our family-related issues didn't just happen in our immediate family; these issues have been passed down through generations, from parent to child to the next generation and so forth.

A note to any reader who is a parent: As your child goes through developmental stages, you will be brought back into your own issues around that developmental stage. If you didn't get your needs met there, it's going to be very hard to meet your child's needs. You will either do to your child what was done to you or just the opposite. Have you ever said something to your child that you swore you'd never say? It's called "reenactment." It's acting out something you swore you'd never do. That's how these dysfunctional systems are passed on through generations. Families fall on a continuum that ranges from nurturing to dysfunctional. Most fall in the middle on this continuum. No family is perfect.

Further on in this chapter, you'll see Table 14.1, which juxtaposes the characteristics of the dysfunctional family against the functional family (which is basically a theoretical model). As I said, all families have some basic dysfunction, some worse than others, but it's important to be able to assess our list of characteristics against some standard.

Where there is addiction in the family, including food addiction, there is a commonality of characteristics. The family attempts to appear to "have it all together," which may look good to the world outside, when in fact there is an internal crisis occurring. (My family was a "looking good" family and made strong efforts to keep that appearance.)

We know from research that children of alcoholics and addicts have higher rates of eating problems. As you will see in the table, the parents in these families generally have high expectations, many rules (which do not change with the age of the developing child), and are often over-protective, perfectionistic, and judgmental. There is often difficulty with communication, expression of feelings, and conflict resolution; lack of boundaries; enmeshment; and physical and/or sexual abuse. Blaming and fault-finding are also characteristic of dysfunctional family systems, and therefore the family members, especially the children, develop and follow the rules shown in the table.

In *Soul Murder: Persecution in the Family* (1973), Morton Schatzman explains that the "murder" of the child's soul results from certain dynamics within the family. These may include inconsistency, unpredictability, arbitrariness, and chaos. Inconsistency and unpredict-ability tend to repress spontaneity and are, in general, "crazy-making." Combined with arbitrariness, these dynamics promote lack of trust and/or fear of abandonment, as well as chronic depression. They result in a chaotic environment. This precludes the development of a safe, secure, and reliable foundation from which to learn about ourselves through risk-taking.

Before we look at the table, we need to examine an underlying thread that has, over the last number of years, become a way to view these dys-functional dynamics. It's the idea of shame. John Bradshaw, author and TV personality, brought much public and clinical focus to this concept. There are different kinds of shame, as he and others have described. He says that healthy shame is that which prevents us from running naked through the supermarket. As has been described, healthy shame gives us "the permission to be human." Natural shame is an auxiliary feeling that signals limits and monitors our pleasure, excitement, and interest. It lets us know we are limited and imperfect beings. As such, it gives us permission to make mistakes and ask for help when we need it. In an article titled "The Shame of Toxic Shame," written for *The Meadows Cutting Edge* newsletter, Fall 2001, author John Bradshaw states:

> "Everyone needs a sense of shame but nobody needs to be ashamed. A natural sense of shame is when you are able to concede that you have made a mistake and that you will make mistakes. Healthy shame lets you know you are not God."[108]

Natural shame is essential to the development of a moral life. When natural shame is nurtured in a healthy way, it develops into guilt (i.e., moral shame). Guilt is the guardian of conscience.

Bradshaw also says that natural shame becomes toxic when children interact with source figures who are immature (developmentally arrested) and morally shameless. The caretaker's shamelessness may take the form of the more-than-human, character-disordered control freak or the perfectionist who chronically judges, blames, criticizes, beats, punishes, or sexually uses his or her children. Or it may take the form of the neurotic character type who feels worthless and less than human, who treats his or her child as superior or worthless. In either polarized character form, the caretaker acts shamelessly and immorally.

The shame we want to examine in this dysfunctional family system is toxic shame, to understand how it has been transferred from parent to child so that the children have the burden and pain of "carried shame." Toxic shame prevents a person from showing her humanness; she has to be perfect; she can never make a mistake. Toxic shame is induced inside children by all forms of child abuse.

> *"What lingers from the parent's individual past,*
> *unresolved or incomplete, often becomes*
> *part of her or his irrational parenting."*
> —VIRGINIA SATIR

Family Systems
Intergenerational
Passed Down from Parent to Child

It's important to understand that Family Systems are evolutionary and can be traced back many generations. The characteristics, beliefs, and behaviors have been embedded in the structure of the family and have been accepted as the norm to the point that the flaws are unseen and there is, therefore, no opportunity for change. Notice the disparity between the dysfunctional and functional family in Table 14.1.

TABLE 14.1. DYSFUNCTIONAL FAMILY VERSUS FUNCTIONAL FAMILY

Note: *While many of these characteristics of troubled or dysfunctional families are common, all may not be present in every troubled family.*

DYSFUNCTIONAL FAMILY	FUNCTIONAL FAMILY
Individual awareness is based on denial, delusion, and shame. The individual serves/exists for the system.	Individual awareness is based on an expanding reality. The system serves/exists for the individual.
Delusion	**Reality-Based**
Delusion is a false belief held with absolute conviction, despite clear facts to the contrary. In a dysfunctional family, delusion operates to shield the members from the reality of abuse, abandonment, and enmeshment. The child has the experiences but does not assign the proper meaning to them. The (adult) child says those experiences were not painful or scary. In *Facing Codependence*, Pia Mellody states, "Like all the other defense mechanisms, delusion is invisible to us, making it a serious problem: we don't know we are deluded. We live in an unreal world based on our delusions, but we see that unreal world as reality. Because we can't afford to hear the facts about our lives as they really are, we often get very angry with people who try to point out any fallacies in our delusions. This position leaves us very vulnerable, since both reality itself and anyone with a strong sense of reality tend to threaten the view we have of our world."[109]	Healthy families exhibit warmth, camaraderie, and cohesiveness. They establish healthy priorities. The family is the top priority. The needs of the family outweigh all other activities. Healthy families ask for and give respect. Members know that respect is a two-way street. Healthy families communicate. Healthy families foster responsibility. Healthy families are not perfect; they may have yelling, bickering, misunderstanding, tension, hurt, and anger—but not all the time, and not for long periods of time; the child's basic sense of security is not threatened. In healthy families, emotional expression is allowed and accepted. Family members can freely ask for and give attention.

Self-Esteem and the Family System

Destruction	Love/Worth
Family members, because of the rigid rules, abuse, shaming, poor communication, prohibition against having and talking about feelings, addictions, anger, and guilt, often behave in self-destructive ways and can be destructive toward one another.	Love is characterized by a healthy expression of putting others first without denigrating one's own view of and responsibility to self. It is the continual learning and putting into practice the pleasure of giving to others, and of knowing other family members well enough that what is provided is consistent with who they are and what they like and need.
Idealization	**Belonging/Freedom/Fun**
Parents are seen as "gods" without imperfections. As children are abandoned through neglect, abuse, or enmeshment, the more they create the illusion of connection with the parent (Robert Firestone calls this the "Fantasy Bond"[110]). In *Healing the Shame That Binds You*, author John Bradshaw states: "In order to create the fantasy bond the child has to idealize his parents and make himself 'bad.' The purpose of this fantasy bonding is survival. The child desperately relies on his parents. They can't be bad. If they are bad or sick, he can't survive. So the fantasy bond (which makes them good and the child bad) is like a mirage in the desert. It gives the child the illusion that there is nourishment and support in his life."[111]	**Belonging:** Unity takes into account individual differences, prerogatives, and boundaries of each person within the family and respects individual right and responsibilities. The family is experienced as being the unifying force for each member within it and, as such, becomes a whole that is greater than the sum of its parts. Individual members are clearly committed to one another in positive ways because of their inherent family strength yet have permission and encouragement for individual creativity and pursuits.

Freedom: All members can freely and appropriately express their perception, feelings, thoughts, desires, and fantasies. Each family member has the freedom to:
• see and hear (perceive) what is here and now, rather than what was, will be, or should be
• think what one thinks, rather than what one should think
• feel what one feels, rather than what one should feel
• ask for what one wants instead of waiting for permission
• take risks on one's own behalf instead of choosing to be secure and always playing it safe

Fun: According to Johan Huizinga, art historian, fun is "an absolute primary category of life, familiar to everybody at a glance right down to the animal level."[112] Family fun (functional family)—enjoyment of activities (taking into account tastes/preferences of each family member):
• provides pleasure
• provides merriment
• provides leisure
• involves looking forward to being together
• is not "mandatory" activity
• offers pleasure as a family unit
• is not forced
• includes fun activities that take everyone's interest into consideration
• creates an atmosphere that is fun and spontaneous |

Approval/Love Must Be Earned	Love Is a Free Gift
Parent(s) who are perfectionistic (as a maladaptive mechanism to deal with their own experience of being shamed) fixate on order, prestige, power, and/or perfect appearances, while preventing their child from failing at anything, and they use the power of granting or withholding approval, validation, support, and love. The message is: "If it's not perfect, people won't love you. No matter how good it is, it's never good enough . . . but keep trying!" **A Note to the Reader:** Look at the hopes and expectations and the hopes and dreams you had for your children and your parents had for you. How did you measure up? Could you ever measure up? Did you get shamed if you failed? Did you hear things like "You'll never accomplish anything," or "You're not good enough," or "What's wrong with you?" or "Can't you do anything right?" Do you remember your quest for approval? What were the conditions? How did you feel when you didn't get it? Were your parents deficient, controlling, or neglectful and uncaring parents, letting you know that approval was an unattainable goal? Did they suffer from their own feelings of inadequacy that they layered onto you? We all have an innate need to be loved and accepted from our birth to the present. If that need is not met in our early years, we believe that there is something defective or unacceptable about us and we will be on an eternal quest for approval. We become people-pleasers as a way to get approval and acceptance. Were you approved of if you got good grades, were popular, pretty/handsome, a cheerleader, and/or helpful at home or to others? If other people praised you? If you were well behaved, compliant? Needless (self-sufficient) or worthless (not materialistic)? Was approval based on losing weight? If you didn't lose the weight, were you a failure in their eyes?	Parents are mature and healthy enough to give love with no strings. Love/approval is given unconditionally and not based on performance or other conditions. Carl Rogers, a founder of humanistic psychology and a major influential psychologist, examined the conditions needed for a person to achieve their full potential. In the process of the development of the self, he believed that at the time the self begins to develop in infancy, the infant learns to need affection, approval, and love from other people, which Rogers termed as "positive regard." The main requirement for a healthy personality is receiving unconditional positive regard, which develops when the mother or caregiver offers love and affection and the attitude it represents become an internalized set of norms and standards for the infant. Children growing up with the feeling of unconditional positive regard will not develop conditions of worth, including feeling a sense of worth only under certain conditions, generally when behavior is not disapproved or rejected. Instead, they feel themselves worthy under all conditions, have no need for defensive behavior, and will not have incongruence between the self and the perception of reality.

Self-Esteem and the Family System

Human Doer/Doing	Human Being
Love is contingent upon achievement. In *Healing the Shame That Binds You,* author John Bradshaw states: "Toxic shame turns you into a human doing because toxic shame says your being is flawed and defective. If your being is flawed and defective, nothing you do could possibly make you lovable. You can't change who you are." Children who were made to take care of their parents emotionally, physically, or sexually and to meet their parents' "childish" needs for power, attention, sex, and belonging were manipulated to do so to avoid physical and emotional abandonment/harm by their parents. In an attempt to be the "good," approved-of child, where there is parental inadequacy, children tend to take on adult responsibilities from a young age. Then parental emotional needs tend to take precedence, and children are often asked to be their parents' caretakers. Children are robbed of their own childhood, and they learn to ignore their own needs and feelings. Because these children are simply unable to play an adult role and take care of their parents, they often feel inadequate and guilty. These feelings continue into adulthood.	Child is loved for being! Loved for who they are, not for what they do.

Closed/Censored/Secret	Open
The unexpressed message is that no one enters or leaves from "our inner circle." Individual boundaries are missing. • "We don't air our dirty linen in public!" • "You keep your mouth shut—it's nobody's business!" • "What goes on in this house STAYS in this house!" There is little opportunity for true expression of ideas and feelings with the family, and strong structures may require its members to maintain a certain image to those outside (mine was a "looking-good family"). Its unhealthy habits and patterns, often seen by the children, must be denied within the family ("elephant in the living room") and protected from disclosure to others. An unhealthy family rarely discusses sensitive areas such as the addiction or mental illness of a family member, money, unemployment, past criminal records, sexual orientation, chronic illness, death, or handicaps. Instead, they are dealt with in one of three ways: they are denied, they are lied about, or they are hidden away as secrets.	Nothing to be ashamed of. Nothing to hide. Individual boundaries are supported. Lines of communication are open between parents and children. Children have input into family matters, but parents make the final decisions. The family unit is characterized by a sense of family wholeness. Each family member has a feeling of belonging which contributes to their personal self-esteem. Friends can be invited into the home without the family's feeling they must protect themselves. Family members talk and listen to each other. They respect the other person's point of view even when it differs from their own. Individuals are allowed to express feelings and needs without fear of reprisal, ridicule, or retaliation from other family members.

Closed/Censored/Secret (continued)	**Open** (continued)
The other rule that comes out of a closed family system is that you don't ask for help. If you asked for help, you would have to reveal the family secrets. So, that's out! The message of the closed/censored/secret system keeps the family isolated from resources that may intervene or provide support. To talk about feelings or disclose a secret only brings up pain, which the family feels is unsolvable and unbearable. Family members learn explicitly or unconsciously that they should never be vulnerable, never open up to "outsiders," and do their best to stuff any feelings that are deemed unacceptable. Family members choosing not to operate in the mode of dependency are maligned with judgment, guilt, alienation, and/or rejection. The rule that the child develops from living in this closed/censored/secret system is: **DON'T TALK** (Or, maybe the child wasn't **told** to keep her mouth shut; maybe her experience was somewhat similar to mine: Due to my mother's unpredictable alcoholic episodes and suicide attempts, I felt so ashamed and fearful of being seen as abnormal or crazy that I never talked about my home life or risked asking anyone over to my house because I never knew when there would be an explosion.)	Family members are allowed to need help and support and communicate problems and conflicts openly. Openness is shown in the willingness to disclose to one another, to be open to new experiences and events, and to receive from others expressions of joy and sadness, excitement and fear—virtually anything one needs or wishes to express. This interfamily openness translates to an outward openness to others beyond the family. At the same time, boundaries are acknowledged and respected as prerogatives of individuals both within and outside the family. In a healthy family, sensitive issues are discussed with all family members, even though the truth and the acceptance of it may be difficult.
Dishonesty	**Honesty**
The unhealthy family accepts lying and keeps secrets. Children may learn how to lie from their parents. They may hear their parents telling lies to employers, friends, customers, or family members. They may even be asked to lie to cover up or confirm their parents' lies. In addition, secrets are common in dysfunctional families. Because there is no open and honest communication, it becomes easier for the family to hide behind lies as well as secrets. Growing up in lying, secretive families, children learn to lie and keep secrets.	A functional family shares openly and honestly with each member of the family. All members are included in open and honest communication. Therefore, children learn to tell the truth, no matter how painful that may be, because the family accepts honesty and frowns upon dishonesty. Healthy families don't have secrets. Of course, age appropriateness is considered in the level of communication.
Rigid Rules (Shame-Based Family Rules)	**Flexible Rules**
In dysfunctional families, one or both parents may insist that the children adhere to rigid rules and that they conform entirely, often with threats of punishment or withholding of customary and healthy activities.	A healthy family maintains authority, but also has flexibility. (Authority means others are heard before a choice is made that will affect them.)

Self-Esteem and the Family System

Rigid Rules (continued)	**Flexible Rules** (continued)
The unhealthy family is autocratic and inflexible. The ruling of the parent(s) is usually irreversible and may not consider the good of all. Or, the system may be permissive with wide boundaries so the family has little sense of unity or cohesiveness.	The parent(s) listen to each individual in the family and reach a compromise based on the good of everyone involved. Rules adjust as the family grows. Healthy families have the ability to overcome conflict and the potential to develop alternative solutions if necessary. They are not impulsive; they negotiate and compromise.
Addicts (to alcohol, drugs, food, gambling, sex, work, rage) generally feel inadequate and shameful about themselves and also feel guilty, are acting shamelessly, and are filled with toxic shame. They want to prove that they can never make a mistake. And because of that, are very perfectionistic and demanding of perfection in others.	The system is able to accommodate changes and role diversity without becoming rigid or intolerant. Rules tend to be made explicit and remain consistent, but with some flexibility to adapt to individual needs and particular situations. Healthy families allow for individuality; each member is encouraged to pursue his or her own interests, and boundaries between individuals are honored.
When the parent(s) carry toxic shame, they have to cover it up. Feeling flawed and defective as human beings, they cover it up by being very demanding and perfectionistic and running the family with a lot of rules (which keep changing) to accommodate how they are feeling about themselves. Suffering from toxic shame, they are rigid, blaming, righteous, moralistic, and controlling. They never want you to see their flaws, so they will control you so you will never see their imperfections. As the result of the need to appear perfect, the rigid parent often cannot tolerate a child's ideas differing from theirs.	When the rules that govern behavior within the family system are nurturing and healthy, the child learns that it's OK to be who she is and that the child is a valuable human being just the way she is.
The child will then be attacked or ridiculed for her thinking. There is little room for individuality or creativity, and individual differences may be ignored. Family dynamics often dictate that family allegiance always be put first in such a way that individual expression and creativity are thwarted and high dependence on the family is created. Children are denied the opportunity to pursue the usual developmental independence that is important to healthy growth and necessary for later healthy independence. (See "Family Rules" on page 329.)	Clear rules are discussed, e.g., hours, respect for property, telephone use, chores, etc. This family gives the child the message that her ideas are sound and complete even though the child has much to learn. The child is not attacked for lack of knowledge but is treated respectfully and, at same time, maybe overruled to enforce a rule valued by the family. (See "Family Rules" on page 332.)
No Sharing of Time	**Sharing Time**
An unhealthy family has very little time for anyone. Oftentimes, plans made or promises given are changed or broken. Requests to spend time together are usually rejected, or invitation to events important to an individual are rebuffed. Mixed messages may be given; while parents say they're interested in what the children do, they rarely share such opportunities. In these families, children learn that their interests or needs aren't important.	A healthy family makes times for everyone in the family. Time is set aside for individuals to be together. This family considers everyone important, parent and child alike. A healthy family knows time needs to be budgeted or shared in order for everyone to get a chance to feel they are special members of the family. This time can be vacation time, a family hour, or time given to encourage or share in another family member's hobby, sport, or event.

Distorted Balance Between Work and Play	Responsibilities and Recreation
A dysfunctional family knows no balance between recreation and responsibilities. This family rarely has a balance between work time and play time. One or more of the children in the home may be very responsible, assuming tasks and obligations for the adults. Other times children are given large amounts of idle time, or money, or both, and ordered to get out of the house. Or children may be brought up in a chaotic home where no one takes any responsibility, nor has any fun—where meals are sporadic, food shopping rarely done, the house seldom cleaned, and the clothes rarely washed. In each of these instances, there is little or no balance between work and fun/play time, and there's no equal sharing of responsibilities. Children in these families learn one of two things: there's no time to relax, or responsibilities are taken care of by others.	A functional family encourages play time as well as responsible time. This family understands children need to be brought up in an atmosphere that has a balance between work time and time for relaxation. It encourages playtime and fun activities as a reward for attention paid to household chores, family obligations, school work, and jobs outside the home. In these families, responsibilities are divided up equally among all the members.
Mistaken Sense of Quality Time	**Quality Time**
A dysfunctional family doesn't understand what quality time is. A family that spends a great deal of time together may not be sharing quality time. The parent who thinks an afternoon in front of a TV is quality time with her child isn't in touch with how to identify or even share meaningful moments. In these families, parents and children rarely spend time together. When they do, the times may be marred by any number of negative situations: criticism, feelings of guilt, anger or fighting, unhappiness, controlling behaviors, and lack of communication. When that happens, children don't learn what quality time is. In these homes, children may learn to accept that the little time given to them is all they really deserve.	A healthy family shares quality time. It includes those moments when parents and children exchange thoughts, feelings, and opinions. It's a time when fun activities are shared or when the family can do something together.
Frozen (Stifled) Feelings	**All Feelings Are Acceptable**
An unhealthy family discourages any display of feelings. The system controls which emotions are allowed. • "Boys don't cry! Don't be a crybaby!" • "Only babies are afraid." • "You're crying. I'll give you something to cry about!" • "You better wipe that smile off your face!" • "You shouldn't feel that way!" In other words, if you're having a feeling, you'd better get rid of it.	A healthy family acknowledges, accepts, and shows feelings. All emotions are allowed and shared. In a healthy family, members are encouraged to feel a wide range of feelings: happiness, sadness; anger, peace; pain, joy; jealousy, pride; fear, courage, love, and hate.

Self-Esteem and the Family System

Frozen (Stifled) Feelings (continued)	**All Feelings Are Acceptable** (continued)
In an unhealthy family, members may only know how to feel one or two feelings, such as anger or sadness. The rule of "It's not OK to talk about or express feelings openly" gives the message that some feelings are bad and family members cannot express or even tolerate these feelings. When a "bad" feeling occurs, such as anger, a person is also likely to feel guilt and shame. In an unhealthy family, expression is discouraged. Even when an emotion is expressed, it may not be acknowledged. Instead, the child may be punished for simple, natural expressions of feelings, such as crying, asking for help, or even happy excitement. The method of functioning in the dysfunctional family is experienced as "normal" for those born into it. Communication wears a veil of defensiveness, alienation, fear, denial, or anger. These feelings are rarely expressed out loud—but tend to form undercurrents within the family. Feelings are instead channeled into behavior patterns that keep the sick family system functioning as smoothly as it can under the circumstances. These dysfunctional patterns, the rules and beliefs we're discussing for all the characteristics, become normalized and part of the basic survival mechanisms which are carried through into adult relationships. That no one should talk about their feelings becomes the unwritten rule because the dysfunctional family members believe they are dependent upon their unhealthy relationship patterns in order to survive. Talking about feelings would only bring up pain which the family feels is unsolvable. The child in this family is left with a constant level of anger, fear and shame as a result of the lack of communication and these feelings become the norm. Over time, the child learns to replace feelings with the simple statement, "I'm fine," which means "I am shut down," "I don't want to talk." In a 1997 article for *Paradigm* titled "Food Addiction," authors A. Leary and A. Meyer state: "Food addicts learned in their families that painful feelings should be avoided. They learn to pretend everything is fine, while hiding their true feelings. They learn not to trust others and to get rid of feelings by bingeing, purging or restricting food."[113]	Members are encouraged to express their feelings, but not only in words. While talking is encouraged, so are the natural expressions of feelings such as crying, a need to be held, or a need to yell. A Robin and Foster study of families found that in solution-focused families, members are able to share their feelings without offending others.[114] David Reiss, who studies family relationships, observed that healthy families speak clearly.[115] They are not rigid in their discussions with each other, nor are they confused and chaotic. They are able to express happiness or sadness to each other. They have a good sense of humor and the ability to laugh at themselves. They respect each other's need for privacy. Problems and troubles in the family are freely and openly discussed or explored.

Frozen (Stifled) Feelings (continued)	All Feelings Are Acceptable (continued)
The rule the child develops from having his feelings denied/demolished/annihilated is: **DON'T FEEL** And what is the best way to numb, sedate, deaden, stuff, etc. feelings? FOOD! Either overeating, under-eating, or eating and purging. Purging certainly is a way to get rid of the anger and sadness that this child feels. Divert the feelings inward; it's easier/safer to feel bad about your behavior than about what is causing it. (See Chapter 13 for in-depth discussion.)	
Chronic Anger and Fear	**Anger and Fear That Resolves**
As a result of the lack of communication and the existence of shameful secrets, family members live with a constant level of anger and fear. Anger and fear become a part of the fabric of everyday life to an extent that family members no longer even notice it. However, they pay the emotional and/or physical price associated with constant anger and fear in terms of their health, their relationships outside the family, and their self-esteem. The environment is one of insecurity. An unhealthy family holds onto anger. In this family where it may not be acceptable to express feelings, emotions are given the chance to build up. Rather than releasing feelings and letting them go, members tend to hang on to feelings much longer. An unhealthy family usually accepts anger as an emotion. In fact, it may be the only emotion that parents will openly express. Because of this, an unhealthy household may be full of angry people with angry feelings. There is rarely any understanding of expression of forgiveness. Anger cannot be released in healthy ways but continues to build. Growing up in this family, children learn that it's better to hold on to anger than to work through it and forgive.	The individual family members feel comfortable and safe to be themselves. A healthy family doesn't stay angry for long. Members are encouraged to express their feelings as a way of working through them. Once the feelings are expressed, there is less tendency to hold on to them. Anger is understood to be an acceptable emotion, freely expressed. Working through anger means learning how to forgive someone. At times, fear exists in a healthy family system but it resolves with communication and concern for each other.

Self-Esteem and the Family System

Punishment/Shaming	Discipline/Forgiveness

If a child makes a mistake, she is punished, judged, and shamed. According to Bradshaw, another side of toxic shame will say, "If I can't be human, I'm less than human. I'll be a slob, incest my children, beat them up, rage at them." The polarities of the condition are all or nothing, black and white, perfect or the worst of the worst! According to Bradshaw, when healthy shame is internalized, it becomes toxic and destroys all balance and boundaries. You become grandiose: either the best or the "best-worst." With toxic shame, you are either more than human (super-achieving) or less than human (underachieving). You are either extraordinary or you are a worm. It's all or nothing. You either have total control (compulsivity) or you have no control (addiction). They are interconnected and set each other up.
 	
Debra L. Kaplan writes, "When a child's emotional needs are not met, she will experience shame by way of abandonment. If that emotional neglect endures, then the child will ultimately internalize that shame, along with any unresolved loneliness, pain, and fear. In the presence of physical, sexual or emotional abuse, the child will develop a level of toxic shame that remains a defining element of her inner self. Should the child not address or successfully challenge the shame core, she will carry that shame core into adulthood and, in turn, pass it along to the next generation, where the cycle begins anew."[116]
 	
Shaming has two forms:
 	
Overt (<u>out</u> in the open, obvious, abject):
• corporal punishment (besides inflicting bodily harm, beating up on a child is very shaming.)
• telling a child any of the following:
  – You're worthless, useless, stupid, crazy, screwed up. What is wrong with you? "Labeling a behavior as 'crazy' is a particularly destructive form of emotional abuse that makes you question your reality and intuition. It is almost always present in rigid and shame-based family systems."[117]
  – How could you think that? Where'd you get that idea from?
  – Why aren't you more like your brother, sister, cousin, kid next door or down the street? Comparing the child to other children
	Goal: Self-discipline and responsible behavior. In families that function effectively, grudges are not held very long. Arguments are short and followed by more friendly interactions.
	In healthy families, the fact that everyone makes mistakes is acknowledged and accepted; mistakes are allowed. Perfection is unattainable, unrealistic, and potentially dull and sterile.
	Children are given age-appropriate responsibilities and are not expected to take on parental responsibilities. Discipline in a healthy family is provided by creating guidelines. Children develop feelings of self-esteem, competence, independence, cooperation, and responsibility when they grow up with guidelines.
	
	Reward (praise, nurturing touch, privileges) are used to reinforce appropriate behavior. Rewards help children learn right from wrong.
	
	Punishment is a penalty for purposefully doing something inappropriate. The purpose of punishment/discipline is to reduce the likelihood that inappropriate behavior will happen again— not to hurt children. Punishment is seldom directly related to misbehavior and includes an action that induces discomfort or pain. In contrast, discipline teaches a child acceptable behavior. Punishment/discipline in a healthy family is in the form of loss of privileges, being grounded, parental disappointment, restitution, and timeout.

Punishment/Shaming (continued)	Discipline/Forgiveness (continued)
(usually by a parent struggling with their own feelings of shame) creates shame by mirroring to the child that they always come up short in the comparison. – You're just like your father/mother! – You're not my kid. – You're not good enough. – Shame on you! – I wish I never had you. – Your needs are not all right with me. – Hurry up and grow up! – Be dependent! – Be a man! – Big boys don't cry. – Act like a nice girl (or a lady)! – You lousy rotten kid! (I heard that one a lot!) – You don't feel that way. – Don't be like that! – You caused it. – You owe it to us. – Of course we love you! – I'm sacrificing myself for you. – How can you do this to me? – We won't love you if you . . . – You're driving me crazy! – You'll never accomplish anything! – It didn't really hurt. – You're so selfish! – You'll be the death of me yet! – That's not true. – I promise . . . (Followed by the breaking of that promise.) – You make me sick! – We wanted a boy/girl. – I hope you have a child just like you. – You're killing me! – It's your fault that . . . – You don't measure up. – You're not what we expected. – What did I do to deserve this – You cost too much. – You (*fill in the blank*). **Covert**—hidden, less obvious: neglect, any form of abuse. A parent's role is to be a positive/affirming mirror for feelings, needs and drives. Throughout each stage of development, the parent can either mirror positive/affirming or negative/shaming ways. These early relationships are the key to developing a self-affirming identity, or not.	

Self-Esteem and the Family System

Punishment/Shaming (continued)	**Discipline/Forgiveness** (continued)
In **infancy** (preverbal stage of development) if the parent is unavailable (because of anger, depression, mental illness, divorce, the effects of any addiction, etc.) and does not touch the child, which serves to make the child feel secure, a betrayal of trust occurs when these intrinsic human needs, feelings, and drives are not affirmed.	
In the next stage of development, **early childhood**, if the parent is contemptuous of the child or punishes by withdrawing love, this represents negative mirroring. The message to the child is that she is a burden, a bother, and will be abandoned if the child is not good enough. The child feels like a burden, too much, too heavy, that her needs are too big. This sets up the child to experience shame when abandonment is perceived.	
In **later childhood**, if a parent creates enmeshment with the child by needing the child to be an extension of themselves, the child begins to take responsibility for the parent's comfort and feeling worthless (shame) when that can't be accomplished.	
In **adolescence**, the most self-conscious developmental stage, if there is not the stability, support, validation of the significant adults, the potential for the disruptive consequences of shame is greater.	
An in-depth analysis of shame follows this table on page 333 . (See also the discussion of shame in Chapter 3: Little Food Addict in Training.)	
Unpredictability	**Reliability/Predictability**
If the parent(s) were addicts, gamblers, rageful, depressed, angry, anxious, stressed out, mentally ill, had serious financial issues, etc., the child most likely lived in an emotional minefield. She couldn't count on consistent mood or attitude or behavior. She never knew who would show up as her parent (i.e., the caring, loving, attentive parent or the nasty, angry, mean, abusive, aggravated, frustrated, impatient, intolerant, drunk, high, stoned, violent, uncaring, neglectful, depressed, isolated one.)	In functioning families, parents can be counted on to provide care for their children. Consistent caregiving fosters secure attachment, which allows children to believe their behavior affects their environment. Thus a sense of environmental predictability is established at an early age. Family behavior, interaction, and customs/traditions are consistent and predictable while allowing for spontaneity. In healthy families, these interpersonal connections are stable and predictable even in difficult times. Everyone knows they can count on each other.

Unpredictability (continued)	**Reliability/Predictability** (continued)
And she was always careful, vigilant, trying not to step on a mine and create an explosion. When the explosion did happen, she probably got blamed for it anyway. Alcoholic families tend to be chaotic and unpredictable. Rules that apply one day don't apply the next. Promises are neither kept nor remembered. Expectations vary from one day to the next. Parents may be strict at times and indifferent at others. In addition, emotional expression is frequently forbidden and discussion about the alcohol use or related family problems is usually nonexistent. Due to the nature of addiction, sporadic and erratic behavior on the part of the "addicted person" results in instability within the entire system. Decisions are made whimsically or based on a reaction rather than a proactive course of rational action. All this results in the child feeling insecure, frustrated, and angry. The shaming message with unpredictability is that: • the child's needs don't matter, • the child's feelings don't matter, • the child doesn't matter. • There's no room for the child's needs; they're too big, and she'd better get rid of them. Certainly the rule that the child figures out from living in a mine-field of unpredictability, broken promises, harsh words and the threat of abuse is: **DON'T TRUST!** *"Living with addiction is a traumatizing experience. We freeze, like deer in the headlights, frightened or even terrified as a family member regularly morphs between a kindly Mr. Hyde into a monstrous Dr. Jekyll. And does this trauma send us into a kind of emotional and psychological shut down that mimics denial or in some way contributes to it?"* —Tian Dayton, PhD[118]	Listening to, spending regular time with, playing with, validating, respecting, and empowering a child will build a positive connection. Trust in a healthy family is built by predictability, kept promises, and fulfilled expectations, as well as honesty in communication about events, relationships, and feelings takes place. It is in this sense that Mom and Dad will be there when needed and trusted to respond in a caring way.

Self-Esteem and the Family System

Unhealthy Competition/ Lack of Cooperation	Respect and Cooperation
As discussed by F. Spencer in *Understanding Children: A Parent's Guide*, "The dysfunctional family often operates within a model of scarcity—that there is a limited amount of love, time, money, food, clothing, safety, etc. The members of the family learn that all of these things must be earned through competition. Rather than developing ways of working together, family members pit themselves against each other."[119] This can result in the child competing with her siblings or vice versa. Or a parent competing with the child.	In healthy families, children are consistently treated with respect and do not fear emotional, verbal, physical, or sexual abuse.
	Strong, secure families stress a sense of personal responsibility and appropriate obligation toward others. Such families have the ability to work together and support each other, no matter how busy and hectic individual schedules may be.
An unhealthy family focuses on only one or two people. In this family, the primary focus is on the dysfunction, the dysfunctional parents, or both. All else becomes secondary, making it difficult for the family to function as a unit. These family members can be seen as spokes on a wheel, with the hub being the dysfunctional parent who demands and requires so much time and attention. Since one or two members are usually the focus most of the time, the family can rarely cooperate as a unit.	In healthy families, there is consistent cohesiveness with one another in meaningful relationships that are stable. These families cooperate with each other as a team. The members of that team sees it as a group of individuals who need to cooperate with one another in order to live and grow effectively as a unit.
	Individuals are conscious of commitments made to family members. One person may be the focus of the family at certain times, but not all the time.
Rigid Roles	**Roles Chosen/Flexible**
Roles are assumed by members of the dysfunctional family to allow them to tolerate both the root problem (e.g., dad's drinking, mom's compulsive eating or starving or purging), and the other symptoms of dysfunctions (e.g., non-communication, anger and fear, etc.). These roles are assigned by the system. These roles help the family members maintain the appearance of equilibrium but allow the core reasons for the dysfunction to remain unchallenged.	Each individual chooses their role in the family. Each personality is allowed to flourish and grow without the bondage of dysfunction. Roles are chosen/ flexible because the family system is what protects each member, rather than roles being the protection against the family system.
Because of emotionally destructive enmeshments in these families, the members develop "roles" that furthers the enmeshment and loss of self. The roles of "hero," "scapegoat," "lost child," or "clown/mascot" create an image to maintain. Thus there is loss of being one's true self. The children fear getting close to others for fear of abandonment.	
(See roles described in Chapter 15: Family and the Food Addict.)	

Opposition to Growth	Encouragement of Growth
The dysfunctional family discourages individual growth and rarely nurtures its members. Unhealthy families are usually so wrapped up in the results of the dysfunction that they don't notice or take an interest in each other. What is important to one family member should be important to the focus of the entire family, or else support will most likely not be given. Nurturing may be nonexistent because no one may know how to nurture. Oftentimes, negative behaviors are used in place of encouragement, support, and love. The unhealthy family may view individual opportunities for growth and challenge as disruptive to the routines of the dysfunctional member and will seek to discourage individual growth. Children brought up in homes that discourage individuality learn to keep the focus on others and not on themselves.	A healthy family has room for individual growth and nurtures this growth. While a healthy family cooperates as a unit, it also recognizes that the unit is made up of individuals. It's important to the family as a whole that individuals be allowed to grow and mature. It's also important that individuals are given encouragement, support, and love—all the elements of nurturing—to help in this growth process. The healthy family recognizes the contributions of each member and realizes that being allowed to be themselves is critical to the health and happiness of the entire family. This family knows that when an individual in the family is happy and able to take advantage of an opportunity for personal growth and challenge, then the family as a whole will benefit.
In summary, all of these characteristics leave the child feeling that there must be something wrong with her that makes her parents behave this way, and they feels powerless to change the parents, the family dynamic, and/or themselves. Mistrust of others, difficulty with emotional expression, and difficulties with intimate relationships carry over into adulthood.	In summary, in a healthy family, the child sees herself as part of a whole, unafraid to express her true feelings and emotions, comfortable asking for information and guidance without fear of being shamed. She feels her worth is unconditional. She knows that her opinions are of value and feels respected and encouraged to learn and grow.

Self-Esteem and the Family System

FAMILY RULES
SHAME-BASED RULES VERSUS HEALTHY RULES

Let's take a look at shame-based family rules versus rules in a healthy family. To start, review the following shame-based family rules to see if you relate to any or all:

- Always do the right thing.
- If it doesn't go as you planned, blame someone.
- Always be in control. If you're not, it's your fault; therefore, use whatever works to get back in control again.
- Never talk about it.
- Don't expect accountability or consistency.
- Stay out of touch with your feelings—Deny! Deny!
- It's not okay to talk about problems.
- Don't trust your instincts or other people.
- Unpleasant feelings should not be openly expressed; keep your feelings to yourself.
- Don't ever talk about your negative emotions. (They really don't mean anything; They're a sign of weakness; They're shameful.)
- Don't get angry.
- Don't get upset.
- Don't cry; it shows weakness. (What do you have to cry about anyway? Do something positive instead. No one really cares. It's a turnoff.)
- Emotions? *Pheh!* Ridiculous! You have a home, food, clothes, school—what is there to be unhappy about? (Translation: Don't have emotions.)
- Be seen and not heard.
- Don't ask questions.
- Don't admit you need help—ever, in anything.
- There is no such thing as "needs." That is just self-indulgent.
- Don't think or talk; just follow directions.
- No back talk.
- Don't contradict me.
- I'm always right; you're always wrong.

- Communication is best when it is indirect—don't address issues or relationships directly.
- Don't talk directly to another person; use another family member as a messenger between two others.
- Always be good, strong, right and perfect, or at least act it. Be strong; you are strong; you are a "good horse"; you can handle anything and you have to handle everything because no one can or really wants to help you.
- Make us proud beyond realistic expectations. You have to be the best.
- Be good, "nice," perfect.
- Do well in school.
- You're not doing your best. Do better.
- You aren't as good as everyone else so you have to work harder. Be more, drive yourself to measure up. You are different.
- Don't be selfish; take care of others and their feelings.
- Do as I say, not as I do.
- Avoid conflict (or avoid dealing with conflict).
- If we disagree with each other, we are attacking or abandoning each other.
- It's not OK to be playful.
- It's not OK to shine or excel too much. Never talk about your positive qualities; that's showing off. Never talk about your negative traits; no one wants to know about them. (*Translation:* Never talk about yourself.)
- Don't call attention to yourself. Don't stand out. Don't laugh too loud. Don't cry too loud. (*Translation:* You're not here. You don't exist. You're invisible. You have no voice.)
- You're the one that has to set a good example and you can if you want to. When you don't, it's because you're being rebellious.
- Good behavior won't be rewarded. Rebellious behavior won't be noticed. (*Translation:* You don't exist.)
- Don't rock the boat.
- Disaster is always lurking just around the corner, so tread lightly; be prepared for whatever could possibly happen. (*Translation:* Spend all your time and energy avoiding possible disasters [cover all the bases]).
- Don't make plans. Don't hope, don't dream. It'll never work out anyway.
- Pretend there are no problems.

Self-Esteem and the Family System

- If you show weakness you're a "throwaway," expendable (like a flimsy paper towel).
- Guard the family secrets, don't discuss the family with outsiders—no one must ever know what's going on at home. Present a pretty picture to the outside world. What goes on at home stays at home!
- Don't betray the family.
- The only thing that gets noticed is weight gain. The only thing that gets rewarded is weight loss and good grades.
- Drinking (or other troubled behavior) is not the cause of our problems.
- Everyone in the family must be an enabler.
- Always maintain the status quo.
- You should feel guilty or scared to say "no."
- Nice people are boring.
- Control others by manipulating with threats, fear, guilt, or pity.
- If you need attention, be overly dramatic to get it.
- Set off others' emotional temperatures to see how it is you feel.
- Always be in control. If you control things and people, you will be safe.
- Don't talk about sex.[120]

With unhealthy rules like these, family members learn to believe they're not valued for who they are but only for their ability to live by the unhealthy rules. Growing up in this landscape is choking. It discourages open and honest communication between family members. Since communication is the lifeblood of relationships, these family members often relate ineffectively with one another. They also have trouble relating to people outside of the family.

Such rules also teach family members that being perfect is more important than being real. When they make natural human mistakes, they experience guilt and shame. Their real self, or true self, is no longer acceptable because it is less than perfect. Gradually, they deny their real selves and develop false selves to try to deal with the guilt.

Finally, the rules of dysfunctional families do not allow members to take care of themselves. They sacrifice personal needs for the needs of others or for the needs of the family system. Others may consider it selfish to concentrate on personal wants and needs. And, of course, they see selfishness as negative. And of course, where there is this rigidity, which has the purpose of control, there will be resistance. Who in your family was the "bad" kid—being defiant and breaking the rules (whether overtly or covertly)?

Now, for the other side of the coin, let's take a look at healthy family rules.

HEALTHY FAMILY RULES

Rules in a healthy family system include the following:

- Situations and circumstances are explained to the child (at her level).

- Problems are acknowledged and resolved.

- All members can freely and appropriately express their perception, feelings, thoughts, desires and fantasies.

- All relationships are dialogical (two-way).

- Each person is of equal value as a person.

- Children's developmental limits are taken into account.

- Communication is direct, congruent and sensory based—i.e. concrete, specific and behavioral.

- Family members can get most of their needs met.

- Family members can be different.

- Parents do what they say. They are self-disciplined disciplinarians.

- Family roles are chosen and flexible.

- Atmosphere is fun and spontaneous.

- The rules require accountability and consequences.

- Violation of others' values leads to guilt (it is expected that people will feel guilty if they do not respect another member).

- Mistakes are forgiven and viewed as learning tools.

- The family system exists for the individual's well-being.

- Parents are in touch with their healthy shame.

Self-Esteem and the Family System

333

Tables 14.2 through 14.5 present a useful way to understand shame:

TABLE 14.2. UNDERSTANDING SHAME		
Shame: What Is It?	**Healthy Shame: A Normal Human Emotion**	**Functions of Healthy Shame**
• <u>Who you are</u> is wrong, bad (guilt: <u>what you did</u> was wrong).	• An emotion that teaches us about our limits; it keeps us grounded; it is a "yellow light."	• Keeps us grounded • Affect auxiliary.[122]
• Person feels "seen in a painfully diminished sense."[121]	• The basic "metaphysical boundary" for human beings.	• Healthy inferiority. • Permission to be human.
• The feeling of an awareness that we are painfully deficient or lacking as a human being.	• Allows us to know our limits, and thus to use our energy more effectively. We have better direction when we know our limits; We don't waste energy on goals we can't reach and things we can't change. Allows for energy to be integrated rather than diffused.	• Source of creativity, generativity.[123] and learning. • Healthy guilt. • Connecting behavior and attachment/love.[124]
• Anger and rage can be a secondary reaction. When rage follows the shame experience, it serves to insulate and protect the self against further exposure and serves to alienate others by keeping them away to avoid feeling shame (shame/rage cycle).	• Signals to us that we are not God; we make mistakes; we need help. • Gives us permission to be human. • Shame is the root feeling of humility.	• Awe and reverence; numinous and source of spirituality.[125] • Healthy shame reminds us of our essential limitations—that we are not God—and points us in the direction of some larger meaning.

TABLE 14.3. UNHEALTHY SHAME

Unhealthy Shame: Toxic, Life-Damaging, Dehumanizing Shame	Shame: Originates Via Fracture in the "Interpersonal Bridge"	Shame-Inducing Process
• When healthy shame is transformed into shame as a state of being. • Shame as an identity is to believe that one's being is flawed, that one is defective as a human being. • Requires a cover-up—a false self—where one tries to be more than or less than human. • Feeling which is the source of many difficult inner states: depression, alienation, self-doubt, isolating loneliness, paranoid and schizoid phenomena, compulsive disorders, deep sense of inferiority, inadequacy, or failure. • Narcissistic deprivation. According to Alice Miller most of us don't get our need for love met. By conforming and adapting to their parents' expectations, children unwittingly begin repressing or forsaking their own inner truth. The child develops a false self (overachieving), attempting to gain love by winning approval from others. • Shame internalized when child is abandoned; feelings, needs, and natural instinctual drives become shame-bound: • The necessary affirming mirroring of child's emotions is absent (parents physically present or absent) • Through abuse and neglect of developmental dependency needs, needs become shame-bound • Sexual abuse—shame binds sex drive • Emotional abuse—shame binds feelings • Enmeshment into the covert/overt needs of the parents or the family system needs • Shame-bound. Whenever the person feels any feeling, any need or any drive, they immediately feel ashamed. • School system/religious system—Shaming is an integral part of the school system. Perfectionism denies healthy shame. It denies that we will make mistakes often and that it's natural to make mistakes. The school system promotes a shame-based measure of grading people's intelligence. Many religious systems too teaches the concept that man is wretched and stained with original sin, that nothing man can do that is of any value, that he is flawed and defective, shame-based to the core. Perfectionism is a tool to deem man sinful because he can't measure up to the standard.	• The interpersonal bridge is the emotional bond that ties people together. • Involves trust, vulnerability, an openness • Catalyst for mutual understanding, change, and personal growth • Emotional disruption of the interpersonal bridge has the most significant potential for inducing shame	• Takes place when one's needs are not responded to appropriately by a significant other. • Can be benign or more destructive. • Destructiveness includes disparagement, humiliation, ridicule, or transfer of blame. • Responding appropriately entails having the need understood and openly acknowledged, whether or not it is gratified. • Internalized shame tells you nothing about you is OK. The person feels flawed and inferior; having a sense of being a failure.

Self-Esteem and the Family System

TABLE 14.4. SHAME, IDENTITY, AND TRAUMA

Shame and Identity	What Counts as Trauma?	Stigma as Trauma

• Personal identity is the result of the process of identification.
 	
• Internalization is the link through which identification leads to identity development.
 	
• Identity development involves three dimensions:
  – Internalization of feelings, beliefs, and attitudes from what significant others say.
  – Internalization of the manner in which they are treated by significant others.
  – Internalization of identifications in the form of images, which are generally unconscious (they are taken inside and made their own).
	• Invalidating environment.
	
	• Being heavy in a "skinny-focused" world.
	
	• Being weighed at school.
	
	• Being told you are too big, too fat, too much.
	
	• Overt and covert abuse.
	
	• Being teased.
	
	• Doing the "presidential fitness test."
	
	• Being an "outsider"; pressure to fit into "the image."
	
	• Perfectionism/Shame/Trauma.
	
	• If it leads to internalized, unhealthy shame, it is trauma.
		• Weight discrimination occurs more frequently than gender or age discrimination.[126]
		
		• Weight discrimination has increased 66% in the last decade.
		
		• Peer victimization can be predicted by weight.[127]
		
		• Obese youth who are victimized by their peers are 2–3 times more likely to experience suicidal thoughts and behaviors than those who are not victimized.
		
		• It is the stigmatizing experience (because it induces shame), not the weight itself, contributing to the psychological outcomes.

TABLE 14.5. SHAME SYMPTOMS, CHARACTERISTICS, AND DEFENSES

Shame and Psychological Symptoms	Characteristics of People Who Feel Shame	Defenses for Shame
• Shame is associated with secretiveness; there is a need for increased assertiveness in the face of fame, power, privilege. • Shame is often cited as the buried emotion in eating disorders, compulsive eating, substance abuse, and other addictive behaviors. • It is not easy to get "in" to the buried emotion. • Besides brain chemistry, all addictions are driven by shame, lack of connectedness, and suppressed emotions.	• Frozen speech • Urgency to hide • Profound sense of being alone • Sense of transparency; thinking someone can see through you • People shamed for feelings, get numbed out; experience "affect-shame bind". To feel anything brings more panic. This leads to internal withdrawal; you go numb and become emotionally dead. • "Needs-Shame Bind"—People are shamed for having needs, and therefore don't want to be around anyone and don't know what needs or feelings are. • People who are shamed for thinking and reasoning become dependent on others for decisions and problem solving. They become approval seekers, self-doubters. • To be shame-bound means that whenever you feel any feeling, any need, or any drive, you immediately feel ashamed. The dynamic core of your human life is grounded in your feelings, your needs and your drives. When these are bound by shame, you are shamed to the core.	• Repression: A way to numb out so the emotions are not felt. • Denial. • Grandiosity: Feeling you are better than the rest. • Power: The more power I have (e.g., making money), the less shame I feel. • Overcontrolling behavior: *I'm going to make you _____. If you don't, it's a reflection of me.* • Blame. • Ambition • Compulsivity: Look at me as I want to be, not as I am. • Dissociation: A form of instant numbing involving denial, regression including elements of distracting imagination. • Projection: If I can't own my own needs, I'll put them on you. • Conversion: If I can't own the need to be touched, I'll convert it into something else.

If you identify with some or all of the characteristics of dysfunction to any degree, you join many other food addicts who also identify. You share one thing in common—that you survived these difficult, traumatic, and debilitating experiences. How did you survive? You developed, like I did, rules to live and survive by. It seems so interesting that we all figured out the same basic rules:

- From the Closed Censored Secret family system we developed the rule: **Don't Talk.**

- From the Frozen Feelings and the messages to get rid of feelings, we developed the rule: **Don't Feel.**

- From being Punished/Shamed and living with Unpredictability, in the minefield, we developed the rule: **Don't Trust.**

Of course, the food (overeating, eating/purging, restricting/starving) was the major support for the entire family to hold everything in, zip the lip, stuff the feelings, and not rely on anyone or anything except one's own distorted, delusional thinking, which is, by definition, non-functional, unrealistic, and faulty. The best summary of dysfunctional family rules I've come across is from Alice Miller who calls them **Poisonous Pedagogy**:

1. Adults are the masters of the dependent child.

2. The adults determine in godlike fashion what is right and what is wrong.

3. The child is held responsible for the parents' anger.

4. The parents must always be shielded.

5. The child's life-affirming feelings pose a threat to the autocratic adult.

6. The child's will (spirit) will be "broken" as soon as possible.

7. All this must happen at a very early age so that the child "won't notice/ realize" and will therefore not be able to expose the adult.[128]

These characteristics of dysfunction and its rules send messages of shame to family members that they are not good enough no matter what they do, that they are not really feeling what they are feeling, that expressing feelings is dangerous and inappropriate, that "appearances" mean everything and, if they are physically or sexually abused, that their bodies are not their own. These messages can contribute to the development of a food addiction and/or serve to maintain one that is already present.

In the dysfunctional family, most likely everyone is "using" food to deal with the pain of these shaming messages, either eating to medicate and/or eradicate the feelings of shame, worthlessness, fear, sadness, guilt, powerlessness, inadequacy, and rage; or trying not to eat to feel, deceptive as it might be, a sense of power and control; or eating and (secretly) purging to feel some sense of control and to discharge the rage of *not* being in control.

Children from dysfunctional families are more likely than others to have low self-esteem. (You will see how this is developed as you proceed through the chapter.) They often experience emotional instability, depression, and anxiety. They have difficulty with peers. They are more likely to develop anorexia nervosa or bulimia or binge eating disorder. They are prone toward alcohol or chemical dependence. And they are more likely to attempt suicide.

As we describe a dysfunctional family, it can be seen to be an indictment of the parents. But it's not meant to be. Parents did the best they knew how to do. If you have children, you know that you love them. You loved them when they came into your life, and as time went on, you continued to love them, even though at times you didn't like them.

Most parents love their kids and genuinely want what is best for them, yet that message often becomes convoluted, inconsistent, and sometimes nearly nonexistent when addiction, mental illness, or other major stressors begin to infiltrate the family system. Maybe the parents lacked the ability to consistently show that love. If they did not love their kids, it was because they didn't know how to love; it was not because of the children. They wanted it to be different, but they did not have the ability to make it different, nor were they able to ask for help or accept help. Think about those moments (maybe few) when your parent(s) showed you care and attention. The problem is that this dysfunction, these messages/behavior patterns have been passed down from their parents to them to you, and most likely it goes back for generations. Maybe in an attempt to deal with their own functional deficits, there was an overfocus on appearance and dieting. The point is that these intergenerational, passed-down messages, and behavior patterns that are abusive and shaming are:

Inadvertent

Unconscious

Unintentional

These messages weren't meant to beat up on the child. It's just that everyone is caught in the dysfunction. This understanding, though, is not meant to relieve the caregivers of having the responsibility for providing

Self-Esteem and the Family System

good care and healthy nurturing and not fulfilling their responsibility, but to show how they did not do their job. They did not fulfill their responsibilities as parents.

"WHY? WHAT DID I DO?"

Quite a few years ago, I had the privilege of facilitating an early recovery food addiction group for ten ultra-orthodox Jewish women for two years. These women were strong, responsible, caring, overworked, sometimes overwhelmed, and very committed to their faith. They were wonderful, and I loved being with them and working with them. They worked very hard to achieve and live in abstinence. These women belonged to a community of Hungarian and Romanian Hasidic Jewish Holocaust survivors and their descendants. They came from difficult European backgrounds with histories of oppression and poverty.

They were very challenged by their lifestyle and responsibilities, which required them to constantly be involved with meal planning and meal preparation for their very large families. They used food for comfort and relief from their stressful and demanding lives, which had many rules they had to live by, including—especially—rules, expressed and implied, against expression of feelings.

During many of our group sessions, there were discussions about the clients' feelings surrounding their relationships with their many children. During one particular session where we were talking about communication within their families, I asked one of the group members, Chava, if she ever told one of her sons that she loved him. She nervously answered, "Ooh, No! I couldn't do that!" Note that these women came from generations of loss, extreme efforts to survive persecution, to survive in general, and heroic attempts to keep their faith and traditions alive. Their culture is not one that fosters the acknowledgment of feelings, let alone their expression. In part, their food addiction was fueled by their inability to know and express their feelings, so they use food to numb, medicate, stuff, and deaden them.

When Chava said she couldn't tell her son she loved him, it became clear what her assignment had to be for the week. If I remember correctly, upon hearing her assignment, she closed her eyes, raised her eyebrows, took a deep breath and said, "OK."

When the group came together the next week, I asked everyone about how they did with their various assignments. When it was Chava's turn, she sheepishly told the group that she tried to find the right moment to talk with her son but couldn't bring herself to do it. The group was supportive and identified with her and expressed understanding of how hard it was for her. I told her that she had to

> repeat the assignment. She took more deep breaths and shared that she understood how important it was for her to succeed and how impossible it felt.
>
> The following week, Chava related her renewed efforts to the group, stating that she waited for the right opportunity to be with her son, Aaron, in the right place at the right time. He was standing in the kitchen, and she was sitting at the kitchen table, and she said, "Ari," and he said, "Yeah, Ma?" She then courageously blurted out, "I love you!" and he answered, "Why, what'd I do?" Chava and the entire group were silent and then couldn't stop talking about how sad they felt for having given their children the message that they had to DO something in order to be loved.
>
> Think back: Did you ever hear "I love you" or "I don't like your behavior—but I love you"? Was your message that you had to DO something in order to get the "I love you" or "You're loved" message?

SELF-ESTEEM

Now let's connect our discussion of dysfunctional families to the concept of "self-esteem." Self-esteem has two components. First, the idea of <u>self</u>:

- An individual person as the object/subject of their own reflective consciousness.
- The union of elements (body, emotions, thoughts, and sensations) that constitute the individuality and identity of a person.
- Having a distinct personality.

The second part of the concept, "<u>esteem</u>," can be defined as:

- To have a high opinion of; to hold in high regard.
- To look upon with appreciation and/or respect.
- To have value and worth.

The implication is that "self"-esteem needs a strong, solid, positive sense of self, which does not develop growing up in a dysfunctional family. The experience of surviving in this type of family renders the food addict—the food addiction developed as a mechanism to survive living in this family—"self"-less. Without much of a self, "esteem" has no base or foundation to attach to. Add to that, addiction, which brings its own level of shame to layer on top of the toxic shame one experienced in their dysfunctional family, further drives down "self" to low depths.

All addicts experience self-esteem issues—food addicts especially, because of the nature of their behavior, and the failed attempts at control find them-"selves" lost in the abyss of a shameful, fraudulent existence. Another thought is that many (food) addicts actually lack a sense of self that goes far beyond low self-esteem. They do not "know" their authentic selves and are unable to recognize or properly express their true feelings. While we are using food, it is impossible to have a clear sense of self, and without clear sense of self, it is impossible for a person to relate to another human being in an open and honest relationship. This is one of the reasons 12 step programs advise against starting a romantic relationship during the first year of recovery.

The "self" gets lost when we people please or assess other people's needs and turn ourselves into pretzels to be what we think they need us to be. Then there is no individual with a distinct personality. We become a part of other individuals and their personality. When in your life did you get the message you were not allowed to be an individual with a distinct personality? Or perhaps you were brought up in a home where you could only be an individual as long as it was what your parents had decided you would be. If you didn't comply, you were chastised and rejected. When was the last time you had a high opinion of yourself and looked upon yourself with appreciation and respect, and felt like a worth-while human being?

The flip-side of low self-esteem is arrogance and grandiosity. The person believes they are above or better than other people. In some family systems, children are taught to see others' mistakes and to find fault with others. They tend to believe that they are superior to others, giving them a false sense of power. In these families, the children are treated as if they can do no wrong.

Regardless of the type of esteem that codependents display, it is not self-esteem. (For a discussion codependency, see page 298.) It is better defined as **other-esteem**. It is based on external things—how they look, who they know, how large their salary is, how well their children perform, the degrees they have earned, or how well they perform activities. The codependent person becomes a human "doing" rather than a human "being." Their esteem is not self-based; it is based on the opinions of others. The problem with other-esteem is that its source is outside of the person and thus vulnerable to changes beyond the codependent's control. Other-esteem is fragile and undependable.

When we people-please or just are not honest about what we think and how we feel in situations, our feelings of being worthwhile and having appreciation and respect for ourselves are just not there. What is there is anger and the feeling that we have no value and are unimportant.

Just know that there is not much "self" in existence at this point. The little food addict lacks a cohesive sense of self. So the idea of self-care, which should be developing, is nowhere on the horizon; it just doesn't exist.

SELF-CARE

The concept of self-care is an important one because it totally relates to one's willingness/ability to follow a plan of eating, which requires planning, shopping, preparing, cleaning up, and being involved in a recovery process, which includes attendance at 12 Step meetings and being connected to others in the recovery process.

It is impossible to teach self-care to a child who is unwilling to delay gratification because she is terrified of abandonment. Self-esteem, on the other hand, makes the child confident that abandonment does not lie waiting in the shadow of delayed gratification.

Teaching self-care may appear to a child as the withdrawal of his parents' support. M. Scott Peck, in his book *The Road Less Traveled*, says that self-care is impossible unless the child feels that she is valuable: "The statement 'I am a valuable person' is essential to mental health and is a cornerstone of self-discipline [delayed gratification]."[129]

It's no wonder that putting down the food and becoming abstinent is so much of a challenge; for many of us, it's the equivalent to "leaving home." Becoming abstinent/embracing abstinence is all about self-care, which, in effect, is making the statement that, "I'm leaving home. I know Mom is not going to do it for me. I have to care for myself. I have to give up the illusion that she'll take care of me. I'm willing to grow up!"

In the article "Fear of Abandonment: Some Lessons from M. Scott Peck and Pia Mellody" by Lawrence S. Freundlich on the Meadowlark website, we learn a valuable insight: An infant is totally dependent on her parents for fulfillment of her needs, and the child expects that the world exists for that purpose. This instinctual expectation of immediate satisfaction is unreasoning, uncivilized, and innocently selfish. She totally lacks the skills for self-care and has no conception that the environment has no other purpose than to care for her. She demands everything, and if it is refused or unavailable, she will presume that she is being abandoned.

According to Peck, young children, if they are to emotionally survive, must learn "delayed gratification." Peck equates delayed gratification with discipline, the discipline forced on every child when she recognizes that she is part of a social system and not "God the Baby." As stated in the article: "Self-care, or the ability to recognize that you will get what you want only if you do some of the job yourself, is learned in the face of the child's basic desire to be totally cared for—'I want what I want and I want it now.' The parental challenge is to teach the child discipline without implying abandonment. In order for a child to grow up, she has to learn that delayed gratification is not the same as abandonment—a big order for a child growing up in a dysfunctional family."[130]

According to Pia Mellody, self-esteem is the first core issue. She says that when we believe we are valuable, we do not have to depend on the opinions of others to verify our value. We are in touch with our inherent worth. Then, because we value ourselves, caring for ourselves becomes an act of self-esteem, because it is natural to care for someone we like.

I think it's useful to note that Pia Mellody points out in her book, *Facing Love Addiction*, the only proper use of the word "abandonment" is in the context of childhood. The child who is without the ability to self-care can, indeed, be abandoned—left with no resources. Adults, who have presumably learned to care for themselves cannot be abandoned; adults have resources even when they are rejected or disappointed in relationships. Adults are responsible for their own self-care.

Developing Healthy Self-Esteem

According to Pia Mellody, healthy self-esteem is created within an individual who knows that she has inherent worth that is equal to others' worth. It cannot be altered by her failings or strengths, which Mellody calls a person's humanity. Parents who are able to affirm, nurture, and set limits for their children without disempowering or falsely empowering them create children who can functionally esteem themselves.

So we can say that self-esteem is evident in an individual with a distinct personality and a high regard and opinion of herself, treating herself with appreciation and respect and feeling worthwhile.

If we don't treat ourselves with appreciation and respect and we don't consider ourselves worthwhile, how will anyone else get the message that we are?

We teach people how to treat us. It depends on our boundaries or lack thereof, what we will tolerate and put up with. If we are "doormats" for others, we will be treated that way. If that's the case, is it any wonder we are so often taken for granted and feel we are last on their list? When were you first on your own list? In *Facing Codependence,* Pia Mellody[131] writes:

> "Children learn to self-esteem first from their major caregivers. But dysfunctional caregivers give their children, verbally or nonverbally, the message that the children are 'less-than' people. These 'less-than' messages from the caregivers become part of the children's own opinion of themselves. Upon reaching adulthood, it is almost impossible for those raised with 'less-than' messages to be able to generate the feeling from within that they have value."

The codependent individual relies on others to determine their worth or gets it from comparing themselves to others, so their self-esteem does not question their own worth or value.

So we've examined the problem "self-esteem" through the lens of dysfunctional family systems, shame, and survival rules. How can it change? How can we get self-esteem? Of course you're probably thinking, *esteemable acts or changing old behavior.* Good answer, but there's more. The following idea was presented to me when I was taking a course on the psychobiology of alcoholism.

When I first saw it, I didn't understand it. Maybe you'll have the same reaction. The way to self-esteem is **IMPULSE CONTROL.**

Babies are in a primitive stage of being. They need instant impulse gratification. Waiting or delaying having needs met is a more mature, grown-up state of being. When adults surrender themselves through impulse gratification, there is guilt, anger, fear, despair, shame, and a loss of self and of self-esteem. I'd like to explain this in the form of two scenarios. The premise of these is that you've been to at least one 12 Step meeting of any fellowship.

Scenario 1

You're sitting at a fairly large 12 Step meeting. There's a speaker who starts sharing their story, telling what happened, what it was like, and what it's like now (it's called "qualifying"). As they're speaking, you're amazed at how much you identify with their story, but more than that, they're almost telling your story but with a different perspective and different insights than you've had. As you're listening, you're feeling very touched and moved and even changed by having a new clarity about your history. You feel very filled and uplifted, actually overflowing with new understandings about yourself.

The speaker ends, there's applause, and then the chairperson asks for a show of hands.

You feel an overwhelming need to share what you've just heard and experienced and you start to raise your hand, and at the same time, the **"Itty-Bitty Shitty Committee"** in your head starts telling you:

- *Don't bother, it will come out stupid.*

- *Other people have more important things to share.*

- *You'll make a fool out of yourself.*

- *Everyone will know you're an embarrassment.*

- *They won't understand you; you won't be able to explain your experience.*

- *You'll be judged and be found unworthy.*

- *No one wants to hear you. You don't matter. You don't make a difference*

- *Don't bring attention to yourself*

- *You don't belong here; you're separate.*

- *No one cares; no one's interested.*

So, your committee wins and you pull your hand down. The meeting ends and you walk out feeling . . . what do you think? Disappointed, angry at yourself, sad, less than, hopeless?

Scenario 2

This is the exact same scenario as number one. This time you have a different response to your **"Itty-Bitty Shitty Committee."** This time, for some reason, you're able to overcome the pressure of the committee and you send your hand way up. I believe that when you triumph in this struggle, a light goes on around you and you'll always be chosen. You share, it's okay—you make sense, you get your point across, and you're able to let the people in the room know what you felt. The meeting ends and how do you think you would feel? Proud of yourself! Pleased with yourself. Maybe . . . SELF-ESTEEM?

Because you resisted the IMPULSE to follow your dysfunctional rules of: 1) **Don't Talk, 2) Don't Feel, and 3) Don't Trust.**

By sharing, you broke the **Don't Talk** rule; by sharing about and exploring your feelings, you broke the **Don't Feel** rule; and by sharing your feelings in front of others, you broke the **Don't Trust** rule by sharing a real part of yourself with other people. Wow, what a stand against your history! Even if you experienced some "share shame" afterward, the act of sharing made a dent in the armor of your maladaptive survival defenses. Every time you go against your rules, you will heal in some fashion, and, at a minimum, experience some self-esteem.

WHAT IS "SHARE SHAME"?

Share shame is a term that was coined in 12 Step programs to explain the feeling of shame that washes over a person who has just shared openly in a group of people, some feelings, and/or thoughts. The subsequent thinking that "What I said was stupid," "I didn't explain_____ well enough," "I made a fool of myself," or "OMG, why did I say that?" gives rise to feelings of humiliation. It is common to have these feelings and thoughts, and they will continue if these feelings and thoughts are kept a secret. What a relief to find out that others identify with this experience!

Becoming abstinent, following the food plan, and going to meetings, which are acts of good self-care, is all about breaking these rules. It presents the only opportunity to truly recover—to reclaim your true "self."

According to Pia Mellody in *Facing Codependence*, "Healthy self-esteem is the internal experience of one's own preciousness and value as a person. It comes from inside a person and moves outward into relationships. Healthy people know that they are valuable and precious even when they make a mistake, are confronted by an angry person, are cheated or lied to, or are rejected by a lover, friend, parent, child, or boss."

These feelings of preciousness and value are born out of abstinence! They cannot exist if one is still in her addiction and abusing herself with food.

AFFIRMATIONS FOR HEALING

Many of us in recovery, especially in early recovery, as clarity begins to take hold, become aware of the internal dialogue that serves to dampen our spirits and contaminates our joy. These self-critical messages and insults often seep into much of our waking moments. This internal attack is an accumulation of stored-up negativity that came to us at a young age, maybe from parents, teachers, or even bullies on the playground. Because children don't have clear emotional boundaries, these messages lodge themselves in our limbic brain and we play them back on a regular basis. Then we become our own abusers, perpetuating the shaming messages of our childhood.

We have to keep in mind that the recovery is not just from the food addiction, but from everything that happened to set us up for the illness.

Positive affirmations serve to feed our brain with different thoughts in order to see the world in a new way. They are the antidote to the toxic messages in our limbic brains. See the list of positive affirmations at the end of this chapter on page 350.

In *Daily Affirmations: For Adult Children of Alcoholics,* Rokelle Lerner explains that our storehouse of shame accumulates over a lifetime and it takes more than a couple of times using this tool (affirmations) to change the neuronal firings in our limbic brain. But with proper and regular use, within a month's time, we can expect to start feeling better; the "voices" get quieter and we start feeling more optimistic and energized.[132]

For healing to take place, it is essential to practice patience, persistence, compassion, and discipline. These are all the ingredients we would hope for in a loving parent.

In essence, by using this tool, we're learning to re-parent ourselves. Not only that, but we're taking charge of our own healing and relieving others of the responsibility of doing this for us.

How we feel about ourselves dictates how we behavior, operate, recover and how we relate to others. The development of self-esteem is an internal one. Real self-esteem stands firm against outside forces. It is knowing our rights as a human being and upholding healthy boundaries. The following essays, which I have accumulated over the years from anonymous sources unless otherwise specified, offer some insight.

* * *

My Bill of Rights

I have the right to be treated with respect.

I have the right to say no and not feel guilty.

I have the right to experience and express my feelings.

I have the right to take time for myself.

I have the right to change my mind.

I have the right to ask for what I want.

I have the right to ask for information.

I have the right to make mistakes.

I have the right to do less than I am humanly capable of.

I have the right to feel good about myself.

I have the right to act only in ways that promote my dignity and
self-respect as long as others' are not violated in the process.

Love Unlimited

* * *

Statement of Personal Rights—Boundaries

<u>Physical Boundary (external boundary)—Protects my body</u>
I have the right to determine when, where, how, and who is going to touch me and how close to me they are going to stand.

<u>Sexual Boundary (external boundary)—Protects the sexual aspects of my body</u>

Self-Esteem and the Family System

I have the right to determine with whom, where, when, and how I am going to be sexual.

<u>Emotional Boundary</u> (internal boundary)—Protects my feelings
My reality (what I think and feel, do or don't do) is more about me and my history than what you are saying or doing or have said or done in front of me. And conversely, your reality (what you think and feel and do or don't do) is more about you and your history than what I am saying or doing in front of you.

I am not responsible for your reality, but I am responsible for noting the impact of my behavior on you. If I have offended you by punching through your boundary system, I am accountable for the effects on you.

<u>Intellectual Boundary</u> (internal boundary)—Protects my thinking
I have the right to think what I want to think. I need only face the consequences of my own thinking. I have the right to decide if information is true, not true, or questionable and to choose to act or not act on the basis of that decision. I need only face the consequences of my choices and actions.

<u>Spiritual Boundary</u> (internal boundary)—Protects my spiritual life
I have the right to think and believe the way I choose about God or my Higher Power. I know that my faith or lack thereof is mine and I do not have to justify it to anyone. I am responsible to live within the bounds of my spiritual beliefs and accept the consequences when I do not. I have a personal relationship with the God of my understanding.

<u>Financial Boundary</u> (internal boundary)—Protects my financial life
I am responsible for my finances. My worth as a person has nothing to do with how much or how little money I have. My relationship with money is simply as a medium of exchange. I know that there is always enough. I love me for who I am, rather than what I have.

* * *

As a Person, I Have the Right to . . .

Be myself.

Refuse requests without feeling selfish.

Be competent and be proud of my accomplishments.

Feel and express anger.

Ask for affection and help. (I may be turned down, but I can ask.)

Be treated as a capable adult.

Be illogical in making decisions.

Make mistakes—and be responsible for them.

Change my mind.

Say "I don't know."

Say "I don't agree."

Say "I don't understand."

Say "I don't care."

Offer no reasons or excuses for justifying my behavior.

Have my opinions respected.

Have my needs be as important as the needs of others.

Tell someone what my needs are. (They may not care to do anything about it.)

Judge my own behavior, thoughts, and emotions and be responsible for their initiation and the consequences upon myself.

Judge if I am responsible for finding solutions to other people's problems.

Take pride in my body and define attractiveness in my own terms.

Grow, learn, change, and value my age and experience.

Sometimes to make demands on others.

* * *

Positive Affirmations

These affirmations are offered as a tool to aid in replacing the negative messages of the past with positive messages of recovery.

1. I am a unique and precious human being, always doing the best I can, always growing in wisdom and in love.

2. Just for today, I will respect my own and other's boundaries.

3. I am in charge of my own life.

Self-Esteem and the Family System

4. My number-one responsibility is my own growth and well-being. The better I am to me, the better I will be with others.

5. I refuse to be put down by the attitudes of opinions of others.

6. I make my own decisions and assume the responsibility for any mistakes. However, I refuse to feel shame or guilt because of them.

7. I am not my actions. I am the actor. My actions may be good or bad. That doesn't make me good or bad.

8. I am not free as to the things that will happen to me. But I am 100% free as to the attitude I have toward these things. My personal well-being or my suffering depend upon my attitudes.

9. I do not have to prove myself to anyone. I need only to express myself as honestly and effectively as I am capable.

10. I am free of animosity or resentment.

11. My emotional well-being is dependent primarily on how I love me.

12. I am kind and gentle toward me. I am whole and good. I am enough.

13. I deserve to be treated with consideration and respect.

14. I live a day at a time and do first things first.

15. I am patient and serene, for I have the rest of my life in which to grow.

16. Every experience I have in life—even the unpleasant ones— contributes to my learning and growth.

17. No one in my world is more important than I am.

18. My mistakes and non-successes do not make me a louse, a crumb, or whatever. They only prove that I am imperfect—that is, "human." And there's nothing wrong with being human.

19. Just for today, I will be vulnerable with someone I trust.

20. Just for today, I will take one compliment and hold it in my heart for more than just a fleeting moment. I will let it nurture me.

21. I am not alone; I am one with God and the universe.

22. I am a precious person.

23. I am a worthwhile person.

24. I am beautiful inside and outside.

25. I love myself unconditionally.

26. I can allow myself ample leisure time without feeling guilty.

27. I deserve to be loved by myself and others.

28. I am a child of God and deserve love, peace, prosperity, and serenity.

29. I forgive myself for hurting myself and others.

30. I forgive myself for letting others hurt me.

31. I forgive myself for accepting sex when I wanted love.

32. Just for today, I will act in a way that I would admire in someone else.

33. I am loved because I deserve love.

34. I am willing to accept love.

35. I am whole and good.

36. I am capable of changing.

37. I am enough.

* * *

Risk Taking Is Free

To laugh—is to risk appearing the fool.
To weep—is to risk appearing sentimental.
To reach out for another—is to risk involvement.
To expose feelings—is to risk exposing your true self.
To place your ideas, your dreams before the crowd—is to risk their loss.
To love—is to risk not being loved in return.
To live—is to risk dying.

Self-Esteem and the Family System

To hope—is to risk despair.
To try—is to risk failure.
But risk must be taken, because the greatest hazard in life is
   to risk nothing.
The person who risks nothing does nothing, has nothing, and
   is nothing.
He may avoid suffering and sorrow, but he simply cannot learn,
   feel, change, grow, love, live.
Chained by his certitude, he is a slave, he has forfeited freedom.
Only a person who risks . . . is free.

* * *

The Unbroken

Rashani Réa, 1991, founder of
Kipukamaluhia Eco-sanctuary in Hawai`i

There is a brokenness
out of which comes the unbroken,
a shatteredness
out of which blooms the unshatterable.
There is a sorrow
beyond all grief which leads to joy
and a fragility
out of whose depths emerges strength.
There is a hollow space too vast for words
through which we pass with each loss,
out of whose darkness we are sanctioned into being.
There is a cry deeper than all sound
whose serrated edges cut the heart
as we break open
to the place inside which is unbreakable
and whole,
while learning to sing.

* * *

My Declaration of Self-Esteem

Virginia Satir

I am me.

In all the world, there is no one exactly like me. There are persons who have some parts like me, but no one adds up exactly like me. Therefore, everything that comes out of me is authentically mine, because I alone choose it.

I own everything about me—my body, including everything it does; my mind, including all my thoughts and ideas; my eyes, including the images of all they behold; my feelings, whatever they might be—anger, joy, frustration, love, disappointment, excitement; my mouth, and all the words that come out of it, polite, sweet, or rough, correct or incorrect; my voice, loud or soft; and all my actions, whether they be to others or myself.

I own my own fantasies, my dreams, my hopes, my fears.

I own all my triumphs and successes, all my failures and mistakes.

Because I own all of me, I can become intimately acquainted with me. By so doing, I can love me and be friendly with me in all my parts. I can then make it possible for all of me to work in my best interests.

I know there are aspects about myself that puzzle me, and other aspects that I do not know. But as long as I am friendly and loving to myself, I can courageously and hopefully look for the solutions to the puzzles and for ways to find out more about me.

However I look and sound, whatever I say and do, and whatever I think and feel at a given moment in time is me. This is authentic and represents where I am at that moment in time.

When I review later how I looked and sounded, what I said and did, and how I thought and felt, some parts may turn out to be unfitting. I can discard that which is unfitting, and keep that which proved fitting, and invent something new for that which I discarded.

I can see, hear, feel, think, say, and do. I have the tools to survive, to be close to others, to be productive, to make sense and order out of the world of people and things outside of me.

I own me, and therefore I can engineer me.

I am me and I am okay.

* * *

The Golden Eagle
Anthony de Mello, The Song of the Bird

A man found an eagle's egg and put it in the nest of a backyard hen. The eaglet hatched with the brood of chicks and grew up with them.

All his life the eagle did what the backyard chickens did, thinking he was a backyard chicken. He scratched the earth for worms and insects. Her clucked and cackled and he would thrash his wings and fly a few feet into the air like the chickens. After all, that is how a chicken is supposed to fly, isn't it?

Years passed and the eagle grew very old. One day he saw a magnificent bird far above him in the cloudless sky. It floated in graceful majesty among the powerful wind currents, with scarcely a beat of its strong golden wings.

The old eagle looked up in awe. "Who's that?" he said to his neighbor.

"That's the eagle, the king of the birds," said his neighbor. "But don't give it another thought. You and I are different from him."

So the eagle never gave it another thought. He died thinking he was a backyard chicken.

Often it is easier to think of ourselves as "backyard chickens" because that is the way we were treated and told we were.

Our goal is to be able to see ourselves as we truly are. That can only happen when you are living in abstinence.

* * *

Who Is The Enemy?

Who is the enemy? We carry him around with ourselves wherever we go. He robs us of our dignity, self-worth, hopes, and freedom. He destroys our potential for happiness, fulfillment, and human growth. He stands as a barrier between ourselves and other human beings. Who is the enemy? The enemy resides within all of us to some degree. The enemy is our own negative self-image and low self-esteem.

Our self-image can be our best friend or worse enemy, depending on its strength or weakness. The need for a positive identity and healthy self-esteem is common to all human beings. This need includes the fundamental achievement of self-acceptance, self-respect, self-confidence, self-reliance, and self-worth. Knowing and believing that our self-image can change for the better is the first step in the human growth process. It is no exaggeration to state that acquiring a positive self-image and authentic self-esteem is essential to self-worth and healthy personal adjustment.

It is essential for self-esteem that we never forfeit appreciation for ourselves and our sense of self-worth. To maintain our self-approval, we must continue to work to achieve our values and human potential. If we keep our self-approval, no matter what other objects of value we may lose, we will still be rich. In an ever-changing and depersonalized world, we must build sufficient self-confidence and self-reliance to weather life's storms and to ward off assaults to our self-esteem.

Obviously, it is impossible to go through life without some negative experiences, experiences that can create self-doubts and put questions in our minds about our abilities and sense of self-worth. These kinds of life circumstances can contribute to a negative self-image and low self-esteem if we let them. Blows to our self-respect and self-esteem can heal more slowly than do bodily injuries and can leave scars that are even more lasting. It is through the building of a more positive self-image and self-esteem that we can meet the many challenges of life and fulfill our basic needs of self-worth, self-acceptance, and personal happiness. We can conquer the enemy of negative self-image and low self-esteem by achieving out potential self—by becoming what we can become.

CHAPTER 15
Family and the Food Addict

In Chapter 2, I illustrated and described the process by which the "Little Addict in Training" becomes a full-fledged addict. We looked at the influence of the family in launching and supporting a fragile and susceptible, vulnerable child into (food) addiction. Now we want to unveil the particulars of the experience of this little being in terms of her positioning in her family. An understanding of the different roles available to this child and what happens when and why she settles into one or more of those roles is critically important, because it sets the stage for the child's beliefs about the world and herself as she grows into adulthood.

A member of Adult Children of Alcoholics, a wonderful 12-Step program, wrote the following with regard to childhood in an alcoholic home:

"From what I can remember of my childhood and from what I have heard at meetings, many families of alcoholics [addicts, including food addicts] seem to live every day with a mixture of intense anxiety and deep, resigned sadness. Often this forms an undercurrent that nobody dares speak of directly. Indeed, many of these miserable, crumbling families try very hard to maintain the pretense that theirs is an acceptable, normal, or even superior family life. Absolute loyalty to this crazy belief system is then made compulsory for the children. Any unhappiness that ever is openly expressed has to be blamed on other targets of opportunity, ones that don't contradict or hit back. Many of us became these targets, and our identity became frozen in this stigmatic role.

The unacknowledged, unmet needs within us could be so readily manipulated; most of us would have made even greater sacrifices if they would have made the family whole. Many of our brothers and sisters came to believe that they really were the problem and did not survive the guilt. Many of us still live in fear of imminent total blame in any situation. We may find it hard to believe that this force, which once nearly killed us, does not objectively exist.

. . . From a child's point of view, however, the pretense of responsibility helps keep a sense of fairness, order, and hope intact. Powerlessness in a disorderly emotional universe threatens us far more than steady, featureless, permanent self-hatred.

. . . Personal autonomy depends largely on how a person develops; rarely did our parents provide much of a model. Alcoholics often have what they think is a very clear sense of order and hierarchy, which they maintain through deadly assaults on the self-esteem of the people closest to them."

Growing up in an environment where there is no understanding and no sense of being known or that you matter is essentially growing up in a wasteland. There is no feeling of safety or being anchored –being unmoored and adrift. The focus is on survival rather than the family being a soft place to land. What an empty state for a child to live in!

The following is, in part, discussed in an article about codependency from the Treatment4Addiction website.

"The family is a system with each individual affecting the other. All the parts are linked and react and interact with each other. It is a system just as the human body is a system. For example, if an individual were to fracture a bone, the other parts of his or her body would have to adjust to prevent putting pressure on the hurt limb, and so the system is then organized around the injury and its adjustments. In the case of alcoholism and addiction, mental illness, or other major problem creating high stress, the family system organizes itself around the disease, and all members are profoundly affected and take on roles or positions that allow them to feel safer and lessen the tension.

Any system is made up of three components:

1. individual parts

2. linked together

3. to accomplish something that no individual part could accomplish on its own

In a family, the parts are the family members. They are linked by rules and boundaries and by their emotional investment in one another. The primary goal is to maintain balance within the system in order to survive."

For any system to function, it must be guided by rules governing how the parts interact, roles that each part assumes in contributing to the

Family and the Food Addict

whole, and other aspects. When the family system operates in unhealthy ways, because one of the parts is "broken" or "sick," it supports maladaptive behavior and the development of addictions.

When problems and circumstances such as parental alcoholism, drug addiction, food addiction, gambling, rage, mental illness, child abuse (emotional, physical, or sexual), or extreme rigidity and control interfere with family functioning, the effects on children can sometimes linger long after these children have grown up and left their problem families. People who grow up in dysfunctional homes and reach adulthood without dealing with the effects of a non-nurturing/abusive childhood are called "adult children." According to Claudia Black, a Ph.D. and addiction recovery expert:

> "In an addictive or depressed family system, the disease becomes the organizing principle. The affected person becomes the central figure from which [around which] everyone else organizes their behavior and reactions, usually in what is a slow insidious process.
>
> "Typically family members do what they can to bring greater consistency, structure and safety into a family system that is becoming unpredictable, chaotic or frightening. To do this they often adopt certain roles or a mixture of roles."[133]

Original work regarding family roles was by Virginia Satir, then adapted by Claudia Black and Sharon Wegscheider-Cruse to fit the addictive family. Over the course of years, the labels vary, yet the descriptions still fit. This chapter is based on the work of these experts, especially the work of Sharon Wegscheider-Cruse. Our discussion here examines a family system where one of the parents, if not both, is in a lot of pain, particularly if addiction is present. Do not dismiss a parent suffering with food addiction; it creates the same dysfunctional dynamics that alcohol, drug addiction, sex addiction, gambling, and mental illness do.

As Sharon Wegscheider-Cruse notes, the family where addiction is present tends to deny in a much greater way what is happening to them than the family where there is no addiction.[134] As we know, denial is an integral part of the disease of addiction. And the family members have a much harder time choosing to change because of the compulsive reactions they learn to have to a person who is compulsively using a substance, including food.

A major need for all people, addict and non-addict, is to feel safe. In the dysfunctional, unhealthy families, which the previous chapter discussed in depth, it's clear that the territory within the family is unsafe and scary. Family members treat the person with the addiction with "kid gloves" to avoid arguing or physical violence. The family members may be frightened for their safety because the addicted person is unpredictable.

Various roles, which are discussed in the following sections, offer the children a way to find a position of some modicum of safety. If you are an only child, you will probably identify with all the roles. If you have siblings, you will most likely see them in these various roles. The following is a model; you may fit perfectly within it or you may see yourself and your siblings in parts, here and there. In any event, it is very important for you to see where and how you do fit into your family to understand more of yourself and your behavior and to be able to change. Please keep in mind that in a dysfunctional family system, most likely everyone is "using" food to deal with their discomfort, frustration, fear, anger, shame—in fact, all their feelings.

CHARACTERISTICS OF THE PARENTS/CAREGIVERS IN THE ADDICTED FAMILY

The Addict

The parent(s) who has become the addict is using a substance and/or behaviors to medicate their feelings. Because of the illness of addiction, the addict experiences feelings of inadequacy, guilt, fear, anger, and hurt. As self-worth diminishes because of feelings of inadequacy, the addict becomes more and more perfectionistic and demanding of those around them. The perfectionism also gives rise to rigidity. As the addictive disease progresses, there is more and more blaming, which pulls the family into the disease. Family members lose trust in one another as the addict experiences lapses in memory and doesn't keep commitments or promises and is unpredictable in their behavior. The addict, in response to the family criticism, begins a process of withdrawing from the family system.

Tables 15.1 to 15.6 present an at-a-glance picture of each family member in their various roles.

Family and the Food Addict

TABLE 15.1. THE ADDICT AT A GLANCE							
Addict	Addict's Behavior	Inner Feelings	Family Members' Feelings	Characteristics	Future Characteristics Without Help	Future Characteristics With Help	Needs in Recovery
Affected person	Rigid Blaming Perfectionism Withdrawing Anger Lying Abusive Hiding	Pain Shame Inadequacy Guilt Fear Anger Loneliness Sadness, Grief Low Self-Esteem Self-Hatred Secrets	Guilt Self-Hatred Helplessness Hurt Loneliness Rejection Low self-worth	Grandiosity Intellectualizes Sarcastic Self-Righteousness	Blackouts Hallucinations Delusion Insanity Distorted Reality Death	Heightened awareness Gutsy Sensitivity to pain Empathy	Need to get out of their head; not intellectualizing Develop awareness of how others feel To become flexible. To work through problem. To express anger without blaming.

The Prime Enabler

The person closest to the addict, most attached to them, is the first person who is directly affected by the addict's illness. Usually we're talking about a spouse or parent, the witness to the self-destructive behavior of the addict and who can see the addict's pain. The spouse may or may not say, "Can't you see what you're doing to yourself?" and is thwarted or ignored because the addict can't see what the spouse sees. The spouse begins to feel rejected and left out. This is the beginning of the spouse's disease of enabling or codependency.

Enabling is doing for others what they are capable of doing for themselves. When a person/addict is enabled, they are prevented from experiencing the consequences of their own actions. By enabling the person/addict, the addict is discouraged from learning from their own mistakes which, in turn, prevents them from realizing they have a problem.

The enabler reacts to the symptoms of the dependency disease in such a way that the addict is shielded from experiencing the consequences of his or her behavior. Shielding occurs when the enabler becomes overly careful in what they say and do so as not to upset the addict and cause more drinking or using or to get the addict angry. Enabling behavior will eventually come in conflict with the enabler's basic values (e.g., honesty). When it does, the enabler develops anger and resentment toward the addict.

The spouse becomes fearful of confronting the addict, saying what they really see and what they really believe, fearful that the addict may leave them. The spouse begins to mirror the addict's belief that the right way to live is to keep their feelings bottled up inside.

The enabling process parallels the downward progression of the dependency disease. As the addict/user's behavior becomes more and more self-destructive, the enabler experiences increased feelings of guilt, shame, and low self-worth.

We know so well that "food" (eating/not eating, eating/purging) is an effective method to find relief from the pain of this situation—to deal with the painful feelings and to try to numb out. In so many families with addiction, we find the addict's significant other looking to food for relief and comfort.

The spouse works hard and takes on the responsibility of keeping up with everything, trying to hold the family together. Many times, they will take a first or second job to pick up the slack. They also try to keep the family "looking good" by making excuses, filtering out what's happening between the parents, not wanting the children to know, not letting the neighbors know, keeping up a front, protecting the addict, shielding the addict from the outside (e.g., job, school, extended family), and becoming overly responsible.

Within this family system, the enabler is the recipient of most of the blaming and begins to experience physical and emotional pain. They try so hard and they don't seem to do anything right.

Unspoken family rules that foster codependent behavior are:

- Don't talk about problems.
- Don't express feelings.
- Don't trust ("Do as I say, not as I do").
- Don't be "selfish"; take care of others and their feelings.
- Don't talk directly to another person; let someone act as a messenger, instead.
- Don't play or be playful.
- Don't rock the boat.

Codependents find themselves mostly identified with the following internal struggles. See if you identify with any of the following statements. Answer yes or no for each.

Are You Codependent?

1. I have lived with someone with an alcohol, drug, or eating problem.

2. I have lived with someone who has hit me or belittled me.

3. I guess at what normal [behavior] is.

4. I suffer from denial. (It used to be thought that only the addict in the family was in denial. What is known today is that all members of the alcoholic/dysfunctional family suffer from denial. Denial is about unawareness. While being "unaware" protects them from the pain, it also keeps the dysfunction going.)

5. I often make decisions for others but have a terrible time making decisions for myself.

6. I have difficulty forming and maintaining close relationships and have grown to expect, often from experience, people to leave me.

7. I fear rejection and abandonment, yet I am rejecting of others.

8. I have an unhealthy dependence on relationships. I will often do anything to hold on to a relationship, to avoid the feelings of abandonment. I am extremely loyal even in the face of evidence that loyalty is undeserved.

9. I have to be "needed" in order to have a relationship with others.

10. I tend to confuse love and pity, with a tendency to "love" people I can pity and rescue.

11. I tend to attract people with many problems in hopes that I will help to "fix" them and help them live happily ever after.

12. I am hypersensitive to the needs of others. (Survival in a dysfunctional family frequently means being constantly aware of the most minor shifts in moods of adults, leading the child to be far more aware of what others were doing and feeling than what was being felt inside.)

13. I have a compelling need to control others. (Fearing normal feelings leads to compulsive needs to control and live life "in a constant rehearsal for living."[135]

14. I believe most other people are incapable of taking care of themselves. I think people in my life would go downhill without my constant efforts to take of them and their responsibilities.

15. I am either super responsible or super irresponsible, and sometimes both.

16. I have an exaggerated sense of responsibility for the actions of others. I believe I am responsible for other people's feelings and/or behaviors.

17. I lack trust in myself and/or others.

18. I minimize, alter, or deny how I truly feel.

19. I have difficulty identifying my own feelings; my sense of how I "feel" is in response to the feelings and/or behavior of others. (Expressing feelings or allowing feelings is often not safe or comfortable in the dysfunctional/alcoholic family. Children often are only allowed particular feelings—"happy," "fine," etc. If other feelings are expressed, they risk abandonment or angry outbursts from parents. Because they learned to numb out feelings in early childhood, they have lost the ability to feel or express emotion. Frequently good feelings, such as excitement, joy, and happiness, are sacrificed, as well as feelings of anger or sadness. Some can cry but never allow feelings of anger; others can allow anger but never risk tears.)

20. I tend to be very critical and judgmental of myself (I judge myself without mercy). I fear criticism and judgment yet I criticize and judge others.

21. I have difficulty setting goals for myself, placing the needs of those around me first.

22. I have low energy from the "struggle" of living.

23. I have an extreme need for approval and recognition. I constantly seek approval and affirmation. I'm always worried about others' opinion of me.

24. I have a fear of being my real self. (If a person is liked, they feel that "I'm fooling you," because children from dysfunctional families early

Family and the Food Addict

on learn to please and relate to the world with acceptable images rather than true selves. There tends to be a felt discrepancy between what is felt inside and what is shown outside, thus leading to the belief that "if others really knew me, they wouldn't like me.")

25. I have a tendency to become hurt when people don't recognize my efforts.

26. I use sex to gain approval and acceptance.

27. I do not perceive myself as a lovable or worthwhile person. I have a poor self-image and struggle with self-worth.

28. I have a compulsive need to be right. (Life is thought of in terms of "right" and "wrong." Often the need to be always correct, appropriate, and "right" replaces an original desire to be loved.)

29. I live in a black-and-white world. (It is as if the addiction/dysfunction kills all the gray cells in the brain, leaving only the black and white. Rigidity and black-and-white thinking are learned from the parents.)

30. I have problems/difficulty with intimacy/intimate relationships/ boundaries.

31. I have repetitive relationship patterns. (Internal beliefs and filters lead adults from dysfunctional families to pick spouses and friends whose behavior replicates their childhood interactions with parents. They frequently find themselves re-creating the painful experiences of their childhood. Why? They are drawn to what is familiar and to what is known. There is a sense of the need to overcome, of, for example, "trying to get my father to not drink or to love me." So, they pick an alcoholic to marry. Children from healthy families work out childhood traumas in the playroom, while children from dysfunctional families find themselves working out painful traumas of the past in real life.)

32. I have difficulty/feel embarrassment receiving recognition and praise/compliments or gifts. I have difficulty hearing the positives. (Because of poor self-images developed in childhood, children from dysfunctional families either discount positive feedback from others, feel a sense of distrust for those complimenting them, or feel a deep sense of pain or loss upon hearing positive things about themselves.)

33. Early in life, I developed the attitude that I have no needs; I can do it myself, thank you. I, therefore, do no ask others to meet my needs or desires.

34. I have grown up with a sense of total helplessness or a sense of total control. (Frequently, these children gain this control in their lives by believing that they caused the responses and behaviors of others. They may feel the victim's feelings and try to rescue one parent from the other. This creates, paradoxically, both a sense of helplessness as well as an inordinate sense of control over their environment.—e.g., "It's my fault that Mom and Dad drink. If I was only better . . ." (See the discussion about caretaking in Chapter 3: Little Food Addict in Training: An Illustration of How Food Addiction Develops.)

35. I have trouble asking for help.

36. I have poor communication skills.

37. I fail to recognize my accomplishments.

38. I compromise my own values and integrity to avoid rejection or others' anger.

39. I have a sense of guilt when asserting myself.

40. I am uncomfortable expressing my true feelings to others. I value others' opinions and feelings more than my own and am afraid to express differing opinions and feelings of my own.

41. I have trouble saying "no" when asked for help. I put aside my own interests in order to do what others want.

42. I value others' approval of my thinking, feelings, and behavior above my own.

43. I have developed patterns of placation, seeking approval, or isolation when faced with conflict because of fears of destructive anger or threat of violence experienced in my childhood, and also because of fear of my own unexpressed rage.

44. I keep quiet to avoid arguments.

45. I am often angry.

Family and the Food Addict

367

46. I often lie/am often dishonest when it would be just as easy to tell the truth. I lie out of self-preservation and usually about my feelings.

47. I have difficulty following projects through from beginning to end.

48. I overextend myself. I have a tendency to do more than my share, most of the time. I often have so many things going at once that I can't do justice to any of them.

49. I manage my time poorly and do not set my priorities in a way that works well for me.

50. I have problems with my own compulsive behaviors and addictions. (Often, in attempts to continue delaying grief and pain from the past, adults from dysfunctional families work compulsively, spend money, eat/starve, exercise, indulge in sex, gamble, become addicted to relationships, or behave in other compulsive ways. Sadly, many adult children begin their own patterns of compulsive drinking or drug use.)

51. I have a need for perfection. I judge everything I think, say, or do harshly/without mercy as never "good enough." I often feel inadequate. I feel like a "bad person" when I make a mistake.

52. I fear failure but sabotage my success.

53. I am uneasy when my life is going smoothly, continually anticipating problems.

54. I feel more alive in the midst of a crisis. I seek tension and crisis, then complain about the results.

55. I avoid conflict or aggravate it; rarely do I deal with it.

56. I am impulsive. I tend to lock myself into a course of action without giving serious consideration to alternative behaviors or possible consequences. (This impulsivity leads to confusion, self-hatred, and loss of control over their environment. In addition, such people spend an excessive amount of energy cleaning up the mess. Because of the turmoil and unpredictability in their early lives and subsequent survival roles developed, they frequently find themselves more comfortable with chaos than with quiet times. Keeping the chaos going or involving themselves in professions where turmoil exists frequently staves off unresolved grief of the past.)

57. I look for immediate, as opposed to deferred, gratification.

58. I care for other people easily yet find it hard to care for myself.

59. I isolate myself from other people.

60. I have difficulty talking to people in authority, such as police or my boss. I respond with fear to authority figures and angry people.

61. I accept sex when I want love.

62. I am confused about who I am or where I am going with my life.

63. I doubt my ability to be who I think I want to be.

64. I am a rigid person; I have difficulty adjusting to change. I overreact to changes over which I have no control.

65. I have difficulty relaxing, letting go, having fun. (While other children were busy learning to relate, compete, play, and develop social skills, children of dysfunctional families were learning the tough lessons of survival. Living becomes more difficult than continued survival, and playing or having fun becomes terrifyingly stressful. The child inside is terrified still of making a mistake or doing it wrong. Letting go means being out of control.)

66. I tend to take myself very seriously. Consequently, I am overly sensitive.

67. I overreact to changes over which I have no control.

68. I usually feel that I am different. (Terminal uniqueness is the "disease"/belief that "certainly no one is going to understand my behavior or problems.")

69. I feel rejected when my significant other spends time with friends.

70. I feel humiliation when my child, spouse, or parent makes a mistake.

If you answered yes to a number of these, you probably are codependent to some degree. (This last one, number 70, brings to mind some experiences with my father, a simple man not so well versed in the rules of etiquette; when he made a faux pas in public, I would die inside, particularly since my sharp-tongued mother would be right there with ridicule.)

Living in this family becomes a minefield, not just for the spouse/

Family and the Food Addict

369

enabler, but for all family members. They are all caught up in the struggle to survive in a family that's experiencing great emotional pain and stress. As a result, they can develop unproductive, compulsive behaviors. Feelings are not expressed openly, and problems are not discussed directly. Unhealthy rules develop and are perpetuated. Family members learn to believe they're not valued for who they are, but only for their ability to live by these unspoken, unhealthy rules. These rules can develop in response to many types of family problems, such as mental illness, terminal disease, or a handicapped family member. An unhealthy system always develops when one member is alcoholic, chemically dependent, a gambler, or has food addiction.

You may have sought out professional help and/or 12-Step programs to recover from these impediments to living a satisfying, happy, and fulfilling life. If you are still "using" food as a way to cope with these difficulties, the help you look for in therapy or 12-Step programs won't be nearly as effective as it would be if you were abstinent.

TABLE 15.2. THE PRIME ENABLER AT A GLANCE

Role	Visible Qualities	Inner Feelings	What He/She Represents to the Family	Characteristics	Future Characteristics Without Help	Future Characteristics With Help	Needs in Recovery
Enabler (Spouse, Parent, Friend, Coworker)	Physically sick Super-Worker Super-responsible Low self-worth Self-Pity Self-Blaming Haughty Makes more choices and decisions to compensate for the victim's lack of power	Pain Anger Hurt Fear Guilt Shame Low Self-Worth	Provider Responsibility	Martyr "Furious but with a smile on face" Manipulative	Physical and emotional breakdown	Loving Nurturing Self-fulfilling Accepting Forgiving	Let go of responsibility Get in touch with feelings Refocus on self (wants and needs) Become aware of self responsibility and let others do the same Deal with anger w/out blaming or falling apart

SURVIVAL ROLES/ADAPTIVE FAMILY ROLES OF THE CHILDREN

The Hero

The behavior of the older (or eldest) child is different from that of the other children because this child relates more often to the parents and less with the other children. As this is the first child, the marriage changes into a family. This child does not have an automatic peer group as the other children do. They do not have another child to model after. Consequently, older and only children role-model those they are closest to—the adults; they become like little adults. That's why they tend to mature earlier and walk and talk earlier.

In healthy, functional families, children bond and attach to their parents through their feelings, their emotions. Since in the dysfunctional family, there isn't much of a feeling life happening between the parents, they're unable to express their feelings back to the child. And since this child role-models after the parents, the child learns to do what they do: Keep your feelings inside and find some kind of behavior to get relief from the pain that they feel. Certainly food helps the enabler to tolerate their pain, and the "Hero" follows suit.

This older/eldest/only child seeks the approval of the parents because without the healthy, necessary experience of bonding, she feels very alone. This child unsuccessfully tries to change what's happening in the home and soon experiences feelings of inadequacy and guilt. They're the "good kids" who get good grades, become sports heroes, and do great things to make up for the lack of emotional closeness.

Because they didn't have power to change the dynamics of their parents' relationship and were never able to feel close to their parents, they work hard for parent's and teachers' approval to prove that they're worth something, that they're okay. They tend to be successful in their lives. That in itself becomes a trap, because they learn that how they get on with people, how they do well, and how they have any self-worth at all is to work for someone else's approval.

These children tend to go into the helping professions, such as social services, teachers, medical, etc. With the help of food and other compulsive behaviors, as these children perform, do well, and become more and more successful, they turn off more and more of their own feelings. They tend to marry addicts and have children who become addicted because

TABLE 15.3. THE HERO AT A GLANCE

Role—The Mode of Survival	Child's Visible Qualities/Traits: Outside Behavior	What Is Not Seen: Child's Inner Feelings and Responses to Feelings	What Child Represents in the Family and Why They Play Along	Characteristics: Strengths and Deficits	Child/Adult Adaptation Without Help and Beliefs That Drive Behavior	Adult Adaptation With Help	Needs in Recovery
Family Hero Super Kid Usually oldest child	"The little mother" "The little man of the family" Good kid Helpful at home Always does what's right Over-achiever Over-responsible Works hard for approval Non-feeling Serious, not much fun Adult-like Extra mature Helpful within the family and successful outside the family Makes good grades Appreciated by others	Feels responsible for the family pain and tries hard to make things better Inadequacy Guilt Hurt Confused Never good enough Lonely Fearful Angry Low self-esteem Can't do enough Can't do it right Hides feelings **Response to Feelings** "I must stay in control of my feelings."	Provides for family: Self-Worth, Pride Successful child must mean successful family/ parents Someone to be proud of	High achiever High grades Friends Sports **Strengths** Successful Organized Leadership skills Decisive Initiator Self-disciplined Goal-oriented **Deficits/Vulnerabilities** Perfectionistic Difficulty listening Inability to follow Inability to relax Lack of spontaneity Inflexible Unwilling to ask for help Undue fear of mistakes Inability to play Severe need to be in control	Workaholic Never wrong Marries a dependent person Need to control and manipulate Responsible for everything Compulsive Can't say no Can't fail Problems in 30s **Beliefs** "If I don't do it, no one will." "If I don't do this, something bad will happen, or things will get worse."	Good executive manager Can accept failure Relaxes Lets go of controlling others Be responsible only for self OK to say "No"!	Learn to ask for and take what he/she needs. Learn to accept failure Let down, relax, and be. Focus on self Stop "fixing" family

they are willing to keep their own feelings and needs inside and take care of everyone else—which is role-modeling after the prime enabler.

Scapegoat

Usually the next born quickly understands that they can never measure up to the first child, who's getting the approval of the parents and gives the parents most bragging rights. As a result, the next born feels sort of emotionally bruised and hurt, and to have any self-worth at all, this child has to emotionally reject the family. In doing so, this child develops a particular kind of behavior to get attention and focus from the family and is seen as "the bad kid" or "the acting-out kid."

In general, a child would rather be praised than punished, but rather be punished than ignored. This child discovers that acting out bring some attention, albeit negative.

This child, in order to find some relief, goes outside the family for any kind of relief, and often attaches to a peer group, especially a chemical-using peer group. This provides the child with a pseudo-family that provides the acceptance not felt in their own family, and the chemicals used in this group give them short-term relief for the pain they feel in their familial rejection.

For an adolescent girl, pregnancy offers her parental attention of a sort for a while and it gives her something to love, which makes up for the lack of love and affection she feels at home.

If these youths are using chemicals, it interferes with their ability to learn, and they show up as low achievers in school. Again, this behavior gets them (negative) attention from the school and their parents. So what has been building in this child is defiance, their cover for their hurt. Defiance is a way of saying, "Notice me! I hurt. I will hang onto my poor choices because it's the only thing I have. I don't have any other self-worth."

The despair these young people feel makes them high suicide risks.

Lost Child

The child that arrives after the "hero" who's getting the positive attention and after the "scapegoat" who's getting the negative attention doesn't quite know how to get in with the parents and begins to believe in their own unimportance. This child doesn't know how to hook up with this

TABLE 15.4. THE SCAPEGOAT AT A GLANCE

Role—The Mode of Survival	Child's Visible Qualities/Traits: Outside Behavior	What Is Not Seen: Child's Inner Feelings and Responses to Feelings	What Child Represents in the Family and Why They Play Along	Characteristics: Strengths and Deficits	Child/Adult Adaptation Without Help and Beliefs That Drive Behavior	Adult Adaptation With Help	Needs in Recovery
Scapegoat Problem Child May be second child	Rebellious family member who "acts out" the family's pain and is focused on as the troublemaker. Chemical use. Values peer group. Hostile. Defiant. Rebellious. A screw-up. Withdrawn. Sullen. Angry. Puts on a "tough act." Acts out. Troublemaker. May try to compete with the hero but loses out. Stops trying to please family. Runs with peers who are like her. Fails in school	Hurt. Guilt. Abandoned. Lonely. Anger. Rejection. Inadequacy. Low self-worth. No self-esteem. Feels left out of family. Feels like a misfit. Needs attention but can't ask for it. **Response to Feelings** "I am angry about it, whatever it is."	Takes focus off addict. Parents focus on scapegoat instead of own dysfunction. "She's the problem!"	Gets negative attention. Won't compete with "family hero." **Strengths** Creative. Less denial, greater honesty. Sense of humor. Close to own feelings. Ability to lead (just in wrong direction). **Deficits/Vulnerabilities** Inappropriate expression of anger. Inability to follow direction. Self-destructive. Intrusive. Irresponsible. Social problems at young ages, e.g., truancy, teenage pregnancy, high school dropout. Addiction. Underachiever. Defiant, rebellious	Chemical use. Unplanned pregnancy. Trouble maker in school and later in office. Intimacy problems. Job loss. Prison, Trouble. **Beliefs** "If I scream loudly enough, someone may notice me." "Take what you want. No one is going to give you anything."	Accept responsibility. Courageous. Risk taker. Good under pressure. Ability to see reality. Has good insight. Helping professional	Get through anger to the hurt. Learn to negotiate instead of rebel

TABLE 15.5. THE LOST CHILD AT A GLANCE

Role—The Mode of Survival	Child's Visible Qualities/Traits: Outside Behavior	What Is Not Seen: Child's Inner Feelings and Responses to Feelings	What Child Represents in the Family and Why They Play Along	Characteristics: Strengths and Deficits	Child/Adult Adaptation Without Help and Beliefs That Drive Behavior	Adult Adaptation With Help	Needs in Recovery
Lost Child May be third child	Does not form close connections with other family members and spends much time alone or quietly busy Loner No close friends Daydreamer Solitary (alone) Rewards self with food Withdrawn Aloofness Ill at ease with others Drifts and floats through life Not missed Quiet Shy Ignored; unnoticed May read, listen to music or look at TV a lot Tries not to be a bother	Unimportant Not allowed to have feelings Loneliness Hurt Abandoned Defeated Inadequacy Fearful Angry Has "given up" Fantasies Feels different Feels like an outsider Low self-worth Feels forgotten **Response to Feelings** "Why should I take the risk to feel? It's better if I don't."	Easy to ignore Relief; at least one kid not to worry about	"Invisible" Quiet No Friends Follower Trouble making decisions Attaches to things, pets, reading **Strengths** Independent Flexible Ability to follow Easygoing attitude Quiet **Deficits/Vulnerabilities** Unable to initiate anything Withdraws Fearful of making decisions Lack of direction Ignored, forgotten Follows without questioning Difficulty perceiving choices and options	Isolated Indecisive Little zest for life Has no fun Can't be intimate Promiscuous or stays emotionally alone Can't say no Often dies early/ suicide **Beliefs** "If I don't get emotionally involved, I won't get hurt." "I can't make a difference anyway." "It is best not to draw attention to yourself."	Independent Talented and creative Imaginative Assertive and resourceful	To reach out Deal with loneliness Face pain Make new, close relationships

Family and the Food Addict

family and becomes plagued with loneliness. They go outside of the family but do not connect with a peer group. They have no model to use, so they begin to consistently withdraw and become loners and tend to become shy. They learn neither how to make friends nor to become intimate. Their performance at school is poor; they hold back because of their shyness and low self-worth, even though they are often bright children and are often misdiagnosed as having a learning disability. To make up for their lack of relationships with people, they treasure things, such as computers, TVs, electronic devices, toys, and pets. This child develops stress-related illnesses, much like the enabler. They often develop asthma, allergies, and other physical illnesses, and can be bed-wetters. These children most often find comfort in food.

Mascot

The younger or youngest child finds herself in this role. Because this child is the youngest, people tend to protect her and tell them very little about what's happening in the family. However, this child can feel the hurt and pain of the family members who are covering up their feelings with their dysfunctional behavior. This child doesn't know that one parent is lost to addiction, that both parents are in deep conflict with each other because of the addiction, but they do feel the overall tension and emotional pain. This child feels fearful, anxious, and tense because they feel it in the family, but since they have very few of the facts, the child feels crazy. They tend to develop phobias (e.g., of the dark, being abandoned, babysitters, being alone, afraid of going to school), because they can't trust reality. As a result, these kids become hyper, discharging the family feelings and often being misdiagnosed as having ADHD. The hyperactivity gets them the attention they want and need but it becomes a trap, as the other behaviors of the other children in the family become a trap for them.

Their way of fitting in and attracting attention is through teasing, humor, acting out, and being silly and/or obnoxious at school. Like the other children, they are using food (the sugars and quickly converted carbs) for comfort and relief and numbing and, as we discussed earlier, they experience cycling blood sugar levels which, along with their position and experience in the family, diminishes their ability to focus and concentrate. Because of their difficulty in concentrating and paying attention, they become slow learners and poor achievers.

TABLE 15.6. THE MASCOT AT A GLANCE

Role—The Mode of Survival	Child's Visible Qualities/Traits: Outside Behavior	What Is Not Seen: Child's Inner Feelings and Responses to Feelings	What Child Represents in the Family and Why They Play Along	Characteristics: Strengths and Deficits	Child/Adult Adaptation Without Help and Beliefs that Drive Behavior	Adult Adaptation With Help	Needs in Recovery
Mascot Clown Maybe youngest child	Uses charm, humor, or ill health to get attention Teasing, being silly, clowning, acting out as way to discharge a lot of the internal fear and tension Super-cute Immature Anything for a laugh or attention Happy-go-lucky Funny Anxious Fragile Family regards them as being in need of protection Disruptive Hyper-energetic Keeps focus on self Slow learner; finds it hard to focus on any one thing Class "cut-up," class clown	Low self-esteem Fear/Terror Anxiety Confused Lonely Inadequacy & unimportance Insecure May feel crazy **Response to Feelings** "I must take the pain away."	Comic relief Fun Humor Distraction Discharges the painful feelings in the family	Hyperactive Learning disabilities Short attention span **Strengths** Sense of humor Flexible Able to relieve stress and pain of others **Deficits/ Vulnerabilities** Attention seeker Distracting Immature Difficulty focusing Poor decision- making ability	Ulcers Can't handle stress Compulsive Compulsive clown Attention needer People pleaser Cut-up Marries another family's "hero" for care Always on verge of hysterics or mania Instead of learning how to develop relationships with people, they learn how to joke with people **Beliefs** "If I make people laugh, there is no pain."	Take care of self No longer clown Charming host and person Good company Quiet wit Good sense of humor Independent Helpful	To take responsibility Risk being serious Assertiveness

Family and the Food Addict

As they grow older, such people continue the same behavior as a way to get attention, with stories and clowning around. The fact that no one takes them too seriously is a price they pay as adults.

Check off which traits you identify with. Are they clustered within one role or do you relate to parts of different roles?

I specifically identify with two of the roles (hero and lost child), and my brother fits perfectly in the other two (scapegoat and mascot).

Which role(s) do you connect with? Write them down on a piece of paper.

Many of us often say that what happened in our childhood is in the past, over and done with. We say, "The past is the past and it has nothing to do with the present!" How wrong that is. The reality is that we carry the behaviors from our roles with us into adulthood *and* we re-create new systems around us where we can continue a pattern that feels safest:

- The family hero feels safest as caretaker and provider.

- The scapegoat feels safest when defending themselves and being hostile.

- The lost child feels safest when not in close relationships.

- The mascot feels safest if she can keep others laughing.

The common fear for all members of these families is that people will find out how they feel. There is also a common set of characteristics that adult children develop as the result of growing up in a family with alcoholism/addiction and dysfunction, that interfere with being a successful, happy adult enjoying life. Understanding and accepting these characteristics, examining their roots, and becoming abstinent will allow for learning better ways of living and are critical in the process of recovering from them.

Janet Geringer Woititz, author of *Adult Children of Alcoholics,*[136] identified the characteristics as follows.

Adult children:

1. Guess at what normal is.

2. Have difficulty in following a project through from beginning to end.

3. Lie when it would be just as easy to tell the truth.

4. Judge themselves without mercy.

5. Have difficulty having fun.

6. Take themselves very seriously.

7. Have difficulty with intimate relationships.

8. Overreact to changes over which they have no control.

9. Constantly seek approval and affirmation.

10. Feel that they are different from other people.

11. Are either super responsible or super irresponsible.

12. Are extremely loyal, even in the face of evidence that such loyalty is undeserved.

13. Are impulsive; they look for immediate as opposed to deferred gratification.

14. Lock themselves into a course of action without giving serious consideration to alternate behaviors or possible consequences.

15. Seek tension and crisis but then complain about the results.

16. Avoid conflict or aggravate it; rarely do they deal with it.

17. Fear rejection and abandonment, yet they are rejecting of others.

18. Fear failure, but sabotage their success.

19. Fear criticism and judgment, yet readily criticize and judge others.

20. Manage their time poorly and do not set their priorities in a way that works well for them.

HOW THE FOOD ADDICT AFFECTS THE FAMILY

Did you ever tell yourself, or do you tell yourself, that your behavior with food—overeating/undereating, binge eating, starving, purging—only affects you and no one else? If you did or do, you're wrong. Those family members around you who love you (even though you may not feel it) are deeply affected by seeing you hurt yourself with food and by your unavailability to them.

As examined in the previous discussions on self-esteem and the little food addict in training, as people who are dealing with eating issues, we're the product of generations of parents dealing with feelings and

Family and the Food Addict

situations through adaptive behaviors, i.e., escapism. By now, you have probably identified how your parents and other family members used food, alcohol, drugs, and other preoccupations to deal with life, and in doing so, role-modeled unhealthy and unrealistic coping skills for you.

Maybe the only time the family members, especially your parent(s), talked to you or each other was during mealtime. Maybe that was the time that you felt noticed or that you belonged in the family. Maybe that's when and how the family members related to each other: through food, sharing, offering, and allowing you to choose foods, meals, restaurants, and so on.

You may also have had many feelings about your parents and home life that you felt embarrassed, shamed, or guilty to talk to anyone about. Without you realizing it, these same dynamics got passed on to your own adult self and families.

Just as you were deeply affected and damaged by the dysfunctional, addictive behaviors of your parents—because they were suffering with addictions, including food, mental illness, or other preoccupations—you also have an impact on your family of origin and the family you created.

Our families have feelings about our eating problems. They have also seen us use unhealthy and unrealistic coping skills.

There is also a great deal of confusion in the homes where there is an eating problem. No one knows what's wrong, and no one is making the connection. The overeater or starver or purger experiences numerous mood swings, and the family is never sure how the person is going to react to anything. They begin to see themselves as the problem. They tend to walk on eggshells or simply throw up their hands and emotionally withdraw from trying to communicate. This may show up as arrogance or passive silence.

Many families are ashamed at the overweight and/or underweight person and neglect to make them aware of functions and invitations from work or school. The eating problem becomes a family problem. Incentives are offered for weight loss, promises are made ("I promise I'll lose weight this time."), threats are made ("This starving has gone far enough, you will sit here until you finish your meal."). Worry can become the preoccupation of the family. Now everyone is addicted—the problem eater to her eating, purging, or starving, and the family to the problem eater and their inability to stop. Take a look at Table 15.6.

TABLE 15.6. SYMPTOMS OF FOOD ADDICTION AS A FAMILY ILLNESS

Addicted Family Member	Codependent Family Member
1. Increased tolerance for overeating (mostly refined/processed carbs), purging, starving.	1. Increased tolerance for unacceptable behavior.
2. Unwillingness to discuss issues.	2. Unwillingness to discuss issues.
3. Medicating feelings.	3. Denying "stuffing" feelings.
4. Neglecting responsibilities.	4. Taking on responsibilities.
5. Trying to control eating.	5. Tries to control addict.
6. Compromising values.	6. Compromises values.
7. Isolating from family.	7. Isolates socially.
8. Focusing on eating/not eating.	8. Focus on addict.
9. Physical problems.	9. Physical problems.
10. Spiritual crisis; loss of hope and options.	10. Spiritual crisis; loss of hope and options.

Ask yourself, *What has been the effect on me and my family?*

As a result of becoming abstinent and coming into recovery, the declarations in the following Bill of Rights will begin to be realized.

Bill of Rights for Adult Children of Addicts/ Dysfunctional Families

I have the right to make other choices besides the choice merely to run away.

I have the right to say "no" when I feel unready or unsafe.

I have the right not to be molested by fear.

I have the right to feel all feelings.

I have the right to believe I'm probably not guilty.

I have the right to make mistakes.

I have the right not to smile when I cry or feel hurt.

I have the right to terminate conversations with those who put me down or humiliate me.

I have the right to be healthier than those around me without feeling guilty.

I have the right to change and grow.

I have the right to be relaxed, playful, and frivolous.

I have the right to set limits and be selfish.

I have the right to get angry, even at someone I love, without fearing that I and the other person, and/or the relationship, will dissolve.

I have the right to do stupid things without believing I am a stupid person.

I have the right not to be ashamed for what I don't know or can't do.

* * *

Comes the Dawn

Veronica Rodriguez

After a while you learn the subtle difference between
holding a hand and chaining a soul;
and you learn that love doesn't mean leaning . . .
and company doesn't mean security.

You begin to learn that kisses aren't contracts,
and presents aren't promises.
And you begin to accept your defeats with your head up
and your eyes open, with the choice of a woman,
not the grief of a child.

And you learn to build all your roads on today, because
tomorrow's ground is too uncertain for plans,
and futures have a way of falling down in mid-flight.

After a while, you learn that even sunshine burns
if you get too much . . . so you plant your own garden
and decorate your own soul . . . instead of waiting for someone else
to bring you flowers.

And you learn that you really can endure, that you really
are strong, and you really do have worth, and you learn,
and learn . . . with every good-bye, you learn.

This profound wisdom become part of true recovery. They are a natural evolution of the self-esteem that emerges from putting down the addictive behaviors with food and allowing feelings and facing life.

PART FOUR

Treatment and Recovery

CHAPTER 16

12 Step Food Recovery Fellowships and Relapse Prevention
Tools of Recovery

Food Addiction is a disease of isolation. The food addict cannot recover on her own—she must join other food addicts on the journey to recovery, the Road of Happy Destiny.
—DIANNE SCHWARTZ

Recovery is switching from a lifestyle centered on eating, bingeing, eating and purging, restricting, starving, and weight and/or body image issues to a lifestyle centered on healthy living. And that is only possible if the food addict is committed to her recovery, which means following the food plan and meetings, meetings, meetings, and involvement in the 12 Step food fellowships. In time, as the food addict becomes comfortable in food recovery and starts to learn about, understand, and discover herself, her recovery process may require her to seek out other 12 Step programs to further their work on herself—e.g., Al Anon, Debtors Anonymous, Survivors of Incest Anonymous, etc.

It has been said in the 12 Step food fellowship rooms that the program is not really a bridge back to life, but rather a tunnel to another 12 Step program, as the recovering addict develops further insight into other issues.

Recovery means healing.

"The natural healing force within each one of us is the greatest force in getting well."
—HIPPOCRATES

To heal, you must take action. Action is doing something. Thinking about doing it, telling yourself you'll do it someday, or hoping you'll heal spontaneously are *not* actions; they are self-deceptive thoughts. Healing requires hard work. Hard work is facing your own fears and changing your belief systems.

Beliefs are ideas you accept as being true and real. Beliefs form the basis of your behavior. If you hold on to the following beliefs, you will need the courage to not allow them to dictate your actions, or lack thereof. As you take action, these beliefs will be disproven:

- You are less valuable than others.
- You will never heal totally.
- If people really knew you, they'd be disgusted.
- You have nothing to offer.

It is important to remember that healing and recovery are part of a **process**, not an event. Recovery is learning how to live a meaningful and comfortable life without using food or other substances to cope.

TRUE RECOVERY

True Recovery . . . is the healing of the human spirit. It is the recognition that we not only have the right to live, but the right to be happy. It is the ability to have a successful work life and satisfying relationships with family members and other loved ones. People who have reached the state of true recovery feel comfortable with their parents and siblings, find that parenting is an attainable skill not a mish-mash of confusing feelings and responsibilities, and enjoy friendships based on mutual delight and sharing of intimacy, not a pain connection.

True Recovery . . . means being able to experience all the joy of life without dread or a fear that it will end, and that it's too good to be true.

—Marilyn J. White, CASAC, NCAC II, Founder, Realization Center Inc.

Recovery begins when we recognize our need for nurturing and we begin to allow ourselves to relate to others. Using food to nurture ourselves causes intense isolation and deep feelings of loneliness.

When we deal with our feelings openly and honestly in the presence of others, healing begins. We learn that we need to turn to people instead of the food and to begin to work through the 12 Step program and therapy (if we're involved with a therapist) to heal.

Goals and Requirements for Recovery:

- Recognition that food addiction is a disease and understanding its nature.

- Recognition of the need for life-long abstinence, achieved a day at a time.

- Development and use of an ongoing recovery program (12 Step) to maintain abstinence.

- Getting help with the underlying problems or conditions that can interfere with recovery.

Foundations for Recovery:

1. **Discipline:** Doing something that you predetermine/know is good for you whether or not you want to do it. Following the food plan does require effort. Planning, preparing, cleaning up afterward, committing your actions to a sponsor (see explanation later in this chapter), and attending 12 Step meetings, whether or not you want to, are all actions you take because you know it's necessary for your recovery.

2. **Integrity:** Absolute honesty. No rationalizations, no excuses. The weighing and measuring of portions is the opportunity to practice being honest—it's when you're alone in your kitchen with the food scale or cup that your integrity is called upon.

3. **Acceptance:** The realization of a fact or truth and the process of coming to terms with it. To give compliance to or approval of. Not fighting the inevitable. The food addict must take personal responsibility for her disease and accept the fact that she has a chronic illness and, to survive it, she will have to be part of the solution, not part of the problem. To stop trying to behave with food as if you were like others who can eat in moderation and who don't obsess about weight and body image. (See Chapter 12: Compliance versus Surrender.)

4. **Compassion:** Having a conscious sympathy for something or someone, or oneself.

> *"In our culture we are prone to be hard on others and even harder on ourselves. Life is difficult enough without beating yourself up. Instead of beating yourself up, embrace your 'inner goodness' and have self-compassion."*
> —RICHARD FIELDS, PH.D.

*"All beings want to be happy, yet so very few know how.
It is out of ignorance that any of us cause suffering
for ourselves or for others."*
—SHARON SALZBERG, *LOVINGKINDNESS*

Learning how to be more compassionate toward others' suffering, as well as our own, is a much more sustainable way of life and recovery.

PARTICIPATION IN 12 STEP FOOD RECOVERY FELLOWSHIPS

Food addiction is a disease of isolation, denial, obsession, compulsion, and shame. The food addict must create a recovery support system that she uses to address these powerful forces. For many food addicts, this is the hard part of recovery—to come out of hiding and asking for help—but only a focus on ongoing recovery support/management can effectively address the chronic nature of food addiction.

Recovery involves doing whatever it takes to stop our unhealthy eating patterns. We have to accept that we can't get better on our own. Some food addicts, especially those who have reached a point where their physical lives are threatened, require inpatient treatment to begin the process of recovery.

That's the reason why we need to participate in 12 Step food recovery fellowships such as FAA, OA, GreySheeters, CEA-HOW, etc. If a food addict can also participate in outpatient treatment (group and individual therapy) along with 12 Step meetings, that's the ideal. (See Chapter 18: Therapy and Treatment for Food Addiction.)

As discussed in Chapter 1: The Disease Concept of Addiction, what science tells us about the power of memory imprinted deep in the brain and the pursuit of reward/pleasure provides validation for the 12 Step recovery processes. The various processes of sponsorship, self-examination, self-disclosure, learning to depend and rely on others for help, and learning to follow defined structure and spiritual principles actually provide vast amounts of support. This support allows us to change how our brains think while developing new pathways of action than can enhance our lives and health.

To recover, the food addict experiences withdrawal, which leads to the restoration of the deficit or imbalance of the neurotransmitter-receptor processes by stopping the triggering of the brain reward pathways.

This is accomplished by following the food plan and participating in a program of recovery—which is the meaning of abstinence.

To put food addiction into remission, it is necessary to engage in purposeful activity that supports long-term productivity and functioning and disables lingering addictive thoughts and actions. Attending 12 Step food recovery–focused meetings, abstinence, exercising, and participation in meditation and therapy are examples of activities that help heal neural pathways and protect against relapse.

Recovery is more than just bringing your body to 12 Step meetings; recovery requires an entire overhaul of one's values and goals and an entire new way of relating to people, one that evolves from following the plan and full participation with a 12 Step food recovery fellowship (meetings, sponsorship, daily phone calls to other program people, service position, sharing at meetings, reading program literature, keeping a journal).

I believe that following the food plan without involvement in a 12 Step food fellowship is being on a diet. It's like the alcoholic stopping drinking and not going to AA. That's not sobriety; that's being "dry" and with that comes the "dry-drunk" syndrome—being miserable, lonely, angry, lost, unhappy, and hurtful to oneself and others, and not changing and growing as a human being.

After we become abstinent from our former eating behaviors, we can look at what those behaviors represent. Recovery isn't just a matter of picking up a fork or putting one down. It requires us to talk honestly about ourselves, while we continue following the food plan—being abstinent—one meal at a time.

Recovery is grounded in the 12 Steps, in an awareness of a power greater than you, such as God or by whatever title you identify and understand that power greater than yourself. That recovery is rooted in the fellowship of the food addict's fellow travelers, other people who are like you—people in recovery.

The priority in the food addict's life has to be recovery. Every morning, the commitment to recovery has to be put first. And every night, the food addict has to remember to be thankful that she has completed another day of abstinence.

Immersing ourselves in one of these fellowships opens us to change in several ways. Initially, we find something other than using food that will fill our spare time. Becoming active in the program, giving service, step-work, and following a plan for personal development are all constructive activities that foster emotional and personal growth. All of us need to get out of our isolated ruts and interact more with other people.

THE MEANING OF THE 12 STEP PROGRAM

Attending meetings; sharing at meetings about your efforts, your feelings, your thoughts, your struggles; listening to other members; talking with other members about recovery; studying the literature; and doing service are only a part of involvement in the program.

The core/basis of the program are the "12 Steps" as was developed by Alcoholics Anonymous.* They are concepts that are used to create and sustain abstinence—under the broadest of definitions—involving a responsible appraisal of all areas of our life, including our relationships with other people.

Admission (Step One)

1. We admitted we were powerless over our food addiction—that our lives had become unmanageable. (Recommended Reading: *Alcoholics Anonymous: The Big Book,* Chapter 5 through ABC's on page 60, as well as *Twelve Steps and Twelve Traditions,* Step One. You will find many of these concepts in these readings.)

Step One consists of two distinct parts. Part One of Step One is about powerlessness, the admission that we have a mental obsession to eat, restrict/starve, and/or eat and purge and that we have an "allergy" of the body to those culprits/triggers. The obsession can lead us to the brink of death or insanity. We used to delude ourselves that "we could take it or leave it." As stated in the "Big Book"(Alcoholics Anonymous): ". . . this utter inability to leave it alone, no matter how great the necessity or the wish."

---

* Twelve Steps of Alcoholics Anonymous are adapted with permission of Alcoholics Anonymous World Services, Inc. ("A.A.W.S.") Permission to adapt the Twelve Steps does not mean that A.A.W.S. has reviewed or approved the contents of this publication, or that A.A.W.S. necessarily agrees with the views expressed herein. A.A. is a program of recovery from alcoholism *only*—use of the Twelve Steps in connection with programs and activities which are patterned after A.A., but which address other problems, or in any other non-A.A. context, does not imply otherwise.

Taking the first step allows a great weight to fall from our shoulders. We let go of the losing battle we have been waging. We recognize that there is no point in continuing the fight. We surrender completely.

We start to recover or heal when we are willing to admit there's something wrong. This is the only Step that speaks to the substance/behavior. This is the only step that must be done perfectly. This step tells us the reality of our problem. In Step One, we surrender the problem. We surrender the war on reality. We realize that, on our own power, we have little ability to let go or change our behavior.

This doesn't mean that being powerless is the same as being helpless. It means recognizing our human limitations, becoming accountable, and making a different choice by asking for help.

I'm always struck by the first word of Step One, "We," which indicates that we can't get well by ourselves; we *must* join with others. It is in this step that the alcoholic puts the alcohol on the shelf and the food addict puts the alcohol, drugs, sugar, artificial sweeteners, flour, wheat, caffeine, volume, high-fat and high-salt foods, hard cheese, and nuts on the shelf, picks up the food plan, and becomes abstinent.

Part Two of Step One is the admission that our lives have been, are now, and will forever remain unmanageable by us alone.

> *"Every natural instinct cries out against the idea of personal powerlessness. It is only through utter defeat we are able to take our first steps toward liberation and strength."*
> —*TWELVE STEPS AND TWELVE TRADITIONS*
> BY ALCOHOLICS ANONYMOUS WORLD SERVICES, INC., PAGE 21

We must accept this truth and all its consequences. Until we do, our abstinence, if we achieve any, will be precarious.

When Step One tells us our lives are unmanageable, it really means we've lost the ability to think sanely. We've lost the ability to manage our lives all by ourselves. Someone needs to manage them for us.

The precursor to Step One is the experience of "hitting bottom" by experiencing a sense of hopelessness and helplessness about one's behavior with food and their life. This state of mind has been labeled "surrender" by Dr. Harry Tiebout (see Chapter 12: Compliance versus Surrender). Surrender is the first step toward recovery.

Surrender will occur naturally if we get out of our own way. Bill Wilson called it "deflation at depth."[137] "We shall find no enduring strength until we first admit complete defeat"[138] and acknowledge that probably no human power can relieve our food addiction.

Active food addiction is only a symptom. We are victims of a mental obsession, a way of thinking so subtly powerful that no amount of human willpower can break it. When we surrender, we recover our true self and we recover our ability to grow and evolve. Our true nature is restored.

The time it takes for the food addict to "put down" the food is determined by her willingness to let go. For many of us, it's a scary proposition to change from the long-time use of food as a way of dealing with cravings (biology) and life in general. Changing these habits/behaviors and lifestyles requires walking through discomfort! That takes courage, which is not the absence of fear, but the ability to walk through it. The food addiction symptoms—undereating, overeating, purging, etc.—have to be replaced with increasingly stronger, more self-enhancing coping resources.

Being at 12 Step food recovery fellowship meetings allows the addict to hear and identify with others who share in the nightmare of the disease and the miracles of recovery. Working the program allows the food addict to experience the power of the recovery and helps them achieve the strength, willingness, and surrender to be abstinent a day at a time.

It is said in the program that when the pain of the problem is greater than the fear of the solution, the addict takes this first step.

I and many others have always felt a deeper sense of surrender, a more whole and a stronger connection to my true self and my Higher Power, as a result of being at a meeting. This process and experience are awesome.

The next eleven steps are about our character defects, and the slogan "Progress not Perfection" applies. It *never* applies to the first step.

Discover a Higher Power . . . As We Understand Him (Steps Two and Three)

2. Came to believe that a Power greater than ourselves could restore us to sanity.

3. Made a decision to turn our will and our lives over to the care of God as we understood him.

12 Step Food Recovery Fellowships and Relapse Prevention

393

The food addict has lost her sense of a true self, including her spiritual identity. The process of these Steps is meant to help the food addict reacquaint herself with her good heart, with the qualities, strengths, and attributes that she has possessed all along but has lost in the obsessions and compulsions of the food addiction.

These two Steps offer a very freeing and open concept. Our God, Higher Power, or Source need not be religious. The 12 Step program does not belong to any one religion or denomination, it is absent of any dogma or creed, and in this powerful sense, it is seen as a spiritual program.

Cleaning House (Steps Four through Nine)

4. Made a searching and fearless moral inventory of ourselves.
5. Admitted to God, to ourselves, and to another human being the exact nature of our wrongs.
6. Were entirely ready to have God remove all these defects of character.
7. Humbly asked Him to remove our shortcomings.
8. Made a list of all persons we had harmed, and became willing to make amends to them all.
9. Made direct amends to such people wherever possible, except when to do so would injure them or others.

As addicts, food and otherwise, we created a "wreckage of the past." These steps allow us to free ourselves of unhealthy attitudes or behaviors that hurt us and others. Arguments, lies, manipulations, resentments, sarcasm, isolation, and fears all need to be "cleaned up" so that a new spiritual journey of living can begin, and it is certainly true that a new freedom is experienced when sincere amends are made and forgiveness is experienced.

The Journey Continues (Steps Ten and Eleven)

10. Continued to take personal inventory and when we were wrong promptly admitted it. (Therefore, not creating "wreckage of the future.")
11. Sought through prayer and meditation to improve our conscious contact with God as we understood Him, praying only for knowledge of His will for us and the power to carry that out.

Most addictions, personality defects, and life challenges cannot be removed permanently. The 12 Step program shows the value of utilizing prayer and meditation in the ongoing healing process. We know today that people who pray or meditate on a regular basis are more serene, healthy, and at peace in their world.

It is often said in the meetings that prayer is talking to our Higher Power and meditation is listening to our Higher Power.

A Spiritual Awakening (Step Twelve)

12. Having had a spiritual awakening as the result of these steps, we tried to carry this message to other food addicts and to practice these principles in all our affairs.

The last principle reflected in the 12 Step program suggests that after practicing the principles of Admittance, Discovering a God or Higher Power (As We Understand Him), Cleaning House, and Continuing the Journey, we then experience a spiritual awakening. Something happens to us; we recognize that we have changed, we feel better, and we are living the spiritual life in all areas of our lives. This experience is something we need to share in service to others. The recovery paradox is: If you want to keep what you have received, then you must be willing to give it away.

The food addict's understanding of these steps allows her to see a way out of the past trauma and abuse that is a part of most food addict's stories. The weeds of shame are uprooted by the practice of replanting new seeds with affirmations, self-care (following the food plan), nurturance, forgiveness, gentleness, and kindness. This also allows the addict to be of greater service, and what a joy that is!

GUIDELINES FOR PREVENTION OF RELAPSE: TOOLS OF RECOVERY

Involvement in a 12 Step food recovery fellowship is essential. These 12 Step food recovery fellowships are not diet clubs; they do not offer diet tips.

These programs see food and weight as symptoms of the problem. We use food like the alcoholic uses alcohol and the drug addict uses drugs.

12 Step Food Recovery Fellowships and Relapse Prevention

395

While a diet can help us lose weight, it often intensifies the compulsion to use food with overeating, undereating, bingeing, and/or purging.

Members suggest that attendance at weight loss programs is harmful to recovery, since such programs have an effect similar to that of suggesting controlled drinking to an active alcoholic. Most dieters alternate periods of control with periods of unrestrained eating and, because food addiction is characterized by loss of control over eating, the advice "just eat less" is very much like telling an alcoholic or other drug addicted person to "just say no."

12 Step food recovery fellowships give the food addict an opportunity to identify with others who have the same problem. In these fellowships, the members share their experience of both the suffering of addictive behavior and the joy of recovery.

These anonymous programs believe that the problems of overeating, under-eating, and/or purging is a three-fold illness—physical, emotional, and spiritual. What the 12 Step programs offer affects recovery on all three levels. The 12 Steps embody a set of principles which, when followed, promote inner change. Sponsors help members understand and apply these principles.

The elimination of trigger foods, following the food plan to establish abstinence, and involvement in the 12 Step program all work together to allow for old attitudes and beliefs to be discarded, and what evolves is a way of dealing with life without using food as a coping mechanism. In following the 12 Steps and the principles of the programs, we achieve lasting freedom from our food obsession and a new way of life.

There is another reason for continuous involvement with food recovery 12 Step fellowships: Everyone who recovers incurs an obligation to the source of their recovery. Those who recognize their obligation to their particular fellowship, who try to fulfill their obligation by loyal attendance, twelve-step work, and other personal involvement, are usually the ones who are enjoying their abstinence. Abstinence may depend on paying back to others what one has received from their own fellowship.

All of the 12 Step food recovery fellowships include continuous daily contact with other recovering people. These are the recommendations:

- **Attending a minimum of three meetings a week** (at least for the first year).

- Meetings allow members to share their recovery, experiences, strength, and hope with one another. Though there are many types of meetings (beginners, topic, "big book" study, step, qualification [in which a member shares their "story" of recovery], etc.), fellowship with others suffering with the disease is the basis of every meeting type.

- Meetings give us an opportunity to identify and confirm our common problem and to share the gifts and the joy we receive through this program of recovery.

- As was discussed in Chapter 1: The Disease Concept of Addiction, 90 meetings in 90 days is highly recommended to become entrenched in recovery and to begin the work to "rewire" the automatic thinking patterns the addict responds to by using food or starving themselves.

- **Calling others** in the program daily (three calls per day is recommended) and talking about your abstinence, your day, your plans, your feelings, your recovery, how you are doing, etc.

  - **Leaving a message on voicemail doesn't count! Texting doesn't count! Emailing doesn't count!** Since food addiction is a disease of isolation, the telephone and meetings are a major tool to combat the aloneness that the disease thrives/prospers in.

  - A wonderful saying in AA is, "An addict alone is in very bad company!" The phone allows us to share on a one-to-one basis and helps us learn how to reach out, ask for help, and extend help to others.

  - Using the phone to speak with fellow members in recovery is often referred to as "a meeting between a meeting."

  - When you're at a meeting, ask others (before or after the meeting) for their phone numbers and the best time to call.

  - The practice of using the phone and going to meetings helps us address and heal the "social" part of the disease of food addiction.

- **Obtaining a sponsor.** A sponsor is someone who can guide us through the program by sharing their experience, strength, and hope, someone who has had the experience of recovery, is abstinent, is committed to abstinence, works a program of recovery, and has a sponsor. By working with other members, sponsors continually renew and reaffirm

12 Step Food Recovery Fellowships and Relapse Prevention

their own recovery. Sponsors share their program up to the level of their own experience.

- ➤ After attending a number of meetings, you will become familiar with those members who consistently attend meetings.
- ➤ Find a member whose recovery you admire, someone who has "what you want." Ask them how they are achieving that recovery. Ask them if they would be willing to sponsor you, using the food plan you are now following or wanting to follow—the food plan outlined in Chapter 11: Realization Center Food Plan for True Recovery From Food Addiction. If they require that you follow a different food plan, thank them and keep looking. You will find the right person. In time, with your own recovery in place, you will become a sponsor to someone else to reinforce your own recovery.
- ➤ A member may work with more than one sponsor and may change sponsors at will.

- **Planning (and maybe preparing) your meals** for the day the night before or in the morning, which is a very self-nurturing experience.
  - ➤ **Write them down.**
  - ➤ **"Turn over your meals" (commit them)** to your sponsor every day for at least a year. Tell someone what and when you'll eat and the weighed and measured portions you are going to eat for the day establishes accountability and relieves you of the dangerous pressure of spontaneously figuring out what to have as a mealtime approaches.
  - ➤ This requires the planning of meals in accordance with the food plan, which eliminates the "last-minuteness" of putting together a meal. This is an amazing process to insure the commitment to abstinence and removes the "Oh my God, it time to eat and I don't know what to have." It's all planned out in advance so there are no surprises and no slipping back to old behavior.
  - ➤ In short time, this becomes routine and the help/support of a sponsor, who has had this experience, is invaluable.
  - ➤ **No skipping of meals,** which will be a trigger to overeat a later meal, justifying it as "making up for" that missed meal.

- **Sharing at meetings** about how you are feeling and how you are doing with your recovery.

- **Participating in fellowship.** Go out after the meetings and talk with others from the meeting.

- **Taking a service position at the meeting,** be it treasurer, literature person, chairperson, etc., in accordance with the criteria of the meeting for these positions.

  ➤ "Carrying the message to the food addict who still suffers is the basic purpose of the Fellowship and therefore the most fundamental form of service. Any service, no matter how small that will help reach a fellow sufferer, adds to the quality of our own recovery. Getting to meetings, putting away chairs, putting out literature, talking to newcomers, doing whatever needs to be done in a group or for the Fellowship as a whole, are ways in which we give back what we have so generously been given. We are encouraged to do what we can when we can. . . . 'A life of sane and happy usefulness' is what we are promised as the result of working the twelve steps. Service helps to fulfill the promise. As OA's responsibility pledge states: 'Always to extend the hand and heart of OA to all who share my compulsion; for this, I am responsible.'"[139]—*Overeaters Anonymous: The Tools of Recovery* pamphlet

- **Never saying "no" when asked to do something related to recovery,** even though it scares you. This is how you will grow and learn about yourself and discover the "real" you.

- **Read recovery literature daily.** Reading and studying FAA, OA, CEA-HOW, etc. literature, *Alcoholics Anonymous: The Big Book,* and *Twelve Steps and Twelve Traditions* (the "12 and 12") helps to understand and reinforce our program. Many members find that when read on a daily basis, the literature further reinforces how to live the twelve steps.

  ➤ The literature of FAA, OA, AA, and other 12 Step recovery fellowships and are an ever-available tool that gives the insight into our refined food addiction, the strength to deal with it, and the very real hope that there is a solution for us.

12 Step Food Recovery Fellowships and Relapse Prevention

- **Keep a journal about your feelings and thoughts.** Most members have found that writing is an indispensable tool for working the steps. Further, putting our thoughts and feelings down on paper or describing a troubling incident helps us to better understand our actions and reactions in a way that is often not revealed to us by simply thinking or talking about them. In the past, we used food as the common reaction to life. When we put our difficulties down on paper, it becomes easier to see situations more clearly and perhaps better discern any necessary action. At some point in your recovery, it will be necessary to write a "fourth step" moral inventory of yourself, searching out defects and persons you have harmed. This is the part of the program where one begins to "clean house."

- In the context of your recovery program and in your life, **allowing yourself:**

  - ➤ **to feel your feelings** and sit with them and talk/share about them with safe people
  - ➤ **to be uncomfortable**
  - ➤ **to be honest**
  - ➤ **to be afraid**
  - ➤ **to be vulnerable**
  - ➤ **to take risks**
  - ➤ **to change attitudes**
  - ➤ **to reach out**
  - ➤ **to allow support**
  - ➤ **to change behaviors**
  - ➤ **to take a stand for yourself**

- It becomes easy to sabotage (damage or destroy) our recovery because it is uncomfortable and new to do all these things.

- **Remember HALT.** It is suggested that you not get too Hungry, too Angry, too Lonely, or too Tired—each of which leads to weakened resolve, leading to potential relapse.

- **Understand your triggers** (such as sugar, sugar substitutes, flour, wheat, caffeine, high sugar fruits, hard/soft cheese, volume, high-fat and/or high-salt foods, nuts, alcohol, drugs, and personal triggering foods) and triggering situations (e.g., family gatherings, celebrations) and talk about them with your support system.

- **Dismantle euphoric recall.** Carefully examine past pleasant memories about your active food addiction behaviors and search for both the obvious and the hidden negatives in the experience. Avoid talking about those real or imagined pleasures once derived from certain foods.

- **Stop magical thinking.** It's important to stop magical thinking about future eating or starving and to stop "awfulizing" your abstinence.

- **Stop kidding yourself** that a bite or two would make some bad situation better or easier to live with.

- **Don't weigh yourself** more than one time per month. I personally believe you should throw away your scale. Unless required by your physician, you don't need to know what you weigh!

  - ➤ Your clothes will tell you about your weight loss or gain. I think weighing yourself is most often a set-up to eat or to restrict; the number will often be more or less than you expected, and disappointment or excitement about your weight is a trigger. The idea of weighing yourself also keeps the focus on the physical aspect of recovery. If you remain abstinent, following the food plan, your weight will become what you are supposed to weigh. Your body will find its proper, healthy weight. Your body is very smart and will appreciate your treating it with the care and respect it requires and will return the "favor" umpteen-fold by becoming highly functional and healthy! **Trust the process!**

  - ➤ If you insist on weighing yourself, it should not be more often than once per month, and you need to "bookend" it by calling a program person, ideally your sponsor, before and after the weigh in, or do it while you're on the phone with them and talk about your feelings about the number.

- **Be aware and accept that you will have urges.** It's normal to want to go back to old eating patterns or starving patterns when uncomfortable feelings arise. But since the urges are coming from your feelings, and not because they've been triggered by some triggering food creating cravings, you can:

  - ➤ **Do something else.** Engage in a non-food related activity, e.g. knitting, reading, take a walk, taking a nap, etc.

12 Step Food Recovery Fellowships and Relapse Prevention

> **Talk it through.** If a recovering food addict talks it through, they don't have to act it out. Food addicts need to talk about their urges as soon as they occur to discharge the power those feelings have to sabotage one's abstinence.

> **Go to a meeting.** If not a "face-to-face" meeting, then call in to a phone meeting and make it a point to share.

> **Write about your feelings** in your journal.

> **Pray.**

> **Do some aerobic exercise.** This will stimulate brain chemistry and both reduce and interrupt the physiology of urges, but generally should be limited to not more than forty minutes per day.

> **Try meditation and relaxation exercises**—Urges are worse when a person is under high stress. The more a person can relax, the lower the intensity of the urges.

- **Remember that urges are time-limited** to two or three hours. So you can use any or all of the above list to protect yourself from "picking up."

- **Remember that each time you face a difficult situation without using food, it will make it easier for you to abstain the next time.**

- **Cultivate enjoyment of abstinence** from overeating/undereating/purging by remembering that, as a result, you have found:

> Freedom from guilt, remorse, and self-condemnation about the food you eat.

> Freedom from the power food once had over you.

> The ability to make choices about the abstinent food you eat.

> The gift to eat and sleep normally and wake up glad you are abstinent.

- **Food addiction is a treatable disease.** Like other diseases, food addiction often requires professional treatment. Enrolling in a treatment program, whether inpatient and/or outpatient, can be very valuable to helping you establish and maintain abstinence and recovery. You just have to be careful to know the treatment program you choose understands food addiction. See Chapter 18: Therapy and Treatment for Food Addiction.

- **Psychotherapy.** See Chapter 18: Therapy and Treatment for Food Addiction.

- **Remember to build your life around your recovery, NOT your recovery around your life!**

* * *

I Am Your Disease. . . .

Author Unknown

I hate meetings. I hate your Higher Power. I hate anyone who has a "Program."

To all who come into contact with me, I wish death and suffering.

Allow me to introduce myself. I am the Disease of Food Addiction

Cunning, Baffling, and Powerful—that's me! I have killed millions, and am quite pleased! I love to catch you with the element of surprise. I love to pretend that I am your friend and lover.

I have given you comfort, have I not? Wasn't I there when you were lonely? When you wanted to die, didn't you call me? I was there. I love to make you hurt. I love to make you cry.

Better yet, I love to make you so numb that you can neither hurt nor cry—you can't feel anything at all. This is true glory! I will give you instant gratification, and all I ask of you is long-term suffering. I have been there for you always. When things were going right for you in your life, you invited me. You said that you didn't deserve these good things, and I was the only one who would agree with you. Together, we were able to destroy all the good.

People don't take me seriously. They take strokes, heart disease and attacks seriously; they take diabetes, amputations, and blindness seriously; they take seizures seriously; they even take obesity and emaciation seriously and esophageal tearing and electrolyte imbalance seriously; they take cancer seriously; they take digestive problems, depression, anxiety, mood swings, poor sleep, ADD, low energy, and hopelessness seriously. They take relapse seriously.

Fools that they are, they don't realize that, without my help, many of these things would not happen!

I am such a hated disease, yet I don't come uninvited. You choose to have me! And many others have chosen me over reality, peace, and happiness.

More than you hate me, I hate all of you who have a 12 Step program. I hate your program, your meetings, and especially your Higher Power. They all weaken me and interfere with my ability to kill you.

But don't worry, I'm here, waiting, lying here quietly. You can't see me, but I am growing. Bigger than ever. When you only exist, I may live. When you live in abstinence, I only exist. But I am here, and until we meet again—IF we meet again—I'm ready to strike you with suffering and death the moment you pick up.

12 STEP FOOD-RELATED/FOCUSED FELLOWSHIPS/MEETINGS

All the 12 Step food recovery fellowships are mutual-help support groups that provide fellowship and helps members understand and overcome addictive/compulsive eating behaviors, including overeating, bulimia, and anorexia.

Food Addicts Anonymous (FAA)

Food Addicts Anonymous (FAA) was founded in 1987 by "Judith C." in Florida after she attended a rehab that had a food program. She took this program and modified it to AA's 12 Steps. FAA's basic premise, which differs from OA's, is that food addiction is a biochemical disease and that some people are addicted to refined high-carbohydrate foods and need to abstain from those foods in order to avoid overeating. Sugar, flour, wheat, and caffeine are some of the triggers to out-of-control eating. When consumed in any amount, FAA believes these substances trigger a biochemical response that causes the food addict to crave and ultimately eat inordinate amounts of food.

FAA has established abstinence guidelines and specific eating plan suggestions, but it is not designed as a diet or weight loss program, even though weight loss is a likely result of abstaining from these substances and following an appropriate plan of eating.

As of 2007, it is estimated that there are over 150 ongoing, weekly meetings around the world, in addition to phone and online meetings.

Contact Info

Website: www. foodaddictsanonymous.org
Address:
Food Addicts Anonymous World Service Office
529 N W Prima Vista Blvd. #301A
Port St. Lucie, FL 34983
Phone: (561) 967-3871
See "A Word from Dianne" on page 409.

Overeaters Anonymous

In 1960, 25 years after Alcoholics Anonymous (AA) was founded, Rozanne, a "compulsive overeater," applied the principles of AA to eating problems (initially, "compulsive overeating"). The idea of a 12 Step fellowship for those suffering with eating problems came to her when she saw a "compulsive" gambler being interview on TV about his recovery in Gamblers Anonymous (GA), also an outgrowth of AA. She related her out-of-control eating to his description of his out-of-control gambling, and Overeaters Anonymous (OA) was born.

The idea of abstinence was framed as the action of refraining from compulsive eating. The program took no position on food plans and believes there are no absolutes for abstinence.

"For some, abstinence facilitates working the 12 Steps; for others, it comes from working the steps. As a result of living the OA program of recovery, the symptom of compulsive eating is removed on a daily basis. Ultimately, we are abstinent because we no longer have the desire to eat compulsively."[140]

—OVEREATERS ANONYMOUS:
THE TOOLS OF RECOVERY PAMPHLET

So, what comes out of this concept is that every member can define their own abstinence. There is no objective measure as there is in AA. In AA, you're abstinent/sober if you have "put down" alcohol and are no longer drinking alcohol—it's very clear, with no ambiguity. You are either "pregnant" or not; there are no areas of grey.

Ah, but how can you hold the same yardstick with food? In the early days of OA and as it much continues today, there is a lack of the understanding that our issues with out-of-control eating or starving is the result of a biochemical condition that stems from brain reward mechanisms which involve very specific food triggers, i.e., sugar, sweeteners, flour, wheat, caffeine, volume, high-fat and/or high-salt foods, hard/soft cheese, high-sugar fruits, and nuts.

There was always the acknowledgement that our issues and problems with eating were threefold: physical, emotional, and spiritual. However, OA takes no official position on the necessary presence of physical recovery—meaning that these trigger foods are necessary to be put on the shelf, like the alcoholic has to put alcohol on the shelf and like the drug addict has to put drugs, including alcohol, on the shelf—for the emotional and the spiritual recovery to begin through working the program. As a result, there are members of the program who proclaim recovery but who have not addressed their problem eating and the biochemistry behind it; they have just expanded their definition of their abstinence to justify whatever they eat.

If a person is unwilling to face their out-of-control eating behaviors, it is impossible for them to recover. They will not experience what is promised by the program—physical recovery—which means their weight will not normalize, since normalized weight comes as a result of following a plan of eating that allows for a sane, appropriate, healthy, and serene relationship with food (see the food plan in Chapter 11).

Some others in the program refer to these individuals as having "fat abstinence." Sometimes, members will say that they are "MBA," meaning "messy, but abstinent." This is an oxymoron used to justify continued participation in the disease.

I'm sorry to say this is not recovery. Either we have "put down" our food triggers and follow the food plan, which allows us to have normalized blood sugar levels, which then makes us available for emotional and spiritual recovery, or we are not actually in recovery.

It saddens me to know that OA has not really grown in this area. There are members, however, who understand the biochemical concept and share their recovery at meetings.

Total abstinence—meaning not using any of the triggers so often mentioned throughout the book, including alcohol and drugs—plus personality and lifestyle changes are essential for full recovery.

According to the OA website, there are about 6,500 groups meeting weekly in over 75 countries with approximately 54,000 members worldwide.

Contact Info

Website: www.oa.org
Mailing address:
OA World Services
PO Box 44020
Rio Rancho, NM 87174-4020
Phone: (505) 891-2664
See "A Word from Dianne" on page 409.

Food Addicts in Recovery Anonymous (FA)

Food Addicts in Recovery Anonymous (FA) is a program of recovery based on the 12 Steps of Alcoholics Anonymous. It was born within the OA program and then in 1998 was established as a separate program. The common denominator uniting members of FA is addiction and a relationship with food that parallels an alcoholic's relationship with alcohol. All meetings are face-to-face; there are no phone or internet FA meetings.

The FA premise is that food addiction is "an illness of the mind, body, and spirit for which there is no cure." As is the case with other addictions, food addiction involves physical craving and an ever-increasing dependence upon and struggle with a substance (in this case, food). Overeating, undereating or self-starvation, bulimia (including exercise bulimia), and extreme obsession with weight or food are among the symptoms of this addiction.

A 2009 survey of FA indicated that there were 430 FA meetings worldwide (391 in the US) with a worldwide membership of four thousand, 3,768 of whom are in the US.

Contact Info

Website: www.foodaddicts.org
Address:
FA World Service Office
400 W. Cummings Park Suite 1700
Woburn, MA 01801
Email: office@foodaddicts.org
Phone: (781) 932-6300
See "A Word from Dianne" on page 409.

Compulsive Eaters Anonymous: Honesty, Open-Mindedness, Willingness (CEA-HOW)

CEA-HOW got its start in 1979 when two food addicts decided there was a need for structure and discipline in recovery from food addiction and they established OA-HOW. After some internal disagreement, OA-HOW reformed in the mid-1990s as CEA-HOW.

The CEA-HOW concept is a disciplined and structured approach that offers the compulsive eater the 12 Steps and 12 Traditions as a program of recovery. The program is based on the belief that the disease is absolute and therefore only absolute acceptance of the CEA-HOW concept will offer any sustained abstinence to those whose compulsion has reached a critical level. The CEA-HOW plan of eating, steps, traditions and tools of recovery are not suggested—rather, they have to be accepted as a requirement for recovery.

Contact Info

Website: ceahow.org
Mailing Address:
CEA-HOW World Service Office
3371 Glendale Boulevard, Suite 104
Los Angeles, CA 90039
Email: gso@ceahow.org
Phone: (323) 660-4333
See "A Word from Dianne" on page 409.

Eating Disorders Anonymous (EDA)

Eating Disorders Anonymous (EDA) endorses sound nutrition and discourages any form of rigidity around food. They do not subscribe to the concept of "abstinence" but indicate that "balance" is their goal. They define recovery as living without obsessing about food, weight and body image. EDA suggestions for recovery are to eat when hungry and stop when moderately full.

The problem here is that if we are talking about addiction being the driving force for those with eating problems, then trying controlled eating or not eating with willpower is analogous to asking the alcoholic to have only one beer, one glass of wine, or one cocktail and then stop. It sets up an impossible inner conflict. I believe it gives the totally wrong message to the suffering individual and prevents them from finding the true answer.

Contact Info

Website: eatingdisordersanonymous.org
Mailing Address:
EDA, Inc.
P.O. Box 55876
Phoenix, AZ 85078-5876
Email: info@eatingdisordersanyonymous.org
See "A Word from Dianne" on page 409.

GreySheeters Anonymous (GSA)

GreySheeters Anonymous (GSA) formed when OA removed its official sanction of the food plans and a number of members who were following the Greysheet food plan separated themselves into a faction that ultimately became a separate food recovery fellowship, GreySheeters Anonymous (GSA). That fellowship exists today, following the same food plan that was created thirty-eight years ago.

That food plan was created by a consensus of a group of struggling OA members. (That's similar to creating a horse by a committee—you end up with a camel.) It defines abstinence as three weighed and measured meals a day with nothing in between but black coffee, tea, or diet soda. The allowed fruit on the plan is not weighed or measured, and therefore, the person following the plan searches the world for the largest fruit available. Gum is allowed so, since there is not enough food on the plan, the followers of the plan are always hungry and trying to manage their hunger with chewing inordinate amounts of gum and/or drinking huge amounts of diet soda and coffee.

To me, this is not recovery. As we have discussed and documented, the caffeine in the coffee or tea and the artificial sweeteners in the diet sodas and the gum will keep the cravings alive and well and will keep you their captive. The three meals a day as they are weighed and measured do not provide a sufficient amount of food, and the unmeasured, un-weighed, industrial-size fruit is too much sugar for your body to deal with at any one time.

The positive for the GreySheeters Anonymous fellowship is that it is very strong in its community. The members demonstrate a strong commitment to their recovery and show a tight-knit support for each other. I just wish that it could have grown and evolved as we have learned more about the biological underpinnings of the disease.

There are, however, members who do not use soda, gum or caffeine, and find great relief from cravings by the exclusion of the grains and potatoes. And, some others are drawn to Greysheet believing they cannot "handle" the carbs of potatoes and grains and experience "freedom" from the cravings with following the Greysheet food plan (and also excluding the aforementioned soda, gum & caffeine).

I do support those who want the support of a strong community and are willing to forgo grains and potatoes and not use soda, gum or caffeine.

Contact Info

Website: www.greysheet.org
Mailing Address, Phone and Email: See website

A WORD FROM DIANNE ABOUT FOOD RECOVERY FELLOWSHIP

To my regret, there is not "one" food recovery fellowship like there is "one" AA, which offers a program of recovery from alcoholism.

The early founders of AA discovered that if they did not pick up the first drink, helped another "drunk," got support from each other, and began working on their "character defects," they could stay sober a day at a time. Dr. William Silkworth, the physician involved in this early "experiment," explained that "these people" (alcoholics) experienced what others did not: The phenomenon of craving when they took the first drink. He explained this phenomenon in terms of an allergy. Brilliant and simple: If these people can stay away from the first drink, they won't get drunk! And they learned that if they supported each other and worked on themselves through the Steps, they could, a day at a time, refrain from taking that first lethal drink. Their recovery is based on putting alcohol and drugs on the shelf and learning how to live their lives without going back to the shelf.

In contrast, however, people who suffer from out-of-control eating have searched their entire lives to find an answer to the manifestation of their disease—the weight—by attempting many diets, weight-loss programs, self-help books, psychotherapy, pills, and surgery, but nothing has really worked as a permanent solution. Unaware that they suffered from a biochemical problem like alcoholics do, the early founders of OA initially looked for an answer to their compulsive eating and weight issues. The idea of applying the principles of the 12 Steps of AA gave them hope.

Initially, OA created and adopted three different food plans, printed on different colored paper (orange, blue, and grey), from which the members could choose to define their "abstinence." The plan printed on the grey paper was the most restrictive—low carb, excluding sugar, starchy veggies, and grains. Interestingly enough, those people who chose the Greysheet plan experienced the most relief from their "compulsivity" and the most weight loss. (It is the plan I first used when I started in OA.)

Eventually, however, the board of trustees of OA decided that endorsing any food plan was adverse to the spiritual basis of the 12 Step program and eliminated the food plans. Of course, this gave rise to another problem: those new members who came initially to lose weight were left without a direction.

Of course, the solution to out-of-control eating can't be the same as is the solution to the out-of-control drinking of alcohol. You can't have total abstinence from food as you can from alcohol. The dilemma was there from the beginning.

Also, OA, from its inception, identified the eating problem they were established to deal with as "compulsive eating" or "compulsive overeating." This is also true for Eating Disorders Anonymous (EDA),

12 Step Food Recovery Fellowships and Relapse Prevention

411

Compulsive Eaters Anonymous (CEA-HOW), and GreySheeters Anonymous (GSA). As you would know by now, I believe that this is a poor and inaccurate description of the problem. The problem is food addiction, of which compulsive eating is a symptom.

When "Judith C." was introduced to the concept of "food addiction" as a biochemical illness when she was in treatment at a rehab in Florida, it opened the door for the establishment of another 12 Step food recovery program that had a premise different from OA—Food Addicts Anonymous (FAA). Its understanding that people's problem eating was the result of addiction to refined carbs and personal triggers gave rise to a food plan that promises relief from cravings. **I totally agree with the concept—I just believe that their food plan allows larger than necessary serving sizes.**

The food plan you find in this book has been developed from sound nutritional principles and is grounded in the understanding that refined carbs and some other foods trigger brain chemistry to activate the phenomenon of craving, which sends any addict, including the food addict, "off to the races" with either overeating or undereating. By following this food plan, you will discover what hundreds of others have found: freedom from craving, level blood sugar levels, stable and optimized energy, stable mood, improved sleep, optimum brain functioning, and normalization of weight, if it's an issue, all resulting in higher self-esteem and dignity and the opportunity to be in life, to grow, and to live in your potential.

This food plan is your answer and will be your lifesaver. At the same time, because you need support and a program, you must attend meetings of one of the food fellowships. Please don't be dissuaded or bullied into abandoning the food plan in Chapter 11 in favor of one of the plans of these fellowships. All these other food plans have limitations and will keep you in bondage to obsession, compulsion, and despair.

Remember, this food plan is your key to living the life you want, and you can carry it with you and attend any 12 Step meeting for the message of recovery.

Since OA is the largest of the food fellowships with the most meetings, you are better off finding an OA or (preferably) an FAA meeting. Hopefully, there are some in your area that have a good track record of recovery.

CHAPTER 17
Sabotage and Relapse

Addicts go in one of only two directions:
Recovery and Growth ... or Relapse and Death.
There's no holding pattern over Newark!
—DIANNE SCHWARTZ

The price of active food addiction is the cost of your soul!

The entire process of recovery—putting down the overeating, eating and purging and/or starving, accepting the food plan, finding 12 Step food recovery meetings, attending those meetings, talking to other members, finding a sponsor, and being consistent with it all—is the hardest thing you will ever have to do in your life. Recovery is a journey, not an event, and it requires constant attention and a system of support from those who understand, identify with, and walk with you on this journey. Food addiction is a chronic disease that does not have a one-page, one-time solution. Embarking on the journey and staying the course is a full-time job in the beginning, even if you already have a full-time job, and a continuing, ongoing job as time goes on. Many recovering food addicts express gratitude for the ongoing job; it gives them a chance to slow down, reflect, and appreciate the required work of recovery because it gives them so much.

This path is not treacherous, but it is tricky. What has been said about the disease of alcohol dependence (alcoholism), which is that it's cunning, baffling, and powerful, is triply true for food addiction. I also add "insidious and patient"; it waits until you are not paying attention, not using the tools of recovery, becoming complacent because you feel so amazing, isolating, or any of the other conditions listed below as relapse signs, and then it sneaks into your palace with malicious intent.

It wants to rob you of your life, plain and simple! Any time we go back to "old behavior" (i.e., picking up the food, for whatever reason), we lose "life" time.

The expression "Life is not a dress rehearsal" is relevant, since addicts, including food addicts, work to avoid thinking about the "life" time they are losing while engaging in and being enslaved by their illness. The time we waste—in the obsessions about weight and body image, getting food or avoiding food, getting rid of it once we are overtaken by bingeing, trying to find the "right" answer, acting out in other addictions to have "control" over our appetites and cravings, covering up, and feeling remorse about acting out with food—is all time we will never get back. During my active food addiction, I somehow fooled myself into thinking there was plenty of time for my life, that it was okay to postpone everything, that I would be okay tomorrow or next week or next year, and I could regain the time in which I was consumed by my food addiction. I experienced many relapses in the course of my quest for a solution to my out-of-control eating.

The sad reality is that the time spent lost in the addiction is never recouped. I'd like to believe that since I lost so much time in the early part of my life to this disease, I'm getting some of it back in my later years. My recovery has allowed me to be healthy and highly functional and to pursue the vision I have for my life. In Joyce Sequichie Hifler's book *A Cherokee Feast of Days: Daily Meditations,* the author writes:

If there is one thing that scares us, it is the thought that any part of life has been wasted.

We look back and ask why we let it happen—what was so important that it could steal our youth, our strength, our capacity to be a somebody—to just be happy?

Is it too late to begin again? Never. It may be with a different set of rules, a standard of values that has changed drastically, but begin again? Yes. Many have started over and have had more happiness and contentment in a short time than in all of what was known as the wasted years.

Anyone who has ever traveled a trail of tears wishes they had known then what they know now.

But we did not, and life is not lived by hindsight.

We did what we knew to do—sometimes with great ignorance.

But if we know the difference now and want to begin again—then why not? And why not now?[141]

Copyright © 1996 by Joyce Sequichie Hifler. All rights reserved including the right of reproduction in whole or in part in any form. Any third party use of this material, outside of this publication, is prohibited.

CHALLENGES OF GETTING INTO RECOVERY: CHALLENGES IN EARLY RECOVERY

One powerful reason that recovery is so difficult for the food addict of whatever age is that it requires "individuation" and separation from the addict's mother/family, whether the connection is current or historical. The negative eating behaviors do serve, in large measure, to keep the food addict dependent on and attached to their mother and the family system, which allows the addict to avoid the scary and painful transitions that go along with growing up. One of the goals of treatment is to help the food addict explore her ambivalence and fantasies about what she imagines will happen as she gets older and has to move on with her life and be independent.

The process of acting like an adult, with the major act of self-care, as is required by abstinence, can be a saboteur if the food addict doesn't get the recovery support necessary to make this transition.

Another reason is that the food has been the most intimate relationship the addict has ever had. The attachment to food and the food addiction behaviors (overeating, undereating, eating and purging) has been the addict's most reliable and sustaining relationship. For the food addict, trusting food has been safer than trusting people. Food never abandons you, never rejects you, never ridicules, never abuses. By bingeing, purging, or starving, the addict gets to say when, how much, and where they engage in that relationship. It's the only relationship that complies with one's needs so absolutely. Recovery interferes with the most intimate relationship you've ever had. That's why it takes so much work. That's why recovery is too hard to accomplish alone.

A third reason is that, as food addicts, we are accustomed to instant gratification, using starving, bingeing, or bingeing and purging to put our feelings to sleep. Once the decision is made to not use these behaviors by following the food plan, the addict may experience a lot of exaggerated feelings—not that they aren't real, but they are more exaggerated than

Sabotage and Relapse

415

the situations call for. Why? Because the addict is not used to having them; they are accustomed to having them for a little while and then numbing them. Eventually, if the addict doesn't go back old behavior, these feelings will be assimilated into the addict's life. But it takes time. However, in the beginning, this is unfamiliar, uncomfortable, and scary for the food addict.

In addition, the onset and flood of feelings can overwhelm and frighten this food addict, now in early recovery, and they may say, "I can't do this; I can't handle this; I can't go on like this; I can't feel like this all the time." The truth is that they won't feel like this all the time; they will feel like this in the beginning, and it's vital that they allow themselves a support system to help because they need it, not because they want it.

If the food addict doesn't reach out for recovery support, these newly experienced feelings can act as a saboteur to the freedom this addict so desires.

In recovery, especially in early recovery, changes are made with the food, with behavior, and within the family system. You'll change what you eat, when you eat, and how you eat, and those are only changes you'll have with the food. What begins to happen is, as you begin to feel your feelings on a consistent basis, without putting them to sleep, you will begin to realize that there may be some things in your life outside of your eating behavior that you want to change. That's very scary because you may not know how to change them, and just because you feel you want to change them doesn't mean you have to do anything about it right away. It means that you have time to think about it, you have time to look at these changes, and you have time to talk about it with supportive people who understand you and possibly have felt these same feelings. Remember that when we become aware of something, often it's an exaggerated awareness. Many people with food addiction are compulsive and, when they think of something—anything—that pops up, they have a compulsive reaction to change it right away. That's very scary.

For example, you may be aware of the fact that you always wanted to go to school and now that you're a little clearer, you really want to get on with your life and hurry up and go to school right away. I would encourage the addict to think about it for a while and not go to school right away. Maybe you were afraid to go to school years ago, and just because you're not eating right now and you're abstinent from overeating or starving doesn't mean that the fear of school is not there. It means STOP in recovery, take time, talk about it, and ask yourself this question, "Am I ready enough to go to school and experience this fear and anxiety over school and not eat or starve over it?" If the answer is "no," maybe it's not time to go to school yet. That doesn't mean that the answer will remain "no" forever, but it may be "no" right now.

There is a principle used in AA that I don't think is talked enough about in the 12 Step food recovery rooms: **Do not make any major changes in the first year of recovery—it's a set-up for sabotage/relapse!** I have seen many food addicts with established abstinence, working their program, who jumped into situations too early and end up picking up the food again.

Recovery is a check on reality. "Can I do this now or can't I do this now?" Part of recovery is not being compulsive, not giving into impulse, not doing it right away just because you thought about it. Recovery is sane living. It is not sane living to jump into something that is going to cause you to go back to your addiction. Sane living is not saying, "I want what I want, when I want it, and I don't care how I get it, and I'll break my abstinence if that's what it takes. I don't care." That's not what most people want to do.

RECOVERY AND HOW IT AFFECTS THE FAMILY: CHANGING THE CONTRACT

Another major stumbling block in recovery is that it requires you to change your patterns within your family.

Do you have an eating partner in your family? What has to change with that person for you to have a healthy relationship with them?

Are you a people-pleaser? Do you need permission from everyone in your family to do what you need to do to recover? When was the last time you did something just for you, without any permission from anyone else, that they may not have been too happy about? (Certainly you never needed permission to binge or purge or starve.)

Your family may not be happy about your being out of the home for meetings, on the phone with other program people, refusing to prepare

Sabotage and Relapse

foods that you have finally accepted that you can't handle, not buying your trigger foods even though they want them in the house, etc. Are you going to give them the power over your recovery? How will you negotiate it with them?

Do you have a pattern in your family where you say, "Oh sure, I can handle that," and it sets you up every time, because you don't want anyone to think, *It's only food! How could you not handle that?* Do you ever say, "I don't want to disrupt anybody, so I say I can handle it and I wind up eating it"?

Will you be able to set the boundaries that will be necessary for your recovery? Will you be able to say, "No, I'm sorry, I can't handle it," and either get some help or ask them not to have the offensive food in the home? Or will you throw up your hands in defeat because it's hard to change the balance in the family? Most likely, those pressuring the addict have a food addiction also, and unconsciously they don't want you to "leave them" by changing and getting well, even though they love you and want to see you happy. This is a major challenge.

SABOTAGE

Sabotage is defined as an act of malicious damage or destruction; to damage or destroy; undermining. What must first be considered is: Whose recovery is it? Have you taken the responsibility for your recovery? Or have you given the responsibility to other people or situations in your life? For example:

- *If I don't get the perfect sponsor, I can't possibly be abstinent or work the program.*

- *I could be abstinent from overeating or purging or starving if things in my house were better.*

- *I could work my program of recovery if I had a job that didn't make me so upset.*

- *And so on.*

Recovery begins with a decision to be abstinent, regardless of past or present situations. Once that decision has been made, recovery can begin. **Recovery** means to restore oneself to a natural balance.

"We learn that the need to control or to please others sabotages our recovery and that love, accepting ourselves, and meeting our needs takes the place of our addiction to food."
—JANET GREESON, "IS IT CONTROL OR COMPLIANCE"
(RECOVERY PRESS, 1991)

RELAPSE

Recovery cannot occur until the food addict acknowledges the presence of addictive disease, recognizes the need for total abstinence from all the food triggers, and makes a decision to maintain abstinence with the assistance of a recovery program.

Following a food plan without using the tools of recovery denies the reality of this being an addiction. This denial is yet another symptom of the disease.

The relapse process begins long before out-of-control eating or starving starts. It's an unfolding process in which the resumption of active food addiction is the last event in a long series of maladaptive responses to internal or external stressors or stimuli. In other words, the end of the relapse process is picking up the "first bite." As is said in AA, one (as in one alcoholic drink) is too many and a thousand is not enough. For us as food addicts, it's the first bite of any of our trigger foods that sets our disease in motion with craving, obsession, and compulsion, and then we're back to bingeing and/or purging. Once we pick up any one of the trigger foods or go off the structure of the food plan, we're on a moving locomotive—we can't stop.

Often, if we "pick up" the food, we look for the "why" behind our overeating or undereating. The answer is that it makes no difference why we relapsed into old behavior; what is important is that we stay away from the behavior.

Knowing the signs, symptoms of, and triggers to a potential relapse is vital to maintaining balance and abstinence (especially during the first 90 to 120 days of abstinence). Some of these warning signs have been identified by Terence Gorski, president of The CENAPS Corporation (a training and consultation firm specializing in recovery from addictive disease and relapse prevention therapy), who has written extensively on relapse.

Sabotage and Relapse

Remember that recovery can be sabotaged in very silent and subtle ways:

- **Complacency** when life begins to improve. People in long-term recovery may believe that they no longer need to focus on their recovery efforts; they may be convinced they will never begin using food again.

  - ➤ Food addiction is like a tiger; it waits. It waits for fatigue and the loss of perspective that comes with being tired. It waits for the recovering addict to cast away her support network. It is ready for those who follow the fast lane and for those who mistakenly start to think they can eat and drink like anyone else. It is dangerous to let up on disciplines when everything is going well. Always having a little fear is a good thing. Many relapses occur when things are going well.

- **Lack of self-care** as the person becomes exhausted and develops or returns to poor health habits.

  - ➤ Not getting sufficient sleep; exhaustion. Allowing yourself to become overly tired or in poor health. Good health and enough rest are important. If you feel good, you are more apt to think well. Feel poor, and your thinking is apt to deteriorate. Feel bad enough, and you might begin thinking that any of the trigger foods couldn't make it any worse.

  - ➤ Lack of exercise. Regular aerobic exercise is a protective factor.

  - ➤ Overexercising. Such activity leads the addict to focus on the symptom (the weight) and not the solution (recovery). It precludes normal activities of daily living.

  - ➤ Poor stress management. Regular stress management activities such as meditation, relaxation exercises, and taking regular breaks and rest periods are all protective factors.

- **Pursuing recovery with less energy than pursuing addiction.**

- **Increase in or return to denial.** People in long-term recovery may start ignoring, rationalizing, justifying, minimizing, blaming, or generalizing addictive thinking and behavior.

- When we ignore a problem, we pretend that it doesn't exist. We deliberately refuse to recognize and to honor what is going on inside of us and around us. When we minimize, we mislead ourselves into believing the problem is so small and insignificant that it isn't worth dealing with. When we rationalize, we find good reasons for having the problem and believe that these good reasons will protect us from the damage of our addiction and of relapse. When we blame our problems on other people, we can convince ourselves that since the problem isn't our fault and there is no way it can lead us into a relapse.
- Addiction is a disease of denial. The denial does not go away simply because the food addict is abstinent. The food addict can deny their need for continuing involvement in their recovery program when they begin to feel better as a result of their abstinence.
- Because denial is an unconscious process, many food addicts believe they are doing the best they can in recovery, when, in fact, they are not.

- **Not following/respecting the guidelines of the food plan.** This includes:
  - Changing mealtime.
  - Skipping meals.
  - Not respecting the timing of your meals, including allowing too much time in between meals.
  - Eating too quickly.
  - Sloppy measurements.
  - Failing to plan.
  - Eating while watching TV, using the phone, or reading a book.
  - Not calling in food changes to your sponsor or another program person
  - Reducing or increasing portion size.
  - Neglecting to check labels.
  - Thoughts of eating off the food plan.

- **Dishonesty,** which begins with a pattern of small, unnecessary little lies and deceits with fellow workers, friends, and family. Then comes

Sabotage and Relapse

important lies to yourself. This is called rationalizing—making excuses for not doing what you do not want to do (e.g. working your program), or for doing what you know you should not do.

- **Impatience** when things are not happening fast enough, such as when weight loss is not happening on your schedule, or when others are not doing what you want or what you think they should do.

- **Wanting too much**; setting goals you cannot reach with normal effort. Do not expect too much. It's always great when good things you were not expecting happen. You will get what you are entitled to as long as you do your best, but maybe not as soon as you think you should. "Happiness is not having what you want, but wanting what you have."[142]

- **Argumentativeness** regarding small and insignificant points of view, indicating a need to always be right. "Why don't you be reasonable and agree with me?" Looking for an excuse to eat.

- **Frustration** with people and also because things may not be going your way. Remember, everything is not going to be just the way you want it. This frustration can come from a belief that life should be easy.

- **Cockiness** that you've got it made, that you no longer fear picking up. Going into food situations to prove to others (or yourself) you have no problem. Do this often enough and it will wear down your defenses. *It can't happen to me* is dangerous thinking. Almost anything can happen to you and is more likely to happen if you get careless. Remember you have a progressive disease, and you will be in worse shape if you relapse.

  ➤ As far as going into seductive food situations, like family get-togethers, is concerned, it is said in AA that "if you hang around a barber shop, you'll eventually get a haircut!" Wise words!

- **Isolation** and attempting to solve problems on your own. You may not share what is going on with others, not allowing others to know what you're thinking and feeling.

  ➤ Having something on your mind and not talking about it.

- ➤ Not telling anyone what's going on.
- ➤ Doing things alone.

- **Not tolerating feelings as they surface in various situations** and finding/using something to *make* them go away.

- **Setting unrealistic goals** or wanting too much progress too quickly. The slower you go, the sooner you will arrive.

- **12 Step program Issues**
  - ➤ Not being in touch with what you really need—e.g., a meeting a day. (Those in AA are more connected to this issue than those in food recovery fellowships.)
  - ➤ Letting up on disciplines like prayer, meditation, daily inventory, or 12 Step meeting attendance. This can stem either from complacency or boredom. You cannot afford to be bored with your program. The cost of relapse is always too great.
  - ➤ Eliminating one or two meetings (maybe someone said something at the meeting you didn't like), or worse, discounting or discontinuing a recovery program, such as neglecting to attend 12 Step meetings or counseling sessions.
  - ➤ Not going to meetings when your family thinks you "should" stay home.
  - ➤ Not doing Step work.
  - ➤ Not reading program literature.
  - ➤ Not studying the *Alcoholics Anonymous: Big Book*.
  - ➤ Not "turning over" meals.
  - ➤ Not calling your sponsor daily and not making other daily program calls.
  - ➤ Not making amends once you understand your obligation to do so.
  - ➤ Using the program to try to become perfect.

- **Emotional Challenges and Issues**
  - ➤ Painful circumstances.
  - ➤ Rebellion/defiance.

Sabotage and Relapse

- Self-pity/negativity/looking for pity—"Why do these things happen to me?" "Why must I be a food addict?" "Nobody appreciates all I am doing (for them)." Feeling like a victim, refusing to acknowledge that you have choices and are responsible for your own life and the quality of it.
- Depression—Overwhelming, unreasonable, and unaccountable despair may occur in cycles and should be dealt with and talked about. You are responsible for taking care of yourself.
- Resentment.
- Insecurity.
- Feeling hostility toward people and/or circumstances.
- Being intolerant; putting others down.
- Expecting too much from others—"I've changed, so why hasn't everyone else changed, too?" All you can control is yourself. It would be great if other people changed their self-destructive behaviors, but that is their problem. You have your own problems to monitor and deal with. You cannot expect others to change their lifestyle just because you have.
- Jealousy of others, including of their looks.
- Feelings of worthlessness and/or inappropriate guilt.
- Perfectionism.
- Anxiety/nameless fears.
- Unrealistic/unchecked anger.
- Judgment, criticism, blame.
- Worrying about what others think.
- Returning to obsession about food and weight.
- Not getting help for emotional/relationship problems.
- Confusing self-concern with selfishness.
- Feeling special and unique beyond what is realistic.

- **Euphoric recall or romanticizing the food.** Remembering and exaggerating the pleasurable experiences of using sugar (candy, cake, and ice cream), flour, caffeine, high-fat and high-salt foods, "special" holiday foods, and the family connection to them, while blocking out painful and unpleasant aspects of the memory.

> ➤ Sometimes recovering people talk about memories of the pleasure of certain trigger foods. When this happens, it can trigger obsessive thinking, compulsive behaviors, and urges. We tend to exaggerate the good feelings and the times they're associated with and ignore the consequences.

> ➤ Your addiction may tell you that, just maybe, you can have those pleasant experiences again. You should avoid these self-conversations whenever possible. When you have these times of euphoric recall, it is important to remember the terrible consequences that happened as your food addiction progressed. Remind yourself of how long it has been since you had good experiences from using food.

- **Awfulizing abstinence.** When food addicts awfulize abstinence, they notice all of the negatives and exaggerate them while blocking out all of the positive aspects of recovery. This leads the recovering food addict to feel deprived in recovery and to believe that being abstinent is not nearly as good as eating like a "normal person."

- **Magical thinking** about the eliminated trigger foods (sugar, sweeteners, flour, caffeine, volume, high fat/salt foods, hard/soft cheese, "munchy/crunchy" foods, nuts, gum, mints, etc.) leads the food addict to believe that using these foods again will solve all of their problems. This magical thinking is brought about by the euphoric recall ("Remember how good it was!") and the awfulizing of abstinence ("Look at how awful it is that I can't eat those foods.")

> ➤ Magical thinking is believing that if you use food, it will make the situation better or that it will help you do something that you think you can't do. An example of this is using food to give you courage in a difficult situation.

> ➤ You used eating, not eating, and/or eating and purging to deal with many different problems. When you were angry, nervous, sad, or happy, you have used food to change/numb how you felt or to try to make it even better.

Sabotage and Relapse

425

> When you have these thoughts, remember that this is your addiction talking to you. You can learn how to do these things without using food. Ask your sponsor or other recovering people how they handle such situations.

- **Empowering the compulsion.** The food addict does this by telling herself that she cannot stand not having the trigger food(s) and that there is no way to resist the urge.

- **Lack of communication.** If the food addict stops talking about her experience in recovery, she will get into trouble. Replacing rigorous honesty with superficial communication will isolate her and prevent her from doing a sanity check with recovering peers on her recovery experiences.

- **Not talking about the feelings/emotions** that are experienced because food is no longer being used to medicate the addict's feelings. Urges, as I define them, are provoked by these feelings and the resultant thoughts about eating or starving must be revealed and discussed.

  > When you have feelings of fear, shame, guilt, and hopelessness, it is absolutely necessary to talk to other recovering people about these thoughts and feelings. By talking to others, you will find out that they had them, too. You can ask them what they did about them and try those things yourself.

  > It is important to remember when these thoughts and feelings happen that this is not you but your addiction trying to regain control. By labeling it as, "That is my addiction talking to me," you can let it go instead of trying to fight it.

  > Remember, identify, and label it as, "That is my addiction talking to me," and focus your attention on something else. If these thoughts continue, call or talk to another recovering person right away.

- **Believing that they can handle social situations** with family or "normal eaters" without discussing it with their recovering support system (food sponsor and peers in the program) and without following suggestions (e.g., don't go, bring a recovering peer with you, arrange to call members of your support system during the event ["book-ending"], bring your abstinent meal with you, etc.).

- **Analyzing** what needs to be shared and what doesn't.

- **Holding on to "just one or two" unhealthy attitudes or resentments.**

- **Not being true to your "self."** Saying "yes" when you need to say "no."

- **Staying in the same patterns** you ate, starved, or purged in.

- **Not doing new things** or asking for help when you need it.

- **Not following program suggestions for spiritual practice:**
  - ➤ Not praying or meditating; not staying in contact with your "Higher Power" daily.
  - ➤ Forgetting gratitude. You may be looking negatively on your life, concentrating on problems that still are not totally corrected. Nobody wants to be a Pollyanna, but it is good to remember where you started from and how much better life is now.
  - ➤ Not writing a daily gratitude list.

- **The use of mood-altering chemicals.** You may feel the need or desire to get away from things by drinking, popping a few pills, etc. (remember alcohol is not on your food plan), and your physician may participate, thinking that you will be responsible and not abuse the medication. This is a subtle way to enter relapse. Take responsibility for your life and the choices that you make.

- **Not owning your abstinence and recovery as your responsibility.**

- **Omnipotence.** This is a feeling that results from a combination of many of the above. You now have all the answers for yourself and others. No one can tell you anything. You cease listening to others for direction and guidance. "I've got this and now I can fly on my own."

The Relapse Cycle

In the chapters on the little food addict, self-esteem, and the family, we discussed shame, how neglect and abuse relate to food addiction, the addict's inner relationship with the self, and the significance of shame and the human condition. Self-esteem, identity, and intimacy are all important areas in the personality that are influenced by the experience of shame.

Sabotage and Relapse

As we discussed, inherent in being human is a need to have meaning in our lives, to have a sense of belonging with others, and to feel valued. We want to feel special in some way, to feel useful and to matter to others. Yet there are many times when a sense of doubt creeps into our consciousness.

Some event causes an awareness of exposure, resulting in self-consciousness. We begin to question our adequacy or our very worth as a human being. Individuals with eating problems may outwardly appear resistant, stubborn, or rebellious while inwardly fostering extremely negative thoughts about themselves.

Internally, the food addict remains stranded in a sort of confused twilight zone, feeling torn between desperate shame and intense anger. The anger is usually blocked from direct expression, then turned back on the addict themselves in the form of self-condemning thoughts and self-destructive behaviors.

Let's see how this works in our lives. Think of a difficult situation you were involved with that happened over the last few weeks. What the situation was is not as important as what negative *thoughts* you started to have about yourself—you know, those "I am" thoughts that come from the **Itty-Bitty Shitty Committee** as an inner voice whispering despair. These **THOUGHTS** may sound like this:

I am flawed and defective as a human being and inferior to others.

I am a mistake.

I'm impossible to love/I'm unlovable.

I can't do anything right.

I'm a failure at relationships.

I'm worthless.

I'm a loser.

I'm stupid.

I'm a screw-up/ a f-up.

I effed up again.

I'm ugly/fat.

I am an inconvenience/bother to everyone.

I don't deserve genuine positive attention.

I'm unacceptable.

I don't deserve to feel good because I really am inferior or defective.

I don't deserve any happiness or self-esteem because I'm bad and I deserve to suffer.

Life really is awful. People who feel happy are stupid and naïve.

If I beat up on myself relentlessly, it will motivate me to recover.

Nothing will ever change, so why try? If I don't get my hopes up, I won't be disappointed.

My opinion is not wanted/useless.

I'm different.

No one can understand me.

No one wants to give me time.

I have to fight to be heard.

No one wants me.

No one cares.

It's all up to me.

I gotta keep calm.

I gotta live on the edge of insanity.

I gotta endure mistreatment.

I gotta keep on dancing.

I have to carry all the responsibility.

I have no one to lean on or support me.

When we doubt ourselves in this way, we somehow believe we are to blame for the situation, that it has something to do with our failure as a human being. We often feel an inner pain saying we are simply not enough, and therefore, there is nothing that can be done about it. This is shame.

How about the rest of the thoughts?

I'll never get it/never get it right.

I'm hopeless.

I don't matter.

I'm too damaged.

Sabotage and Relapse

Basically, these thoughts come from core beliefs that have been formed from childhood as we have discussed previously. (See Chapter3: Little Food Addict in Training and Chapter 14: Self-Esteem and Family Systems.)

1. Self-Image: *I am basically a bad, unworthy person.*

2. Relationships: *No one would love me as I am.*

3. Needs: *My needs are never going to be met if I have to depend on others.*

It doesn't stop there though. The thoughts give rise to **FEELINGS**. These thoughts lead you to feel:

Sad	*Disconnected*	*Trapped*
Hurt	*Separate*	*Controlled*
Depressed	*Isolated*	*Forced*
Despair	*Deprived*	*Smothered*
Rejected	*Unimportant*	*Put down*
Abandoned	*Useless*	*Not good enough*
Unlovable	*Worthless*	*Less than*
Inadequate	*Unwanted*	*Mad*
Powerless	*Not understood*	*Angry*
Lost	*Criticized*	*Rage*
Nervous	*Judged*	*Guilt*
Anxious	*Betrayed*	*Loss*
Disappointed	*Overwhelmed*	*Grief*
Empty	*Frightened*	*Shame*
Lonely	*Scared*	*Embarrassment*

What comes next? Only three clients in the over twenty-plus years in which I have presented this lecture have ever guessed the answer.

URGES

To act out—to "pick up" food (eating or restricting), and, if chemically dependent, alcohol or drugs. Next are actions.

ACTIONS

These will be one of three options:

- *Repress the urge*
- *Do something else*
  - *Go to a meeting*
  - *Call a program friend*
  - *Read recovery literature*
  - *Write about feelings*
  - *Anything else recovery related*
- *Act out—"pick up"*

If the food addict "picks up," reverting to old coping behavior by using sugar, flour, or any of trigger foods, then the thoughts above start all over again, and then the feelings, and so on—and the addict is now caught in a relapse cycle.

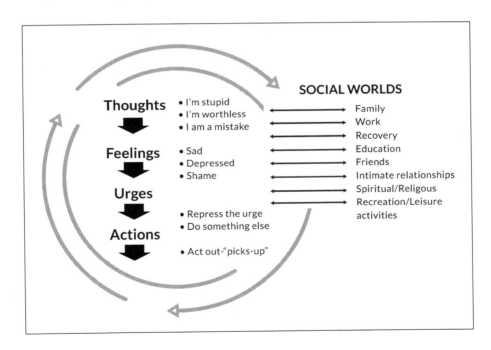

How do we prevent this cycle? By doing the work of recovery, which will begin to change our core beliefs, which are lies anyway. No one is

Sabotage and Relapse

born without value, worth, and preciousness. But our experiences in our families, receiving messages that we're not good enough, being shamed for who we are, using food to comfort ourselves and numb our feelings, and feeling crazed and out of control, all conspire to undermine our inherent, basic sense of worth and preciousness.

Once the food addict is in relapse, every area of her life is impacted. What are the social worlds we live in?

- Family
- Work
- Recovery
- Education

- Friendships
- Intimate relationships
- Spiritual/religious
- Recreation/leisure activities

So when you, the food addict, are having thoughts that you are a "screw-up," "a loser," and/or any of those other negative thoughts you have about yourself, does that affect how you behave and relate to family members? Of course it does. And when there is a difficult situation in your family, do you start thinking, *No one wants my opinion,* or any of the other negative thoughts mentioned above? Most likely yes.

The idea is that there is an interaction between all the social worlds you live in, the thoughts, feelings, and urges living in you, and the actions that you take in response to these. That's how food addiction is a "social" illness.

The problems of food addiction include:

- Malnutrition and metabolic dysfunction

- Medical complications

- Brain dysfunction—Interference with perception, judgment, decision-making, focus, concentration, thought processing, analytic thinking, etc.

- Addictive preoccupation—The food addict's thinking patterns are altered by the addiction as the disease progresses. These changes cause the addict to have strong thoughts, desires, and physical cravings. These processes also change the way the addict sees the world. They lead the addict to believe that using the food is better than not using, despite the consequences that result from using.

See Chapter 2: What is Food Addiction? for an in-depth discussion.

As the physical and psychological problems mentioned above get worse, the addicted person's behavior becomes more antisocial and self-destructive. Frequent social consequences include poor and unhealthy relationships, avoidance of relationships (isolation), occupational problems (poor job performance, taking jobs that the addict is theoretically overqualified for, inability to work, money problems, illness, death), etc.

In addition, most, if not all, food addicts have been raised in families that did not provide proper support, guidance, and values. (See Chapters 14 and 15.) This causes them to develop self-defeating personality styles that interfere with their ability to have healthy relationships and productive lifestyles. Personality is the habitual way of thinking, feeling, acting, and relating to others that develops in childhood and continues in adult life. Personality develops as a result of an interaction between genetically inherited traits and family environment.

Growing up in a dysfunctional family causes a person to have a distorted view of the world. That person learns coping methods, including the "use" of food, that are dysfunctional. In addition, the family may not have been able to provide guidance or foster the development of social and occupational skills that allow a person to fully participate in society. This lack of skills and distorted personality functioning fuel the addictive process and leaves the food addict ill-equipped to live a healthy fulfilling life. But there is upside potential beginning with the development of self-love.

Be in the present—and do the best you can. **Recovery is the ultimate act of self-love!**

CHAPTER 18

Therapy and Treatment
for Food Addiction

We teach people how to treat us.

—ANONYMOUS

Food addiction is a treatable disease that should be treated. Like other diseases, food addiction requires professional treatment in addition to a 12 step program. At some point in your quest for recovery, getting into therapy or treatment, if you can afford it, is important. However, I believe it is necessary to be with a therapist who understands food addiction and will support and respect your abstinence and the need to avoid the triggering substances (sugar, sugar substitutes, flour, wheat, caffeine, etc.) to remain without cravings.

If your therapist believes you should be able to eat everything in moderation, walk away quickly and find someone else. This attempt at moderate eating is what you have been trying to do most of your life, and you're reading this book, looking for a solution, because you have not been able to successfully eat in moderation. *A therapist who does not understand that your addiction is an issue of chronic brain disease of brain reward, motivation, memory, and related circuitry will sabotage your recovery.*

Treatment is typically available on an outpatient basis and should include psychoeducation groups, early recovery groups, individual counseling sessions, and, if appropriate, psychiatric evaluation and medication management. That's the model Realization Center uses so successfully. The treatment program becomes the anchor or mooring from which the food addict can embark on the path to recovery and healing.

Getting into recovery is like learning a second language. It takes concentration and work. But over time, it comes to be second nature, like a well-learned second language. You learn a new language of choice, rather than compulsion. You learn a new language of feelings and empathy for self and others, rather than arrogance and disregard. You learn a new language of boundaries and responsibility, rather than wild wide-openness and impulsiveness. You can become quite proficient and even eloquent in your new second language of recovery. But it will never be your first language. You can either speak the language of addiction flawlessly or speak the language of recovery with an accent. The right therapist/counselor and treatment program can be a wonderful recovery language teacher.

Food addicts have lost clarity about what they truly want, other than a thin body and the supposed acceptance that will come with that body ideal. Most often, they have lost their sense of true self, including their spiritual identity. It is common in therapy to hear that clients are afraid of recovery itself because of who they will be, if and when they let go of the active addiction and become abstinent.

Many therapists believe that if they can help their client unravel their feelings about their history of abuse, neglect, abandonment, and shame, doing so will allow the problematic eating behavior to resolve. Working first on the "underlying issues" gives the client the wrong message.

The food addict suffers from addiction which can only resolve when the behavior is tackled first. The food addiction is interrupted through the use of 12 Step food recovery fellowships; cognitive behavioral therapy, which provides clients with ways to cope with life without using eating/not eating, breaking patterns that support the addiction; and/or motivational enhancement therapy, a combination of client-centered and cognitive behavioral techniques aimed at raising clients' awareness of the consequences of their problem eating behavior in their lives and encouraging them to a make a commitment to change. The therapist and/or treatment program should help the client deal with the fear of letting go of the behaviors that have protected them from their feelings and help the client begin making changes in their eating or not eating using the food plan as the guide.

We work on behavior first, then insight follows. The focus should always be on helping clients manage/resolve their symptoms (overeating, purging, starving) first and acquiring personal insight later in their treatment.

Therapy and Treatment for Food Addiction

Diane Mickley, MD, director of the Wilkins Center for Eating Disorders in Greenwich, Connecticut, says:

"In treating eating disorders in general, one of the common myths is that there are underlying psychological problems, you work them out, and the illness will evaporate. But it's the reverse. If you have an eating disorder, you must first manage food, weight, and eating symptoms if you want to do good work in therapy. The notion that you'll take someone who is throwing up [or overeating] all day and build her confidence makes no sense—the act of vomiting [or overeating] provides her with emotional Novocain, and if you numb your feelings, how are you going to learn what you feel?"[143]

So, abstinence comes first.

The therapeutic relationship serves as an instrument in the healing process by providing an environment where trust and self-discovery can occur. I believe the food addict needs much encouragement, support, loving confrontation, and positive reinforcement of their ability to change and become abstinent.

After some basic education about the concept of Realization Center's Food Addiction Treatment Program (i.e., nature of cravings [brain driven] and the basics of the function of blood sugar levels), I ask clients to try "the breakfast." It's the easiest meal with the least thought and shopping required and it provides immediate positive effects—sustained energy and better mood for three to five hours.

Most clients are amazed that such a "small change," with such little effort, creates such a benefit, and then some clients begin to feel hopeful and encouraged and others get scared. It's all part of the experience, and if they continue to attend, it all usually gets worked out toward abstinence.

> *"A journey of a thousand miles*
> *begins with a single step."*
> —LAO TZU

GOALS OF TREATMENT

The overall goal in treatment is to enable the food addict to work through the core belief of not being good enough as a person and to support their emergence from an identity infused with shame, doubt, and fear, as well as to help reacquaint the food addict with their good heart, with qualities, strengths, and attributes that they have possessed all along but have lost in the obsessions and compulsions of the food addiction.

The 12 Steps, first developed by Alcoholics Anonymous, have become the basis for Overeaters Anonymous and other 12 Step food recovery–focused fellowships. The steps become integrated into one's daily life and the addict begins to grow emotionally and spiritually.

Treatment for food addiction should incorporate the principles of the 12 Step model, which has been so successful in treating other addictions. Hope is created as the disease is arrested and the food addict finds she can live a healthy life without the addictive behaviors, begins to build trusting relationships with others, and sheds the old identity that depends upon the food addiction.

Recovery is a lifelong process.

> *"What would you attempt to do*
> *if you knew you could not fail?"*
> —ROBERT H. SCHULLER

Food addiction reflects the addict's discomfort and dissatisfaction with herself. The addict lacks an enduring sense of a meaningful self and continuously experiences the anxiety of being lost and alone. She frantically escapes the terror of nothingness through what she does to her body—by the mood and consciousness-altering aspects of bingeing, purging, and starving, as well as by using her body as the only measure of her value. The food addict is alienated from others, but especially from herself. She loses any comfortable connection with her community. She loses her sense of effectiveness and control over her life. Her view of herself becomes increasingly distorted through the lens of a misperceived body image.

The therapist has the responsibility and opportunity to direct the client to true recovery—to help the client uncover the truth first by helping

Therapy and Treatment for Food Addiction

the client become abstinent, which will allow for the identification and resolution of those distorted beliefs and feelings which are a direct consequence of the food addiction itself. Self-esteem and a sense of efficacy begin to emerge so quickly when the food addict puts down the behavior and follows the food plan and works though any fears about attending 12 Step food fellowship meetings. As feelings begin to emerge as a result of the addict's no longer anesthetizing herself, then—and only then—can the distorted beliefs the addict has about her worth and meaning can be unraveled. The first year of recovery is a vulnerable time for the newly abstinent food addict. The therapist must be careful not to explore or provoke the recall of early traumatic experiences and memories, which can serve to undermine the foundation of abstinence and recovery the food addict needs to build at this time.

Unfortunately, many therapists, including addiction counselors, who don't understand the true nature of food addiction are often "off course" in their attempt to help their clients. A client presenting with symptoms of overweight, bulimia or anorexia, lethargy, and a general lack of self-care would rightly indicate depression. Yet what is the cause of the depression? The therapist or addictions counselor would do well to look "outside the box." A surprising answer may become clear; the client may be an undiagnosed food addict! The food addiction itself may be the cause of depression!

If the addict continues to use food for comfort, there is a guarantee that her emotional growth will be stunted. Searching for solutions may be distracting the therapist from the immediate and treatable problem: the client is a food addict and needs to abstain from toxic foods! Focusing on early childhood trauma, abuse, alcoholism, abandonment, etc., from the outset may prevent the initiation of food addiction treatment. While the client continues to use, the therapist or counselor will be unable to penetrate the protective shell surrounding the addict's mind and emotions. Food addiction serves as a buffer against the emergence of painful feelings.

Some of the goals of treatment that should only be undertaken after the client has been determined to be medically stable include:

- Psychoeducation about the disease of food addiction with introduction to the food plan.

- Helping the food addict develop abstinence from overeating, bingeing, bingeing/purging, and starving behaviors by replacing those behaviors with healthy eating patterns and nutritional stability—the Food Plan.

- Involving the client in a 12 Step food recovery fellowship and encouraging the client to attend meetings.

- Supporting the client through the withdrawal process.

- Addressing coexisting diagnoses.

- Reducing the effects of trauma.

- Decreasing depression and anxiety.

- Increasing self-esteem, which begins with "putting down" the trigger foods and "picking up" the abstinent plan of eating.

- Identifying relapse triggers.

- Promoting flexibility.

- Clarifying distortions in body image.

- Exercise moderation.

- Improving communication skills and the ability to accurately identify feelings and expression of feelings.

- Improving problem-solving and conflict-resolution skills.

- Establishing appropriate boundaries.

- Identifying the old messages and thought patterns and replacing them with healthy messages and patterns.

- Family therapy.

- Developing a leisure activity plan.

Feelings Buried Alive Never Die

The work you need to do in therapy at this early point in your abstinence is to deal with the feelings that will surface because you're not using food to push them down. Early abstinence is not the time to "dig away" at your abuse issues unless the feelings are interfering with your being

Therapy and Treatment for Food Addiction

439

comfortable in abstinence. Remember, you want to work on changing your behavior with food first.

Therapy, along with involvement with a 12 Step food fellowship, helps the addict to identify and name their feelings as they surface and learn to accept those feelings without self-judgment. Most addicts starting this process don't know anything about feelings; they have automatic responses to them that have been programed since childhood. They don't know that feelings aren't good or bad—they're just feelings. The addict has to learn that how they express their feelings may be helpful or hurtful, but the feelings themselves are okay to have. It's so important to explain to the addict that some feelings are painful, but it is not necessary to eat or starve over them to cover them up. The food addict needs to know and be reassured that it is okay to feel the pain, that they won't die from the feeling, and, alternatively, that it's okay to allow oneself to feel the pleasure of pleasant feelings.

Most food addicts have layers of difficult feelings, anger and rage over sadness and hurt, over anger and rage, over sadness and hurt. A good therapist will help the client identify the anger as it surfaces, even if it has "lace" around it, meaning "anger with a smile."

Anger is probably the most prevalent underlying emotion a food addict knows, yet it is the hardest for most food addicts to express. Many of us have spent years practicing the art of "people-pleasing" so we could be accepted despite our "repulsive" looks and our belief in our worthlessness. We tend to go out of our way to overcompensate for our belief that people have negative perceptions of us. Of course, the people-pleasing started so early in our lives to survive the shaming messages of our childhood.

To recover, we must bring our anger to the surface. It is important for recovering food addicts to be able to vent their rage at their struggles, both with their addiction and with their history. How does this take place? Very little work is required. Usually, when we stop eating compulsively, anger automatically erupts within four or five days. This rage has been festering under the surface, and an effective lid has been kept on the pressure cooker by the self-sedation achieved with food.

In treatment, anger is seen as a positive. It is legitimate and can only be suppressed through return to the abuse of food or other substances.

The Big Book of True Recovery from Food Addiction and Beyond

Indeed, in 12 Step programs, we are encouraged to face our resentments by taking a fearless, thorough inventory of ourselves—the Fourth Step of recovery.

REALIZATION CENTER MODEL

The foundation of The Realization Center Model is the eighteen-week education series. The food addict is concurrently placed in a therapy group, which is specifically targeted to support early recovery. Another necessary component is the individual counseling, which introduces the Realization Center Food Plan for True Recovery; subsequent sessions guide the client as to how to incorporate the food plan into their lives. A 12 Step philosophy is also an integral part of the clinical program.

Food Recovery Education Series

The eighteen-week education series that I have presented over these many years at Realization Center, which is now embodied in this book, serves to lift the veil of the distorted and erroneous beliefs the addict has about herself and the world.

Showing the food addict how they ended up lost in self-destructive, obsessional, compulsive behaviors is the beginning for the food addict finding a way out of their hopelessness and shame. Demonstrating that their circumstance is not their fault but the result of generations of "stuff" is the beginning for the food addict to relinquish their tight grip on the substances and behaviors they use. Offering an alternative (i.e., recovery) to what they falsely believe is the answer becomes a beacon, the "light at the end of the tunnel." In the recovery fellowships, the well-known expression is that, during the darkest hours of the food addict being active in their addiction, the addict believes the light at the end of the tunnel is just another oncoming train!

Johari's Window

In one of the psychoeducation sessions, I explain Johari's Window.

Johari's Window is a graphic way of looking at ourselves in relation to other people. The four panes of the window show the four possible conditions of knowledge about what is "going on" with us.

Therapy and Treatment for Food Addiction

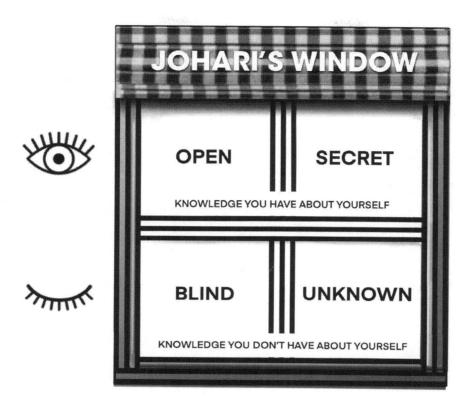

The top two panes, Panes 1 and 2, represent knowledge you have about yourself.

1. The **Open** pane holds those things you do not find threatening and are willing to have others see, like your eye color, hair, and height, or what you're willing to tell others about yourself, such as preferences for food, movies, books you like, work you do, and other superficial information. This pane holds the information you're willing to share about yourself at a party with people you've just met or with acquaintances.

2. The **Secret** pane represents those things you know about yourself that you don't want others to know, things you believe that would cause others to reject you if they knew them (e.g., your feelings!), and behaviors that you find unacceptable in yourself and you assume that others would dislike, mistrust, or be revolted by, etc., if they found out (e.g., your addictions and addictive behaviors).

The bottom two panes, Panes 3 and 4, represent knowledge you don't have about yourself.

3. The **Blind** pane are those things that others perceive about you that you can't see about yourself, things like how you present yourself, such as that you look angry all the time or laugh inappropriately. I'm sure you've had the experience where someone said to you, "You look or seem angry or pissed or sad," and you immediately smiled and said, "No, I'm okay, I'm fine." In a group, if a group member tells you that you seem mad or sad, you have the opportunity not to reject that information, but to say, "Thank you for telling me. I was not aware of that, and I will think about my feelings." When you understand this, you also have the responsibility to tell other group members your observation of them.

4. The **Subconscious** pane are those things neither you nor others can perceive about you. Things in the subconscious are not available to us.

The purpose of group therapy is to help the food addict get rid of as much of the Blind and Secret areas as possible. The advantage to being open is that you do not have secrets you need to hide from others or fears of what others may see in you. You have a better chance for developing and maintaining close interpersonal relationships and experiencing intimacy.

At Realization Center, there are over 150 groups per week in the Manhattan and the Brooklyn Centers that offer the opportunity to work on these areas. The psychoeducation series demonstrates that there is a solution, there is hope and, that itself becomes a motivating force. Often clients become abstinent during the series.

One powerful reason that recovery is so difficult for the food addict is because it requires "individuation" and separation from mother and/or family, whether or not the connection is current or historical. The eating behaviors do serve, in large measure, to keep the food addict dependent on and attached to their mother and the family system, which allows them to avoid the scary and painful transitions that go along with growing up. One of the goals of treatment is to help the food addict explore her ambivalence and fantasies about what she imagines will happen as she gets older and has to move on with her life as an individual without child-like attachments—in effect, "leaving home."

The Benefit of Group Therapy for Food Recovery

Group therapy is a powerful therapeutic tool for the food addict to work through the fear of letting go of their self-destructive behavior and thinking, the fear of being "seen and known" (even though that what we all want so much), and the fear of connecting with others.

Being in a group allows the power of peer influence to facilitate recovery. A successful group is able to engage in a process of working toward a deep level of intimacy and safety. It can create a shift from resistance to working toward mutual recovery.

Clients are challenged to ask for help and to put their struggle into words. By doing so, much of the shame and isolation is replaced by connection, hope, and a willingness to look at themselves in new or different ways.

In the early recovery groups at Realization Center, I encourage each group member to call every other group member once during the week and talk about their recovery process and their thoughts and feelings about it. This helps to break isolation, and promotes a positive response that challenges the beliefs they have, beliefs such as "No one wants to talk with me," "I don't know what to say," "I'll be bothering them," "I feel stupid," or "I am stupid." The client gets to learn they are not alone in these beliefs and feelings, and they begin to feel better about reaching out and talking about themselves. They are also encouraged to attend 12 Step food recovery fellowship meetings.

The clients in the groups focusing on early recovery have the opportunity to talk with each other about their fears of changing, their successes, the "chatter" in their heads, their "missteps," and their resistance to changing, and they get to experience each other's support and validation of their feelings. They also kindly confront each other's denial, mistaken beliefs, and inertia. They get to experience that they are not unique in their feelings and behaviors and beliefs, which help to lessen the shame that all food addicts experience. They arrange to go to 12 Step meetings together—a requirement of being in the group—which makes it easier to get started in the 12 Step food recovery fellowships. The group addresses how to achieve abstinence and the triggers that will sabotage it.

In group therapy, food addicts can practice "using their voice" and stating their needs, which is often a foreign and terrifying experience but is essential to reclaiming their true selves.

At Realization Center, I also facilitate an advanced Food Addiction Recovery Group for clients who are abstinent (i.e., following Realization Center Food Plan for True Recovery from Food Addiction), who attend 12 Step food recovery fellowship meetings, who have a sponsor, and who want support and guidance to address the challenges of life without using food and the underlying issues as they are surfacing. The group becomes a microcosm of their lives.

Addicts tend to re-create their family of origin wherever they go—in their workplace, social life, intimate relationships, and psychotherapy groups. For example, the member that assumes the role of caretaker/fixer in the group is fulfilling the role she plays in the outside world.

This group allows for the members to experience the "transference"[144] that develops in all effective therapy groups and to talk about those feelings in a safe environment. In focusing on underlying issues and not merely the food plan, the facilitator establishes the landscape of the group as that of a safe, trusting environment. In time, members are able to be real and honest with each other and with themselves, responding and reacting in real time, accepting feedback sometimes in the form of criticism in an effort to change self-destructive behavior and distorted beliefs about themselves that no longer fit their picture of recovery. The safe environment of the group allows for an intimacy, maybe for the first time in the addict's life. Often, deep, hidden secrets are uncovered and revealed.

This group is very meaningful for the recovering food addict because it supports the growing awareness and strengths of the group members and because it ensures we are mindful of the potential for relapse and are watchful for relapse signs.

However, treatment is more than symptom management. It must not only help clients understand the meaning of their symptoms, but it must also help them to trust their voices when confronted with silencing forces, such as family and those in authority, and to cope adaptively when those forces will not change.

In group, we explore the various systems the addict lives in—family, social, interpersonal, recovery, occupational, therapeutic, etc.—and work to understand how these systems may be informing the client of their worth, value, meaning, and power. Out of this exploration with clients, we hope to create a new system that will encourage the use of their voice,

Therapy and Treatment for Food Addiction

build up their true self, and provide coping tools to deal with unchanging forces outside the treatment environment.

A "Food Funeral"

Occasionally, we have a "food funeral" in the Early Recovery group at Realization Center. Clients are requested to prepare a eulogy for the substance or behaviors that want to say "goodbye" to and bring it the following week for the funeral. The chairs are set up in a line on two sides facing each other, with a podium at the head and a coffin-shaped box (with a skull and crossbones on the top) on the floor in the middle of these chairs. Candlesticks on either side of the "coffin" are added for effect. Each group member comes up to the podium to share their "goodbye." It's also a wonderful opportunity for the other group members to learn more about each other's real truth about their eating issues.

Here are a few of the latest eulogies:

Pamela's Eulogy

What I am putting in the coffin:

Days of oblivion

Beating the crap out of myself mentally

The terror the next morning after the binge

Lost money to food

The fear of my husband getting home to a lethargic,
non-talkative me

My lying

My not showing up for social things because I binged

The bloat

The bad skin

The false promises I make to myself

The feeling of grandiosity

Andrea's Eulogy

I want to express my deepest happiness over the death of foods that have made me fat and unable to fit in clothes, and make me sad, alone, paranoid, angry, and suicidal. When you were in my life, you insured that my life was one of desperation and sadness. A number of you have gone to hell:

Chocolate—like heroin, you hooked me, and the momentary pleasure of you became my greatest enemy. You lied and pretended to take the pain away, only to replace it with an even greater pain.

Pasta, bread, and pizza—you were not as obvious as chocolate, but your subtle ways took me down. You flooded my thoughts all the time. You became the most important thing. You were all I cared about. Like chocolate, you were devious; you comforted me and then you abandoned me, leaving me in a constant state of wanting more and never having enough.

Nuts, you sat with me during the late night as I mindlessly ate you. You lied, too, because I never got any emotional relief afterward. You are the "Trojan horse" for sugar, flour, and wheat. When I had you, it was just a matter of time before I binged.

Caffeine, you were useless and unnecessary. You made me believe that I need you for energy. Liar! Good riddance.

French Fries, you were sexy and messy, the trophy wife of my food plan. Again, you provided zero sustenance. I have replaced you with a fluffy, enriching potato. Au revoir!

You are nothing but ghosts of a difficult past!

Beatrice's Eulogy

Coffee:

C—chaos

O—ongoing anxiety

F—false energy

F—feelings you helped me suppress

E—endless cycles of energy crashes

E—ecstasy of life without you

OVERCOMING ADDICTION

Overcoming addiction is, in part, a learning process, and people in recovery work to make and maintain healthy changes. In behavioral therapy, clinicians help patients learn techniques to avoid or navigate safely through experiences that evoke powerful urges to use food—stressful situations and the people, places, and things that will trigger powerful urges to return to old coping behaviors with food.

Therapy and Treatment for Food Addiction

The first year of abstinence and recovery present big challenges. The food addict needs to renegotiate their life without using food. The recovering food addict must negotiate their first birthday, Thanksgiving, anniversaries, Christmas, Passover, Easter, long holiday weekends, family events, vacations, etc., without going back to the food. These special events require the food addict to strategize and use their support system with an eye on the time *after* the event when the addict's guard may be lowered because they were successful in staying abstinent through the occasion.

Role of Therapy and Treatment

I see the role of therapy and treatment as complementary and adjunctive to participation in a 12 Step food recovery fellowship. The food addict may initially find the treatment program in her quest for an answer. Besides educating the addict about the nature of the problem, it's also incumbent on the therapist to help the client move through any resistance to participate in a 12 Step food recovery fellowship.

I believe that all resistance to going to meetings and being involved in a recovery program comes from fear—that is, fear of being rejected, fear of being exposed, fear of being seen, of being known and found unacceptable, as well as the fear of being accepted and taken in, which might produce feelings of loss and separation from one's old behaviors and family.

A major goal of therapy is for a person to discover that she is not worthless, not disposable, not rejectable, not inadequate—that who she really is, is "enough." There is no better forum for a food addict to discover the "wonderful" truth about herself than the 12 Step food recovery fellowships. Of course, the food addict may first begin to experience all this in the treatment program with psychoeducation and group participation.

It's interesting to note that a newly sober alcoholic will be told in AA to attend one meeting a day for a year in order to stay sober, and they get to use sugar and coffee to manage their cravings. The food addict, who has a more difficult, challenging addiction because they have to eat and not use any substance to support their abstinence, doesn't receive the same message! Remember, alcoholics can think back to a time in their lives when they weren't using alcohol; the food addict cannot do the same regarding food or eating! The food addict has to deal with their substance four times a day (three meals plus one metabolic adjustment), plus dealing with the rituals and family gatherings. How is abstinence a part of a rainy day? Disappointment? Your birthday?

The addict should never think that therapy or treatment is a replacement for the recovery program. Therapy and treatment programs are not enough to counteract the power of food addiction.

The role of the therapist is to also help the food addict negotiate the challenges and fears that arise in the recovery program, including but not limited to:

- Sharing at meetings.
- Asking for help.
- Allowing themselves to receive help.
- Asking someone to be a sponsor.
- Working with that sponsor.
- "Firing" a sponsor if it's not working out.
- Volunteering to do "service" (e.g., chairing a meeting; taking a service position such as treasurer, literature person, intergroup representative, etc.).
- Reaching out to others with phone calls.
- Socializing after a meeting.

The therapist has the opportunity to help clients find abstinence, to help them use the tools of recovery, and to guide them to actually experience an abundant life, the personal wholeness that comes from acting out the true desires of their heart.

From my own experience, helping food addicts discover and express their authentic selves and identity—to help them become themselves—is a reward beyond words.

CHAPTER 19
Recovery . . . Discovery

*"Man wishes to be confirmed in his being by man, and wishes
to have a presence in the being of the other . . . secretly and
bashfully he watches for the Yes which allows him to be and
which can come to him only from one human person to another."*
—MARTIN BUBER

If you have read through the book to this point, kudos to you. If you have read through the book *and* made some changes with your eating behavior—e.g., eating "the breakfast"—I really applaud you. Change is hard for most people; change for an addict around her addiction is the hardest thing she will ever have to do. If you have the willingness to attend 12 Step food recovery fellowship meetings, you'll be on your way to changing, and if you begin to follow the food plan, you will have an experience of yourself that you have never had before.

As I have said throughout this book, if you use the plan and don't move into recovery by attending meetings, you will have the same result that you have experienced with dieting: eventual failure and defeat. The disease of food addiction will not resolve with a diet.

If you embrace the food plan *and* attend meetings and get involved in the 12 Step program, you will become a star in your own movie. Self-esteem will start to appear. You will begin to get to know yourself differently. This is more a journey of "discovery" than "recovery."

As long as one is active in one's food addiction, one's authentic self is hidden, unknown. Authenticity is based on being real, not running away, not running to a substance, which then creates frustration, self-loathing, shame, despair, hopelessness, and deprivation. Putting down the food and asking for and accepting help through the 12 Step program allows the addict to come alive and begin the journey to becoming real.

Abstinence gives us the courage to be real.

As is beautifully written in *The Velveteen Rabbit*:

"What is REAL?" asked the Rabbit one day, when they were lying side by side near the nursery fender, before Nana came to tidy the room. "Does it mean having things that buzz inside you and a stick-out handle?"

"Real isn't how you are made," said the Skin Horse. "It's a thing that happens to you. When a child loves you for a long, long time, not just to play with, but REALLY loves you, then you become Real."

"Does it hurt?" asked the Rabbit.

"Sometimes," said the Skin Horse, for he was always truthful. "When you are Real you don't mind being hurt."

"Does it happen all at once, like being wound up," he asked, "or bit by bit?"

"It doesn't happen all at once," said the Skin Horse. "You become. It takes a long time. That's why it doesn't happen often to people who break easily, or have sharp edges, or who have to be carefully kept. Generally, by the time you are Real, most of your hair has been loved off, and your eyes drop out and you get loose in your joints and very shabby.

But these things don't matter at all, because once you are Real you can't be ugly, except to people who don't understand."

"I suppose *you* are real?" said the Rabbit. And then he wished he had not said it, for he thought the Skin Horse might be sensitive. But the Skin Horse only smiled.

"The Boy's Uncle made me Real," he said. "That was a great many years ago; but once you are Real you can't become unreal again. It lasts for always."

The Rabbit sighed. He thought it would be a long time before the magic called Real happened to him. He longed to become Real, to know what it felt like; and yet the idea of growing shabby and losing his eyes and whiskers was rather sad.

He wished that he could become it without these uncomfortable things happening to him.[145]

> *"The greatest despair is to not become*
> *the person you were meant to be."*
> —SOREN KIERKEGAARD

Many years ago, a very overweight, unhappy, and poorly functioning woman came to my lecture series in hopes of finally finding an answer to her long-standing eating issues. She had literally tried every diet, weight-loss program, pill, exercise routine, therapeutic intervention, and self-help program, and nothing had worked to help her find peace with her relationship with food. Over time, I began to see her individually. She would very often ask me, "Am I real yet?" and "What if I do all this work and there's nothing there? If I have no soul?"

In finding abstinence, her lifetime of shame, guilt, people-pleasing, false messages, low self-esteem, masks, and poor health was slowly peeled away. And what could not fail to emerge was a sense of self; an understanding of her true value as a human being; the ability to eschew unacceptable behavior toward herself and by others; more energy; better physical health; no more fear of authenticity, her own and that of others; the freedom to express her emotions; and the realization that emotions are neither good nor bad—they just are.

Today, she has a life beyond her wildest dreams. She is of normalized weight, is highly functional, and has become productive and fulfilled in work that she didn't have any idea about when she embarked on her journey of recovery. She understands that being abstinent and working a program of recovery means she cannot stay in her old self; it no longer fits.

John Howard Prin, BA, LADC, in an article for the Summer 2009 issue of *Paradigm* titled "Reclaiming Your Destiny," writes:

> "Sooner or later every functioning adult faces a primal, deep-rooted quandary: 'Why am I alive?' 'What is my purpose in life?' 'What am I going to do about it?' Many people avoid the responsibility of answering these questions by abusing alcohol, drugs, food, gambling, sex, or video games. A great deal of addictive thinking and bizarre, destructive behavior is grounded in avoiding responsibility.
>
> "Once you put down all the substances and behaviors—including, especially, the food—you begin to open yourself to unleashing and radically embracing the most complete version of your authentic self, what I call your 'True You.' This self is essential to your destiny. Rediscovering [or discovering] your 'True You' destiny becomes the foundation of your personal inner journey of recovery, of profound transformation and fulfillment that leads to personal wholeness."[146]

Recovery starts with a willingness to not starve, overeat, or purge. If there is no willingness, there is no book, therapist, or group that can help you. The willingness to participate in making changes is the prime need in recovery. Once you have it, it doesn't make it easier; it just makes it possible. It all begins with a decision.

One of the challenges in recovery is that feelings start to surface. That can be very scary. When you spend so much of your life working to kill off your feelings with the food and with other substances and behaviors (alcohol, drugs, shopping, spending, gambling), *and* you make a decision to not use the food—remember, alcohol and drugs are included in the list of triggers, so if you follow the food plan, they have to be gone also—your feelings will begin to surface. Going to meetings gives you a place to talk about what you're feeling and how you feel about those feelings and to hear others share their experiences with feelings. Therapy can be invaluable at this point, but only with a therapist who will support you in this process and not try to make you "normal" with food. (See Chapter 18: Therapy and Treatment for Food Addiction.)

Recovery is about becoming functional in all of life's areas. Recovery consists of finding healthy alternatives to get from Point A (discomfort) to Point B (comfort) without the use of substances. It's about becoming clear and open and present. If food is in the way, none of that is possible.

What is the work of recovery? It's somewhat simple, but it's big. As I have been saying, it's this: Following the food plan (weighing and measuring portions, respecting the timing of meals, etc.), working with a food sponsor, going to 12 Step food recovery meetings and sharing yourself in this program (getting phone numbers, calling other recovering food addicts daily, working with a sponsor, sharing at meetings, doing service, reading recovery literature), and participation in some exercise routine.

Showing up for recovery is showing up for yourself, showing up for life.

The result of this work is amazing. You discover newfound energy, a stable mood, a positive outlook on life, hope, clear thinking, less codependence since you are no longer abusing yourself with food, and the ability to recognize you don't deserve abuse and to start asserting yourself against the abuse of others in whatever form it was inflicted on you. You begin to set boundaries with others. This all takes time and a lot of support from others in the program.

Recovery . . . Discovery

The food addict must understand that real change takes time; addiction and recovery are both progressive phenomena. Rather than understanding that recovery is a long and progressive process, just as was the development of the disease, the expectation of the food addict is that it will be quick. We must realize that, even when the food addict is abstinent, character traits take time to change. The recovering addict should not lose patience with herself and should certainly not have unrealistic expectations of others. The 12 Steps of recovery are steps, not a high-speed elevator. The slogan "time takes time" means that there is no microwave for recovery.

It's important to remember that recovering people have a long and difficult road to follow. We must learn and practice a way of life that will keep us abstinent. The core of our abstinence is learning new ways of managing our thoughts and feelings that will help us to contribute to life and help others. To do this, we must examine and change how we view ourselves and the way we build and maintain relationships with others.

A big part of recovery is learning nonverbally by finding and watching how others that we admire and respect are living an abstinent life. The 12 Step programs tells us to "stick with the winners." As we get to know the true winners who are living abstinently, we ask them what they do to stay abstinent. We're often told, "If you want what we have, then do what we did/do." Nobody can teach us how to stay abstinent; all they can do is invite us into a culture where we can observe how abstinent people deal with themselves, other people, and the world. We are told to "take the best/what fits and leave the rest." We are also reminded to "keep coming back."

This reminder is important because as we progress in recovery, we will experience new challenges that require new solutions. We also need a place to practice our abstinence skills among others who support our efforts and who share with us the gift of honesty. Remember, abstinence skills are perishable. Unless we practice them every day, we become sloppy and start going back to our old addictive ways of thinking, managing our feelings, and relating to others. Recovery is a group effort. No matter how strong you are or how hard you try, you can't do it by yourself.

This is what the journey of recovery is all about: learning to work in harmony with other people to live an abstinent and responsible life based upon the higher principles embodied in the 12 Step Program. The purpose of recovery is to experience life at all times, to be present for your life, and to be available for what the universe will bring.

A client once said, "Recovery is about becoming right-sized." I think most of us have lived our lives from a "too small" perspective. We don't know how significant we really are. To find our truth and our true self and achieve full recovery, total abstinence plus personality and lifestyle changes are essential.

Recovery means healing.

Spirituality and Recovery

Buddhist cosmology describes addiction as the "Land of Hungry Ghosts" where people have huge appetites that are unable to be satisfied. Buddhism describes addiction as being "a false refuge," a delusional place to try and hide and escape from being present in life with the good and bad. Addiction is viewed as the inability to see the abundance and joy in our everyday lives. Developing a calm awareness can help in not being distracted from life, instead being more present and mindful "in the now."

What true recovery from food addiction offers is a true refuge—a real place, with real people, a community, and principles and guidelines to live by. It allows us to be open to spirituality. In *The Spirituality of Imperfection*, Ernest Kurtz writes that we have suffered *zerrissenheit*, or "torn-to-pieces." Spirituality, as he describes it, is the healing process of "making whole."

Spirituality helps us first to see, then to understand, and eventually to accept the imperfection that lies at the core of our human *being*. Accepting our human limitations brings us inner peace. What a relief it is to put an end to the fight within ourselves! Also, as we find the permission to be the imperfect beings that we are, we become able to let others be who they are.

While we're in the disease of food addiction, we are cut off from all parts of ourselves, including our "spirit." We're unable to access that part of ourselves that is our spirit; we're too caught up with obsession, compulsion, disgust, fear, shame, anger, remorse, craving, guilt, hopelessness, despair, denial, and pretense. We're totally self-involved, self-focused. There's no room for the expression of our spirit. The price of being active in this disease is "the cost of your soul." Or, as *The Big Book* says, we are shut off from "the sunlight of the Spirit."

Recovery . . . Discovery

Recovery is an inside-out journey, as opposed to the outside-in process of food addiction. It means accepting our imperfections, not trying to become perfect. What we need to do is become more human, not perfect. We need to recover our true selves, not immortalize and glorify our false self.

According to John Bradshaw:

"Recovery is about an awakening. Recovery literally awakens us from a restless sleep that has numbed our feelings and left us emotionally and spiritually groggy and exhausted. This awakening begins with the eye-opening experience and recognition of our powerlessness—with the recognition of our limitations and our need for help—and with hard work of transforming our toxic shame into healthy shame. It is this healthy shame that is the source of our spirituality. . . ."

"Spirituality is living each moment of life more abundantly. It is honoring our values in our simplest acts. Spirituality is being present in our feelings. It is being more conscious and more aware of the connection of ourselves to others and all things."[147]

The road of recovery brings us to a new level of awareness and understanding and to a sense of self-fulfillment far surpassing any of the fleeting pleasures or excitement that eating or not eating ever could provide. It is the willingness, determination, and commitment to embrace ourselves and the difficult feelings that we tried to bury with food that leads to a destination of meaning and purpose and that brings a deep sense of self-respect and appreciation for the value of one's own life.

As the food addict participates in her 12 Step food recovery program, it naturally ensues that she begins to share with others in the program and, as recovery evolves, the food addict experiences the exquisite, life-affirming pleasure of being valuable to other human beings.

> *"Each of us is here for a brief sojourn; for what purpose*
> *he knows not, though he sometimes thinks he senses it.*
> *But without deeper reflection, one knows from daily life*
> *that one exists for other people. . . ."*
> —ALBERT EINSTEIN, SWISS PHYSICIST

When I first came into OA in 1976, I felt totally worthless, lost, ashamed of my being, terrified, isolated, totally less-than, hopeless, depressed, and probably passively suicidal (I don't quite remember that). I kept going to meetings despite my feelings. As a result, my journey of recovery has allowed me to be of service, to help thousands of suffering addicts through the program and my treatment center—what a miracle! My life has meaning and purpose and I have a mission and a legacy: this book! Is it any wonder that I am so passionate about real, *true* recovery?

In addition, being in recovery allows for serenity a good part of the time, for relationships with friends and family who are loved and loving, and for a close, ongoing contact with the God or Higher Power of one's understanding. It offers richness in life. The recovering addict can look back on the past and feel compassion for not only the people struggling around her, but also compassion for the naive and addicted person she was. It brings the knowledge that she will always be a food addict, but that she doesn't have to ever again be that self-destructive.

And, in the end, for those who let neither rain, nor snow, nor gloom of night deter their journey, they find themselves able to say, "I am grateful to be a food addict."

In recovery, the little food addict has the opportunity to believe in abundance and her own worthiness. She can begin to understand that miracles can open up in her life in ways never imagined.

Recovery allows the food addict:

- To learn functionality—feeling what you feel, knowing what you feel, and saying what you feel and what you want.

- To no longer be obsessed with food, weight or body image, and to be released from the bondage of food, from the bondage of perfection with your body.

- To let go of and be free of the pursuit of thinness

- To learn and know that you have always had value.

- To learn and know that your self-hatred was based on a longing to have grown up in a whole and connected world where you could have had healthier experience.

Recovery . . . Discovery

- To learn and know that you could not and should not be any different than you are, based on the events along your path.

- To work on loving yourself no matter what.

- To feel whole.

- To learn and know that you have a right to your feelings and you don't have to do anything to deserve love from others.

- To no longer live in the malnourished state of dieting, existing on diet drinks and food substitutes instead of food, creating feelings of deprivation and despair.

- To get rid of your shame and self-hatred.

- To feel much less self-hatred about your body, and to be much more accepting of your body even before experiencing complete physical recovery.

- To be fully conscious as you walk on your path, and to accept yourself in the moment that you're in.

- To learn that you can get through difficult times without using food.

- To not let feelings dictate behavior (e.g., experiencing fear and doing it anyway).

- The ability to step back and not have to act impulsively just because you had a thought.

- To hold yourself to high standards.

- To not beat up on yourself.

- To accept your reality without denying the reality of others and to accept who you are—"I am who I am."

- To walk in harmony with your true self.

- To continue to discover and know your truth—your authentic self.

- To accept and be proud of that truth and to continue to confirm your truth.

- To continue to re-parent yourself.

- To recognize and manage distorted thinking.

- To be honest in your relationships with people and not set yourself or others up.

- To put yourself first some of the time.

- To allow yourself to put somebody else first sometimes.

- To listen to somebody else, to listen to their feelings.

- To not give so much advice.

- To identify what went on in your childhood, talk about the feelings, work through the anger, not eat or starve over it and come to a place of peace and get on with your life.

- To make mistakes and sometimes step backward, but not with the food! (See Chapter 17: Sabotage and Relapse.)

- To practice being imperfect, but not with the food!

- To be perfectly yourself and share in life.

- To be spontaneous, but not with the food!

- To allow others to know who you are, to know that you are vulnerable, to know that you are afraid.

- To make choices and experience feelings.

- To feel comfortable in your own skin.

- To be able to say "no" or "yes."

- To follow your path and learn to accept it fully.

- To experience the beginning of some tranquility in your home and in your life.

Some of us say that were it not for our eating issues, we may not have come to view our lives and the lives of others with empathy or to understand what it means to respect the frailty and vulnerability in all human beings.

There was a quote written on the board in the conference room at Realization Center where I present my lectures. It was put there by another clinician who used the room prior my group. I was struck by its simplicity and truth.

*Affliction comes to us
not to make us sad, but sober/abstinent
not to make us sorry, but wise.*
—H.G. WELLS

Our purpose in recovery is not to feel sorry for ourselves. Rather than self-pity, we must translate our pain into clarity about what matters, into self-knowledge so we do not repeat, and into resilience so we reclaim our strength.

With understanding our pain comes responsibility. Suffering is what calls us to become better people. The undone list naturally leads us to actions we know we must now take.

We know too much to leave things as they are. Our internal guidance systems are fundamentally altered. Self-pity, bitterness, and repression kept us in our old, compulsive ways. Acknowledging our pain brings relief but also new responsibilities. As C.S. Lewis put it years ago when his beloved wife died four years into their marriage, "Pain is what God gave us to grow up."

The Hindu *Bhagavad Gita* suggests we have a duty to act, to realize our full potential in the world, to construct or discover a unique individuality, and thereby to live authentically.[148] Author Stephen Cope explains, "Real fulfillment comes from authentically grappling with the possibility inside you, in a disciplined, concentrated, focused way." That is what 12 Step programs teach us to do.[149]

*"The purpose of life
is to live a life of purpose."*
—ROBERT BYRNE

In *The Way of Man*, philosopher Martin Buber relates a Hasidic parable about one Rabbi Zusya, a self-effacing scholar who has a deathbed revelation that he shares with the friends keeping vigil at his side. "In the next life, I shall not be asked: 'Why were you not more like Moses?'" he says. "I shall be asked: 'Why were you not more like Zusya?'"[150]

A Zen Story

Matajura wanted to become a great swordsman, but his father said he wasn't quick enough and could never learn. So Matajura went to the famous dueler, Banzo, and asked to become his pupil.

"How long will it take me to become a master?" he asked. "Suppose I become your servant, to be with you every minute. How long?"

"Ten years," said Banzo.

"My father is getting old. Before ten years have passed, I will have to return home to take care of him. Suppose I work twice as hard. How long will it take me?"

"Thirty years," said Banzo.

"How is that?" asked Matajura. "First you say ten years. Then, when I offer to work twice as hard, you say it will take me three times as long. Let me make myself clear: I will work unceasingly. No hardship will be too much. How long will it take?"

"Seventy years," said Banzo. "A pupil in such a hurry learns slowly."

Matajura understood. Without asking for any promises in terms of time, he became Banzo's servant.

He cleaned, he cooked, he washed, he gardened. He was ordered never to speak of fencing or to touch a sword. He was very sad at this, but he had given his promise to the master and resolved to keep his word. Three years passed for Matajura as a servant.

One day, as Matajura was gardening, Banzo came up quietly behind him and gave him a terrible whack with a wooden sword. The next day in the kitchen, the same blow fell again. Thereafter, day in, day out, from every corner and at any moment, Matajura was attacked by Banzo's wooden sword. He learned to live on the balls of his feet, ready to dodge at any moment. He became a body with no desires, no thought, only eternal readiness and quickness.

Banzo smiled, and started lessons. Soon Matajura was the greatest swordsman in Japan.

* * *

If Life Is a Game, These Are the Rules
Ten Rules for Being Human

Created by Chérie Carter-Scott, Ph.D. MCC as seen in her
#1 bestselling book, *If Life is a Game, These are the Rules:
Ten Rules for Being Human,* Broadway Books 1998

1. **You will receive a body.**
   You may love it or hate it, but this one body will be yours for the duration of your lifetime on earth.

2. **You will be presented with lessons.**
   You are enrolled in a full-time informal school called "life." Each day in this school you will have the opportunity to learn lessons. You may like the lessons or hate them, but you have designed them as part of your curriculum.

3. **There are no mistakes, only lessons.**
   Growth is a process of trial and error: experimentation. The "failed" experiments are as much a part of the process as the experiment that ultimately "works."

4. **A lesson is repeated until learned.**
   A lesson will be presented to you in various forms until you have learned it. When you have learned it, you can then go on to the next lesson.

5. **Learning does not end.**
   There is no part of life that does not contain lessons. If you are alive, there are lessons to be learned.

6. **"There" is no better than "here."**
   When your "there" has become a "here," you will simply obtain another "there" that will, again, look better than "here."

7. **Others are only mirrors of you.**
   You cannot love or hate something about another person unless it reflects to you something you love or hate about yourself. Each reflection is an opportunity for growth.

8. What you make of your life is up to you.

You have all the tools and resources you need, what you make of them is up to you. The choice is yours.

9. Your answers lie inside you.

The answers to life's questions lie inside you. All you need do is look, listen, and trust.

10. You will forget all this at birth!

Throughout the process of life, you will have opportunities to remember, if you choose.[151]

Here's another way to look at this process of recovery. This poem is well known in the addiction recovering community.

There's a Hole in My Sidewalk: The Romance of Self-Discovery[152]

Portia Nelson

I

I walk down the street.
There is a deep hole in the
  sidewalk.
I pretend I don't see it.
I fall in.
I am lost, I am helpless.
It isn't my fault.
It takes forever to find a way out.

II

I walk down the same street.
There is a deep hole in the
  sidewalk.
I pretend I don't see it.
I fall in again.
I can't believe I am in the same
  place.
But it isn't my fault.
It still takes a long time to get out.

III

I walk down the same street.
There is a deep hole in the
  sidewalk.
I see it is there.
I still fall in . . . it's a habit.
My eyes are open.
I know where I am.
It is my fault.
I get out immediately.

IV

I walk down the same street.
There is a deep hole in the
  sidewalk.
I walk around it.

V

I walk down another street.

CONCLUSION
Last Words

I believe a fitting way to end this discussion on recovery and this book is to list the "promises" of recovery as they are written in *Alcoholics Anonymous: The Big Book*. They are very meaningful, beautiful, and very true.

> If we are painstaking about this phase of our development, we will be amazed before we are halfway through. We are going to know a new freedom and a new happiness. We will not regret the past nor wish to shut the door on it. We will comprehend the word serenity and we will know peace. No matter how far down the scale we have gone, we will see how our experience can benefit others. That feeling of uselessness and self-pity will disappear. We will lose interest in selfish things and gain interest in our fellows. Self-seeking will slip away. Our whole attitude and outlook on life will change. Fear of people and of economic insecurity will leave us. We will intuitively know how to handle situations which used to baffle us. We will suddenly realize that God is doing for us what we could not do for ourselves.
>
> Are these extravagant promises? We think not. They are being fulfilled among us, sometimes quickly, sometimes slowly. They will always materialize if we work for them.[153]

In recovery, the little food addict takes back all that was robbed from her (i.e., feeling precious, lovable, valuable), and lives as a healed whole person. The little food addict, much older now, learns how to live a meaningful and comfortable life without using food or other substances to cope. She learns to grow in individualism and become separate from those upon whom she has become so dependent. The recovering food addict becomes empowered to be a unique individual. She also learns to allow others the freedom to become uniquely who they were created to be. By embracing her individual uniqueness, the recovering food addict develops the ability to accept others' differences and uniqueness. She becomes free to love herself and others.

Recovery is a journey that we'll hopefully stay on for the rest of our lives, a day at a time.

I wish you abstinence, and I wish you freedom from the bondage of food addiction.

God bless you in your journey to and in recovery!

APPENDIX

"Am I Addicted to Food?" Questionnaire

Food addiction is no different from drug and alcohol addiction. Consider the following signs and symptoms of food addiction. Think of your eating behaviors being as honest with yourself as you are able. Use the following questionnaire to assess whether you are, indeed, a food addict.

	YES	NO
1. I eat when I'm not hungry.		
2. I don't eat when I am hungry.		
3. I deny that I am ever hungry.		
4. I go on binges for no apparent reason.		
5. I give too much time and thought to food.		
6. I look forward with pleasure and anticipation to those times I can eat alone.		
7. I eat differently in private than I do in public.		
8. My eating/purging/starving affects how I live.		
9. I resent when others tell me to use "willpower" to stop overeating.		
10. I eat to escape from worries or troubles.		
11. I have been treated for a food-related condition.		
12. My eating/purging/starving make others unhappy.		
13. I use(d) food to help me stop drinking or using drugs.		

14. I overeat/purge/starve when I am angry, lonely or tired.		
15. I bond with food rather than with people.		
16. I can't remember the last time I went several days without overeating/purging/starving.		
17. I have unexplained mood swings.		
18. I constantly think about my eating/purging/starving/weight/ body size.		
19. I don't know when I am physically hungry.		
20. I calculate calories obsessively.		
21. I crave food even after a large meal.		
22. I eat more than I intended.		
23. I crave sugary, starch and/or fatty foods.		
24. I eat to "treat myself" after a long hard day.		
25. I need to feel stuffed.		
26. A "normal size" meal makes me feel stuffed—I need to get rid of it.		
27. I keep eating even after I feel stuffed.		
28. I daydream about food.		
29. I overexercise to compensate for my eating.		
30. I skip meals on a regular basis.		
31. I believe that being" in control" of my food/starving = being in control of my life.		
32. I have taken laxatives or forced myself to vomiting after eating.		
33. I believe that overeating/purging/starving controls my life.		
34. I eat/purge/starve when I am stressed/nervous/anxious or depressed.		

"Am I Addicted to Food?" Questionnaire

35. I think I will feel calmer and more relaxed after I eat/purge.		
36. I think I will feel more energetic after I eat/starve/purge.		
37. I eat so as not to explode in anger.		
38. I eat when I am bored.		
39. I experience low self-esteem as a result of my eating/purging/starving behaviors.		
40. I believe that I will never be thin enough.		
41. I feel shame about my eating/purging/starving.		
42. I avoid socializing because of my overeating/purging/starving.		
43. I make excuses for my weight.		
44. I am uptight (because of my weight) around people to whom I am sexually attracted.		
45. I spend too much money on food.		
46. I have stolen other peoples' food.		
47. I eat until I am physically ill.		
48. My eating/purging/starving impairs my ability to be functional and productive.		
49. I sneak food in secret.		
50. My starving is a secret.		
51. My purging is a secret.		
52. I am a chronic dieter, but always gain back more than I lose.		
53. I feel hopeless about my eating/purging/starving.		
54. There is food addiction in my family.		

A "yes" answer to any one of these indicates the probability of food addiction.

Acknowledgments

Beginning in 1976, I attended Overeaters Anonymous meetings for years, believing the program held the answer to my out-of-control eating. In the process, I learned about a series of educational eating problems workshops presented by Gale Schneider, Credentialled Alcoholism Counselor (CAC) and Credentialled Eating Disorder Counselor (CEDC) (d. 2020), who became a friend of mine. The series became, in part, the outline for the educational series I developed, which eventually evolved into this book. Unfortunately today, as was the case in 1976, it is believed that compulsive overeating is the problem. As my knowledge grew and expanded, I expanded what I learned from Gale to incorporate addiction as the basis of eating problems. I'm so grateful to Gale.

This book had its start in 1988 when I met Marilyn J. White at a bon-voyage party for a mutual acquaintance. At the time, Marilyn was completing her licensing application to New York State to operate an outpatient chemical dependence treatment center—Realization Center. As a person in recovery and an accountant, her work in recovery intrigued me and I offered her some business advice. It soon became clear that as partners we could really grow and develop Realization Center. Marilyn believed I could help her realize her dream of growing a large outpatient addictions treatment center, and together we have surpassed that goal. Needless to say, my gratitude goes to Marilyn for helping me embark on this journey.

My early work at the Center, interacting with clients in a clinical environment, not only educated me about addiction treatment, but also revealed engagement skills I hadn't realized I had. My therapist at the time, Alan Brody, PhD, encouraged me to obtain my CAC—not a small feat!

Following my accreditation, I began running groups and education series on the relationship of food to alcohol and drug dependence. But

468

Acknowledgments

it wasn't until 1995, when I attended a conference at the Robert Woods Johnson Campus in New Jersey, "Food Addiction 2000," that I finally understood eating problems are an addiction in their own right. The conference, orchestrated by Kay Sheppard, MA, included a panel of distinguished, credentialled professionals who presented the case for food addiction. Addiction was the missing link in understanding the nature of eating issues. Kay Sheppard is a pioneer in treating the disease of food addiction. She certainly launched me on my journey to uncover the truth about, and recover from, my addictive eating behaviors.

When I decided to write this book, I shared the idea with my wonderful therapist at the time, Lalitha Devi, CASAC, a very important teacher and healer for me. I told her my clients had been telling me to write a book for some time. Taking a practical approach, she asked me what I would need to do that. I said, "A computer." She asked me when I would have the computer, I think I told her within two weeks. That was the beginning. I bought a laptop, a Sony Vaio, and started with what I thought would be the easiest chapter, Denial.

In 2013, I received a notice that Fordham University's School of Social Work was seeking papers for the NASW Annual Addiction Institute. I mentioned it in passing to our Director of Community Relations, Pia Marinangeli, PhD, LCSW, CASAC, that since I didn't have a masters' degree, my proposal for a workshop wouldn't be considered. Pia said that was nonsense and I should write it. I wrote the proposal and lo and behold, it was accepted! I was shocked! I named the workshop "Exploring the True Culprits in Food Addiction, It's Not Broccoli."

I am grateful to my friend Mary Pender Greene, LCSW-R, CGP, and President and CEO of MPG Consulting. A career and executive coach, consultant, trainer, psychotherapist, and author, she is also the former Assistant Executive Director at the Jewish Board of Family and Children's Services. Mary was the former President of NASW and attended my workshop at their conference. She was enthusiastic about my book and really liked the title of the workshop as a title for the book. Her insight into the publishing world has proved invaluable.

Marilyn encouraged me to show my finished manuscript to friend Suzanne Slesin, Publisher and Editorial Director of Pointed Leaf Press. Suzie is an over-the-top successful editor and author in the world of art and design. Her positive feedback on my then-unedited manuscript gave me the encouragement to send it to publishers in the health, nutrition, and wellness arena.

Fortunately, I was led to the right editor, Carol Killman Rosenberg, who was a great match for the book. She used her good judgement and editorial skills to make my message more readable and understandable.

Michael Allen, my very talented nephew, contributed the illustrations. He's a wonderful and imaginative artist and graphic designer, as can be seen in all the illustrations. I particularly love the alligators in the moat surrounding the Fortress and the Little Addict entering the "Land of Addiction."

My thanks to Ronald Hoffman MD, a major force in the arena of integrative medicine and my trusted physician. I have learned so much from him; he is a walking encyclopedia of health and nutrition. He also generously agreed to write the foreword and guided me to my editor.

I am totally indebted to Marcia Bodenstein for her unwavering support as a champion and protector of the book and its message. She made herself totally available to review the manuscript and to help me respond to my editor's suggestions. Marcia has been a sounding board in the difficult process of getting to publication. Whenever I've been unsure about any changes, her judgment and perspective have been a wonderful guide.

My gratitude to all the players in this exciting venture who have played a role in the birth of what I believe is an important document for the understanding that the eating problems in our society is mainly addiction—Gale, Kay, Marilyn, Lalitha, Pia, Mary, Carol, Michael, Ronald Hoffman, and Marcia—and all the clients who have helped confirm this understanding.

Resources

Realization Center

Website: www.realizationcenternyc.com
Mailing Address:
  New York City
    Realization Center
    19 Union Square West
    7th Floor
    New York, NY 10003-3304
  Phone: (212) 627-9600
  Brooklyn
    Realization Center
    175 Remsen Street
    2nd Floor
    Brooklyn, New York, 11201
E-mail: info@realizationcenternyc.com
Community Relations Department: info@realizationcenternyc.com

Food Addicts Anonymous (FAA)

Website: www. foodaddictsanonymous.org
Address:
    Food Addicts Anonymous World Service Office
    529 N W Prima Vista Blvd. #301A
    Port St. Lucie, FL 34983
Phone: (561) 967-3871

GreySheeters Anonymous (GSA)

Website: www.greysheet.org
Mailing Address, Phone and E-mail: See website

Overeaters Anonymous (OA)

Website: www.oa.org
Address:
  6075 Zenith Court NE
  P.O. Box 44727
  Rio Rancho, NM 87174
Phone: (505) 891-2664

Food Addicts in Recovery Anonymous (FA)

Website: www.foodaddicts.org
Address:
  FA World Service Office
  400 W. Cummings Park Suite 1700
  Woburn, MA 01801
  USA
E-Mail: office@foodaddicts.org
Phone: (781) 932-6300

Endnotes

1 Engber, Daniel. "Unexpected Clues Emerge about Why Diets Fail." *Scientific American*. January 13, 2020. Accessed August 17, 2021. www.scientificamerican.com/article/unexpected-clues-emerge-about-why-diets-fail/.

2 Fox, Robin. "Food and Eating: An Anthropological Perspective." Social Issues Research Center (SIRC). Accessed May 22, 2018. www.sirc.org/publik/foxfood.pdf.

3 This is a Yiddishism intended to offset the "evil eye."

4 DuPont, MD, Robert L. "Addiction in Medicine." *Trans Am Clin Climatol Assoc.* 119 (2008):227–241. www.ncbi.nlm.nih.gov/pmc/articles/PMC2394682/

5 DuPont, MD, Robert. "Addiction: A New Paradigm." *Bulletin of the Menninger Clinic* 62, no. 2 (February 1998):231–42.

6 Silkworth, MD, William Duncan. "The Doctor's Opinion." Silkworth.net. Accessed June 5, 2018. silkworth.net/pages/silkworth/doctorsopinion.php.

7 Prager, Michael. "Food Addiction." *Paradigm* 14, no 3 (Summer 2009):4–5. www.addictionrecov.org/Paradigm/DisplayParadigmIssue.aspx?ID=31.

8 Gold, MD, Mark S. *Eating Disorders, Overeating, Pathological Attachment to Food: Independent or Addictive Disorder?* Boca Raton, FL: CRC Press, 2004.

9 Noble, E.P., R.E. Noble, T. Ritchie, K. Syndulko, M. C. Bohlman, L.A. Noble, Y. Zhang, R.S. Sparkes, and D.K. Grandy. "D2 Dopamine Receptor Gene and Obesity." *Int J Eat Disord.* 15, no. 3 (April 1994):205–17. www.ncbi.nlm.nih.gov/pubmed/8199600; Obesity and Food Addiction Summit. www.foodaddictionsummit.org.; Beitscher-Campbell, H., K. Blum, M. Febo, M.A. Madigan, J. Giordano, R.D. Badgaiyan, E.R. Braverman, K. Dushaj, M. Li, and M.S. Gold. "Pilot Clinical Observations Between Food and Drug Seeking Derived from Fifty Cases Attending an Eating Disorder Clinic." *J Behav Addict.* 5, no. 3 (September 2016):533-41. doi: 10.1556/2006.5.2016.055.

10 Hoebel, B.G., N.M. Aveda, and P. Rada. "Evidence for Sugar Addiction: Behavioral and Neurochemical Effects of Intermittent, Excessive Sugar Intake." *Neurosci Biobehav Rev* 32, no. 1 (2008):20–39. doi:10.1016/j.neubiorev.2007.04.019

11 Madsen, Heather B., and Serge H. Ahmed. "Drug Versus Sweet Reward: Greater Attraction to and Preference for Sweet Versus Drug Cues." *Addiction Biology* 20, no. 3 (May 2015):433–44.

12 Drewnowski, A., D.D. Krahn, M.A. Demitrack, K. Naim, and B.A. Gosnell. "Taste Response and Preference for Sweet, High-Fat Foods: Evidence of Opioid Involvement." *Physiol Behav* 51, no. 2 (February 1992):371-9. www.ncbi.nlm.nih.gov/pubmed/1313591.

13 Colantuoni, C., P. Rada, J. McCarthy, C. Patten, N.M. Avena, A. Chadeayne, and B.G. Hoebel. "Evidence that Intermittent, Excessive Sugar Intake Causes Endogenous

Opioid Dependence," *Obesity Research* 10, no. 6 (June 2002):478-88. doi:10.1038/oby.2002.66.

14 Shell, Ellen Ruppel. *The Hungry Gene: The Science of Fat and the Future of Thin.* New York: Atlantic Monthly Press, 2002; von Deneen, K.M., M.S. Gold, and Y. Liu. "Food Addiction and Cues in Prader-Willi Syndrome," *Addictive Medicine* 3, no. 1 (March 2009):19-25.

15 Mooney, Andrea. "Addicted to . . . Food?" Harvard Medical School. July 3, 2013. Accessed May 23, 2018. hms.harvard.edu/news/addicted-food-7-3-13.

16 Volkow, Nora D., Gene-Jack Wang, Joanna Fowler, and Frank Telang. "Overlapping Neuronal Circuits in Addiction and Obesity: Evidence of Systems Pathology." *Philos Trans R Soc London B Biol Sci* 363, no. 1507 (October 2008):3191-2000. doi: 10.1098/rstb.2008.0107.

17 Dufty, William. *Sugar Blues.* New York: Warner Books, 1975; Appleton, Nancy. *Lick the Sugar Habit.* New York: Avery Publishers, 1988; OA World Service. *Overeaters Anonymous, Volumes I and II.* New Mexico: Overeaters Anonymous Inc., 2002; *Connection: Journal of Food Addicts in Recovery Anonymous,* 2004.

18 Overeaters Anonymous. "Overeaters Anonymous Membership Survey Report." Overeaters Anonymous, Inc., 2004; Kriz, Kerry-Lynn Murphy. "The Efficacy of Overeaters Anonymous in Fostering Abstinence in Binge-eating Disorder and Bulimia Nervosa." Virginia Polytechnic Institute. May 6, 2002. Accessed May 23, 2018. vtechworks.lib.vt.edu/bitstream/handle/10919/11044/Dissertation.pdf?sequence=1&isAllowed=y.

19 Kline, Monte. *The Junk Food Withdrawal Manual.* Denver, CO: Nutri-Books Corp., 1978; Bernard, MD, Neal. *Breaking the Food Seduction; The Hidden Reasons Behind Food Craving—and 7 Steps to End Them Naturally.* New York: St. Martin's Press, 2003.

20 Ludwig, MD, PhD, David. "Effects of Dietary Glycemic Index on Brain Regions Related to Reward and Craving in Men." *American Journal of Clinical Nutrition* 98, no. 3 (September 2013):641-47. academic.oup.com/ajcn/article/98/3/641/4577039.

21 Hoebel, B.G., N.M. Aveda, and P. Rada. "Evidence for Sugar Addiction: Behavioral and Neurochemical Effects of Intermittent, Excessive Sugar Intake." *Neurosci Biobehav Rev* 32, no. 1 (2008):20–39. doi:10.1016/j.neubiorev.2007.04.019.

22 Leshner, Alan I. "Addiction is a Brain Disease." *ASAM News,* Vol. 13, No. 1, January/February 1998.

23 American Society of Addiction Medicine. "Definition of Addiction." ASAM.org. Accessed May 23, 2018. www.asam.org/quality-practice/definition-of-addiction.

24 Sheppard, Kay. "The Biochemistry of Food Addiction." Breaking Free from Food Addiction. Accessed May 23, 2018. kaysheppard.com/articles/the-biochemistry-of-food-addiction/.

25 Crumpler, LCSW, Ann. "Understanding Addictions." *Paradigm* 11, no. 3 (Summer 2006):4-5. www.addictionrecov.org/Paradigm/DisplayParadigmIssue.aspx?ID=19.

26 Obesity and Food Addiction Summit. "Summit Agenda." Accessed May 31, 2018. www.foodaddictionsummit.org/agenda.htm.

Endnotes

27 Crumpler, LCSW, Ann. "Understanding Addictions." *Paradigm* 11, no. 3 (Summer 2006):4-5. www.addictionrecov.org/Paradigm/DisplayParadigmIssue.aspx?ID=19.

28 Campbell, Angelique, "Food as Drug" Metro.us, 2007.

29 American Society of Addiction Medicine. "Definition of Addiction." ASAM.org. Accessed May 23, 2018. www.asam.org/quality-practice/definition-of-addiction.

30 Sheppard, Kay. *Food Addiction: The Body Knows.* Deerfield Beach, FL: Health Communications, Inc., 1993.

31 Fiorentino, N MSW, Regan, K ACSW, CEAP. "Facts on: Food Addiction." New Jersey Alcohol/Drug Resource Center & Clearinghouse, Center of Alcohol Studies, Smither Hall-Busch Campus, Rutgers University, Piscataway NJ. Fact Sheet No. 26.

32 Anonymous. "Letters to the Editor." *The Sun* magazine, October 2005.

33 Per Marilyn J. White, CASAC, NCAC II, founder of Realization Center Inc., the oldest and largest addictions treatment program in Manhattan and Brooklyn, New York.

34 Fiorentino, N MSW, Regan, K ACSW, CEAP. "Facts on: Food Addiction." New Jersey Alcohol/Drug Resource Center & Clearinghouse, Center of Alcohol Studies, Smither Hall-Busch Campus, Rutgers University, Piscataway NJ. Fact Sheet No. 26.

35 Starks, Charles and Starks, Peggy. *Disease Concept of Food Addiction (The Workbook)*, Fairwinds Institute, Inc. 1995.

36 Per research by Linus Pauling, Ph.D.

37 American Foundation for Suicide Prevention "Suicide Statistics." AFSP.org. Accessed May 23, 2018. afsp.org/about-suicide/suicide-statistics/.

38 Sheppard, Kay. *Food Addiction: The Body Knows.* Deerfield Beach, FL: Health Communications, Inc., 1993.

39 American College Health Association, *Eating Disorders: What Everyone Should Know* (brochure). 1999.

40 Katherine, MA, Anne. *Anatomy of a Food Addiction: The Brain Chemistry of Overeating.* Carlsbad, CA: Gürze Books, 1991.

41 Katherine, MA, Anne. *Anatomy of a Food Addiction: The Brain Chemistry of Overeating.* Carlsbad, CA: Gürze Books, 1991.

42 Miller, Kelsey. "Most Girls Start Dieting by Age 8," January 26, 2105. Refinery29. com. https://www.refinery29.com/en-us/2015/01/81288/children-dieting-body-image

43 National Organization for Women. "Get the Facts." NOW.org. Accessed April 4, 2022. now.org/now-foundation/love-your-body/love-your-body-whats-it-all-about/get-the-facts/

44 Polivy, J. and C.P. Herman. "Dieting and binging: A causal analysis." *American Psychologist,* 40, no. 3 (February 1985): 193–201. doi:10.1037//0003-066x.40.2.193.

45 Cabrera, Dena. "Thin to Win." *Together* magazine, May/June 2011.

46 This list was organically developed over many years of presenting the lecture "Little Addict in Training" and from clients who have offered their thoughts about this newborn in the world. Notice their relational groupings.

47 Bowlby, J. *Attachment and Loss 1: Attachment*. New York: Basic Books, 1982, 1969.

48 Markham, Laura. "How to Set Effective Limits for Your Child." *Aha Parenting*. Accessed May 23, 2018. www.ahaparenting.com/parenting-tools/positive-discipline/effective-limits.

49 Ingram, Chip. *Effective Parenting in a Defective World*. Dallas TX: Tyndale House Publishers, 2006.

50 Mahler, M., F. Pine, and A. Bergman. *The Psychological Birth of the Human Infant*. New York: Basic Books, 1975.

51 Grasso, L. Interview with John Bradshaw: The Blind Obedience That Binds Us All. Recovery Networker, September, 1992.

52 Forward, Susan, and Craig Buck. *Toxic Parents: Overcoming Their Hurtful Legacy and Reclaiming Your Life*. New York: Bantam, 1989.

53 Kuntz, Becky, Victor Groze, and William R. Yates. "Bulimia: A Systemic Family History Perspective." *Families in Society* 73, no. 10 (1992):604–12. psycnet.apa.org/record/1993-18141-001.

54 Kristof, Nicholas. "A Poverty Solution That Starts With a Hug." *The New York Times*. January 7, 2012. Accessed May 30, 2018. www.nytimes.com/2012/01/08/opinion/sunday/kristof-a-poverty-solution-that-starts-with-a-hug.html.

55 Schatzman, Morton. *Soul Murder: Persecution in the Family*. New York City, NY: Random House, 1973.

56 To abstain from over- or undereating and/or eating and purging, which requires eating in a way that does not trigger cravings. This can be accomplished only by eliminating all trigger foods—the sugars, sugar substitutes, flour, and all other refined carbohydrates, and eating in a way that normalizes blood sugar levels—i.e., the Food Plan. (See further discussion in Part Two: The Solution: Abstinence.)

57 Turgay, MD, FRCPC, Atilla. "Comorbidity of Dysthymic Disorders in Children & Adolescents." *Paradigm* 11, no. 4 (Fall 2006):6–7. www.addictionrecov.org/Paradigm/DisplayParadigmIssue.aspx?ID=20.

58 Dayton, Tian, PhD. *Emotional Sobriety: From Relationship Trauma to Resilience to Balance*. Deerfield Beach, FL: Health Communications, Inc., 2007.

59 Kase, Aaron. "How Childhood Stress and Trauma Spark Drug Dependence." Reset.me. May 26, 2015. Accessed May 30, 2018. reset.me/story/doctor-explains-how-childhood-stress-and-trauma-sparks-drug-dependence/.

60 Van der Kolk, Bessel. *Psychological Trauma*. 2nd ed. Arlington, VA: American Psychiatric Press, 2003.

61 Sadker, Myra, and David Sadker. *Failing at Fairness: How America's Schools Cheat Girls*. New York City, NY: Charles Scribner's Sons, 1995.

62 Andersen, A., L. Cohn, and T. Holbrook. *Making Weight: Men's Conflicts With Food, Weight, Shape & Appearance*. Carlsbad, CA: Gürve Books, 2000.

63 Holtzman, Shaindy. "Anorexia and Bulimia: Deadly Illnesses," *Jewish Press,* March 1, 2002.

Endnotes

64 The "DMZ" was a term coined during the Korean War that designated a Korean "Demilitarized Zone," with the "good guys" on one side and the "bad guys" on the other. If someone wanted to escape from the "bad guys" [North Korea] and go over to the "good guys," they could get killed in the process.

65 Bradshaw, John. "Our Families, Ourselves." *Recovery Today,* April 2004.

66 Black, Claudia. *It Will Never Happen to Me: Growing Up With Addiction as Youngsters, Adolescents, Adults.* Center City, MN: Hazelden, 2002.

67 Hoebel, B.G., N.M. Aveda, and P. Rada. "Evidence for Sugar Addiction: Behavioral and Neurochemical Effects of Intermittent, Excessive Sugar Intake." *Neurosci Biobehav Rev* 32, no. 1 (2008):20–39. doi:10.1016/j.neubiorev.2007.04.019.

68 Food addiction in men is more hidden—their addiction is often concealed by their exercise.

69 Fiorentino, N MSW, Regan, K ACSW, CEAP. "Facts on: Food Addiction." New Jersey Alcohol/Drug Resource Center & Clearinghouse, Center of Alcohol Studies, Smither Hall-Busch Campus, Rutgers University, Piscataway NJ Fact Sheet No. 26.

70 The definition of "healthy diet" in the United States has been distorted by our nutritional education being provided by Kellogg, General Mills, The Sugar Institute, etc. For example, we are taught that a "healthy breakfast" is a bowl of "Fiber One Cereal" and a banana or a "Hot Pocket" or a sugary "breakfast drink" or "breakfast bar." Many of these ads are directed to kids, who quickly become addicted to the sugars and refined carbs in these products. And then they grow into adults who are slaves to these behaviors with food.

71 Kizilos, P. "Eating Disorders Can Block Recovery from Chemical Dependency." *Hazelden Voice,* Winter 1997.

72 Beasley, J. *How to Defeat Alcoholism: Nutritional Guidelines for Getting Sober,* 1989. Reprint ed. Addictionend.com 2001.

73 Mercola, DO, Joseph. "New Revelations Support Diet and Exercise to Reverse Leptin Resistance, Thereby Promoting a Healthy Weight." Mercola.com. October 29, 2012. Accessed May 30, 2018. articles.mercola.com/sites/articles/archive/2012/10/29/leptin-resistance.aspx.

74 Lustig, R. *Fat Chance: Beating the Odds Against Sugar, Processed Food, Obesity and Disease.* New York: Plume Publishing, 2012.

75 This handout is available as a PDF download from https://cdn.vortala.com/childsites/uploads/2048/files/147_Ways_Sugar.pdf.

76 Lustig, R. "Fructose: Metabolic, Hedonic, and Societal Parallels with Ethanol." *Journal of the American Dietetic Association,* v.110, no. 9 (Sept. 2010): 1307–1321. doi:10.1016/jada.2010.06.008 after -1321.

77 Eight years of data collected by Sharon P. Fowler, MPH, and colleagues at the University of Texas Health Science Center, San Antonio. Fowler, S.P. 65th Annual Scientific Sessions, American Diabetes Association, San Diego, June 10–14 2005; Abstract 1058-P Sharon P. Fowler, MPH, University of Texas Health Science Center School of Medicine, San Antonio.

78 Leslie Bonci, MPH, University of Pittsburgh Medical Center; WebMD News: "Artificial Sweeteners May Damage Diet Efforts;" Davidson, T.L. *International Journal of Obesity,* July 2004; vol 28: pp 933–955.

79 Sinatra, Stephen, Jan Sinatra, and Roberta Jo Lieberman. *Heart Sense for Women: Your Plan for Natural Prevention and Treatment.* New York City, NY: Plume, 2001.

80 Randolph, MD, Theron G. "The Addiction Pyramid." *Noha News,* no. 1 (Winter 1990):1, 3-4. superiorsites3.com/NNW90AddictionPyramid.htm.

81 MedBroadcast. "Addicted to Caffeine." MedBroadcast.com. Accessed August 10, 2018. http://medbroadcast.com/channel/nutrition/diet-and-disease/addicted-to-caffeine

82 Wang, G.J., D. Tomasi, W. Backus, R. Wang. and N. Volkov. "Gastric Distention Activates Satiety Circuitry In the Human Brain," *Neuroimage* Vol 39 Issue 4 15 Feb 2008, pp. 1824–1831.

83 Mason, Michael. "The Energy-Drink Buzz Is Unmistakable. The Health Impact Is Unknown." *The New York Times* on the Web. December 12, 2006. Accessed May 30, 2018. www.nytimes.com/learning/teachers/featured_articles/20061212tuesday.html.; Duke University School of Medicine. "Faculty: James Lane." Duke Psychiatry and Behavioral Sciences. Accessed May 30, 2018. psychiatry.duke.edu/lane-james-dundas.

84 The history of prescription diet pills has been dangerous at best, e.g., Fenfluramine [fen-phen] was pulled from pharmacy shelves in 1997 for causing dangerous and potentially fatal side effects and others with difficult immediate side effects and unknown long-term side effects have taken its place.

85 Kübler-Ross, MD, Elisabeth. *On Death and Dying: What The Dying Have to Teach Doctors, Nurses, Clergy and Their Own Families.* New York City, NY: MacMillan Publishing, Inc., 1976.

86 Rutledge, Thom. *Recovery Today.* Institute of Chemical Dependency Studies, April 2003.

87 See Chapter 11: *Realization Center Food Plan for True Recovery From Food Addiction.*

88 Ross, MA, Julia. *The Mood Cure: The 4-Step Program to Take Charge of Your Emotions—Today.* New York City, NY: Penguin Books, 2003.

89 Ibid3.

90 According to the National Institutes of Health, ADAM Medical Encyclopedia: Diverticulosis occurs when small bulging sacs or pouches of the inner lining of the intestine (diverticula) become inflamed or infected. No one knows exactly what causes the sacs, or pouches of diverticulosis to form. Eating a low fiber diet is one of the most likely causes. People who eat mostly processed food, as many Americans eat, do not get enough fiber in their diet. Processed foods include white rice, white bread, most breakfast cereals, crackers, and pretzels. As a result, constipation and hard stools are more likely to occur—causing people to strain when passing stools. This increases the pressure in the colon or intestines and may cause these pouches to form. Diverticulosis is very common. It is found in more than half of Americans over age 60. Only a small number of these people will develop diverticulitis. Diverticulitis is caused by small pieces of stool (feces) that become trapped in these pouches, causing infection or inflammation. People with diverticulosis often have no symptoms, but they may have bloating

Endnotes

479

and cramping in the lower part of the belly. Rarely, they may notice blood in their stool or on toilet paper. Symptoms of diverticulitis are more severe and often start suddenly, but they may become worse over a few days. They include: tenderness, usually in the left lower side of the abdomen, bloating or gas, fever and chills, nausea and vomiting, not feeling hungry and not eating.

91 Testimonial: After James, a client, had attended a number of my food addiction lectures, he expressed his deep gratitude to me. All his life, he had experienced stomach pain and distress, and no medical person had ever been able to help him. However, he told me that since he started the food plan, he had no more stomach pain.

92 Tiebout, Harry M. (December 1954). "Ego Factors in Surrender in Alcoholism." *Quarterly Journal of Studies on Alcohol*: 610–621. Reprinted in *Harry Teibout: The Collected Writings*; Tiebout, Harry (1949). "The Act of Surrender in the Therapeutic Process, with Special Reference to Alcoholism". *Quarterly Journal of Studies on Alcohol*: 48–58. Reprinted in *Harry Tiebout: The Collected Writings*; Tiebout, Harry (1953). "Surrender versus Compliance in Therapy, with Special Reference to Alcoholism." *Quarterly Journal of Studies on Alcohol*: 58–68. Reprinted in *Harry Tiebout: The Collected Writings*.

93 Tiebout, Harry. *Harry Tiebout: Collected Writings*. Center City, MN: Hazelden Publishing, 1999.

94 Ibid.

95 Ibid.

96 Ibid.

97 Ibid.

98 Bradshaw, John, *Healing the Shame That Binds You*. Deerfield Beach, FL: Health Communications, Inc., 1988.

99 Starks, Charles A. EdD, and Peggy Starks, B MS. *Disease Concept of Food Addiction: The Workbook*. Clearwater, FL: Fairwinds Institute, 1995.

100 Cooper, Rebecca. "Understanding the Binge Cycle." *Recovery Today*. April 2004.

101 Knapp, Caroline. *Appetites: Why Women Want*. Berkeley, CA: Counterpoint Press, 2003.

102 Attributed to Pia Mellody. Definition presented in a lecture at The Meadows—Survivors I Workshop, 2006.

103 Anderson, Dr. Matthew. "Eating to Kill" course, January 7, 2005.

104 Solutions Recovery. "The 8 Core Emotions." Solutions Recovery: An AAC Facility. September 12, 2013. Accessed June 6, 2018. www.solutions-recovery.com/blog/the-8-core-emotions/.

105 Prather, Hugh. *Notes to Myself*. Lafayette, CA: Real People Press, 1970.

106 Crumpler, LCSW, Ann. "Understanding Addictions." *Paradigm* 11, no. 3 (Summer 2006):4–5. www.addictionrecov.org/Paradigm/DisplayParadigmIssue.aspx?ID=19.

107 Stoop, David, and James Masteller. *Forgiving Our Parents, Forgiving Ourselves: Healing Adult Children of Dysfunctional Families*. Ventura, CA: Regal, 1997.

108 Bradshaw, John. "The Shame of Toxic Shame." *The Meadows Cutting Edge* (Newsletter), Fall, 2001.

109 Mellody, Pia, Andrea Wells Miller, and J. Keith Miller. *Facing Codependence*. San Francisco, CA: HarperOne, 1989.

110 Firestone, Robert, PhD. *The Fantasy Bond: Structure of Psychological Defenses*. Santa Barbara, CA: Glendon Associates, 1998.

111 Bradshaw, John. *Healing the Shame That Binds You*. Deerfield Beach, FL: Health Communications, Inc., 1988.

112 Huizinga, Johan. *Homo Ludens: A Study of the Play-Elements in Culture*. Brooklyn, NY: Angelica Press, 2016.

113 Leary, Amy, MS CMHC, and Angie Meyer, LCPC, CADC, CCGC. "Food Addiction." *Paradigm*. Summer 1997.

114 Robin, Arthur L., and Sharon L. Foster. *Negotiating Parent-Adolescent Conflict: A Behavioral-Family Systems Approach*. New York: Guildford Press, 1989.

115 Reiss, David. *The Family's Construction of Reality*. Cambridge, MA: Harvard University Press, 1981.

116 Kaplan, MA, LAC, LISAC, Debra L. "Fabled Truths and Family Lies." October 15, 2010. Accessed May 30, 2018. debrakaplancounseling.com/fabled-truths-and-family-lies/.

117 Ibid.

118 Dayton, PhD, Tian. "Denial: Is It Always Pathological?" TianDayton.com. Accessed May 30, 2018. www.tiandayton.com/denial-is-it-always-pathological.

119 Spencer, Frances. *Understanding Children: A Parent's Guide*. Galashiels,UK: Launchpoint, 2002.

120 Thank you, Marcia, for allowing me to include the rules you grew up with in this inset.

121 Kaufman, Gershen, PhD. *The Psychology of Shame: The Theory and Treatment of Shame-Based Syndromes*. New York: Springer Publishing, 1989.

122 "Shame is called an affect auxiliary because it always involves other affects, namely interest and/or enjoyment. Shame is triggered only after the effects of interest or enjoyment have been activated, and it inhibits one or the other or both." (Hollinger MD, Paul C. "Primary Affects: Enjoyment, Shame, Disgust & Dissmell." *Psychology Today,* Aug 16, 2016. www.psychologytoday.com/us/blog/great-kids-great-parents/201608/primary-affects-0. According to Bradshaw, shame monitors excitement and pleasure. It creates a boundary for our sexual desires. In adolescence, healthy shame is the source of good identity, a disciplined focus on the future and/or studious limits in pursuing intellectual interests.

123 Coined by Erik Erikson to "denote a concern for establishing and guiding the next generation" and is said to stem from a sense of optimism about humanity. Bradshaw says toxically shamed people tend to become stagnant as life goes on—living in a guarded secretive defensive way—trying to be more than human (perfect and controlling) or less than human (losing interest in life or stagnated in some addictive behavior).

Endnotes

124 A securely attached person with a solid sense of self/worth (feeling lovable and wanting to love another) is capable of connecting with another in intimate relationships. Intimacy, which requires vulnerability and a lack of defensiveness, requires healthy shame.

125 "Anyone who has nurtured healthy shame and experienced awe and reverence for the immensity of life must acknowledge the numinous." (idea of the holy—mystery of life—that there is something greater than ourselves) Bradshaw, John. *Healing the Shame That Binds You.* Deerfield Beach, FL: Health Communications, 1988.

126 Puhl, R.M., T. Andreyeva, and K.D. Brownell. "Perceptions of Weight Discrimination: Prevalence and Comparison to Race and Gender Discrimination in America." *International Journal of Obesity (Lond)* 32, no. 6 (June 2008):992–1000. doi: 10.1038/ijo.2008.22.

127 Griffiths, L.J., D. Wolke, A.S. Page, et al. "Obesity and Bullying: Different Effects for Boys and Girls." *Archives of Disease in Childhood.* v. 91, no. 2 (February 2006): 121–125.

128 Miller, Alice. *For Your Own Good: The Roots of Violence in Child Rearing.* New York: Farrar, Straus and Giroux 1983.

129 Peck, M. Scott. *The Road Less Travelled.* Anniversary ed. New York: Touchstone, 2003.

130 Freundlich, Lawrence S. "Fear of Abandonment: Some Lessons from M. Scott Peck and Pia Mellody." Themeadows.com, 2006. https://www.themeadows.com/blog/item/392-fear-of-abandonment-some-lessons-from-m-scott-peck-and-pia-mellody.

131 Mellody, Pia. *Facing Codependence: What It Is, Where It Comes from, How It Sabotages Our Lives.* New York City, NY: Harper and Row, 2003.

132 Lerner, Rokelle. *Daily Affirmations Strengthening My Recovery: Meditations for Adult Children of Alcoholics/Dysfunctional Families.* 1st ed. Lakewood, CA: Adult Children of Alcoholics World Service Organization, 2003.

133 Black, PhD, Claudia. "Family Roles." Guiding Hearts With Hope. Accessed May 30, 2018. www.guidingheartswithhope.org/uploads/8/5/8/7/8587840/familyrolesinaddiction.pdf.

134 Wegscheider-Cruse, Sharon. *Another Chance.* Palo Alto, CA: Science and Behavior Books, Inc. 1989.

135 The quoted phrase is attributed to Sharon Wegscheider-Cruse.

136 Woititz, EdD, Janet Geringer. *Adult Children of Alcoholics.* Deerfield Beach, FL: Health Communications, Inc., 1990.

137 Wilson, Bill. "Alcoholics Anonymous in Its Third Decade: Presented to the New York City Medical Society on Alcoholism by Bill W., April 28, 1958." Silkworth.net. Accessed June 5, 2018. silkworth.net/pages/aahistory/billw2/billwtalk19.php.

138 *Twelve Steps and Twelve Traditions.* New York: Alcoholics Anonymous World Services. p. 22.

139 Overeaters Anonymous. *Overeaters Anonymous: The Tools of Recovery.* Los Angeles: Overeaters Anonymous, 1981. Pamphlet.

140 Ibid

141 Hifler, Joyce Sequichie. *A Cherokee Feast of Days: Daily Meditations.* 1st ed. San Francisco, CA: Council Oak Books, 1992.

142 Schachtel, Hyman Judah. *The Real Enjoyment of Living.* 1st dd. Boston, MA: E. P. Dutton, 1954.

143 HealthyPlace. "Help for Adult Women with Eating Disorders." HealthyPlace: For Your Mental Health. July 11, 2016. Accessed June 6, 2018. www.healthyplace.com/alternative-mental-health/eating-disorders-alternative/help-for-adult-women-with-eating-disorders.

144 Transference refers to the phenomenon in psychotherapy in which there is an unconscious redirection of feelings from one person to another. (Sigmund Freud)

145 Williams, Margery. *The Velveteen Rabbit, or How Toys Become Real.* Garden City, NY: Doubleday and Company, Inc., 1922.

146 Prin, BA, LADC, John Howard. "Reclaiming Your Destiny." *Paradigm* 14, no. 3 (Summer 2009):16–17. www.addictionrecov.org/Paradigm/DisplayParadigmIssue.aspx?ID=31.

147 Bradshaw, MA, John. "Spirituality in Everyday Life." The Meadows Blog. Accessed June 6, 2018. www.themeadows.com/blog/item/402-spirituality-in-everyday-life.

148 Wright, Karen. "Dare to Be Yourself." *Psychology Today.* Last reviewed June 9, 2016. Accessed June 6, 2018. www.psychologytoday.com/intl/articles/200805/dare-be-yourself?collection=144473.

149 Ibid.

150 Buber, Martin. *The Way of Man.* New York: Citadel Press, 1966.

151 Carter-Scott, Chérie, PhD, MCC. *If Life Is a Game, These Are the Rules: Ten Rules for Being Human.* New York: Broadway Books, 1998.

152 Nelson, Portia. *There's a Hole in My Sidewalk: The Romance of Self-Discovery.* New York: Beyond Words/Atria, 1993. Copyright © 1993 by Portia Nelson. Reprinted with the permission of Beyond Words/Atria Books, a division of Simon & Schuster, Inc. All rights reserved.

153 *Alcoholics Anonymous: The Big Book.* New York: Alcoholics Anonymous World Services. p. 83–84. Reprinted with permission from A.A. World Services, Inc.

Index

AA. *See* Alcoholics Anonymous
abandonment, 1, 104, 112, 127, 147, 297, 342
Abrahamson, E.M., x
abstinence, 23, 26, 33, 35, 44, 52, 62–63, 125, 131, 146–147, 153, 219–225, 238, 270, 271–281, 342, 387, 405, 476–56
   awfulizing of, 400, 424
abuse, 95, 99, 105, 107–109, 130, 136, 438–439
   covert, 107
   overt, 107
   physical, 108
   sexual, 12, 108–109, 140, 290
acceptance, 211–214, 264, 265, 266, 274, 277–278, 387
Addiction Model of Treatment, 32–33
addictions, ix–x, 19, 23, 42, 47–48, 143–145, 148–155, 161, 264–267, 290, 310, 426, 454
   biopsychosocial model of, 40–43, 47, 48–49, 80
   definitions of, 40–41 50, 52–59
   disease concept of, 25–26, 31–49, 53
   genetics and, ix, 4, 47, 48
   increased tolerance/less reward cycle, 37, 41, 51, 65–67, 388
   recovery, ix, 3, 24, 25–26, 273–274
   rewards of, xi, 4, 31, 36, 40–41, 47–48, 49, 51, 148–149, 157
   risk mitigation strategy, ix
   social factors, 32, 149
   treatment success rate, 154–155
   withdrawal, 19, 36, 51, 72–73, 80, 144, 154–155, 184–185, 222–225

   See also alcoholism; drug addiction; food addiction; smoking
addicts, 360–361
   characteristics of parents/caregivers, 360–369
   codependency and enablement of, 361–369, 378–380
   family systems and, 48, 106, 148, 357–381
   substance obsessions of, 51, 58, 67–68, 152
   rights of adult children, 380–381
   roles of children of, 370–381
adolescents, 64, 104, 143, 325, 480
adrenal glands, 165, 183, 184
adrenaline, 43, 183
adult children, 359, 377–378, 380–381
Adult Children of Alcoholics (Woititz), 377–378
affect auxiliary, 333, 480n121
affect-shame bind, 336
affirmations, 224, 347–356
agave, 179
aging, 3
Ahmed, S.H., 36
Al-Anon, 15
alcohol, 46, 175–176, 177, 254
alcoholics, 33–34, 45, 143, 264–265, 266, 326, 409–410, 447
   children of, 326, 357–358, 377–378
Alcoholics Anonymous, ix, 11, 45, 53, 150, 274, 390, 403, 404, 405, 409, 416, 418, 421, 447
Alcoholics Anonymous: The Big Book (Alcoholics Anonymous), 26, 65, 150, 155, 398, 422, 454, 463

alcoholism, ix, xi, 33–34, 45, 53, 66–67, 80, 143, 266, 409–410
  relapses, ix, xi, 161
  relationship with food addiction, 148–155
  sobriety and, 219, 410, 447
  substance substitution, ix, x, 45, 150, 447
American Academy of Pediatrics, 115
American College Health Association
  Eating Disorders, 68
American Society of Addiction Medicine, 40–41, 48–49, 53
amino acids, 227
amphetamines, 10–11, 12–13, 14, 15, 17–18, 153
amygdala, 46
amylopectin A, 182
Anatomy of a Food Addiction (Katherine), 69–70, 71
Andersen, Arnold, 141
Anderson, Matthew
  "Eat to Kill," 299–300
Andrea's Eulogy, 446
anger, 124, 127, 135, 208–209, 267, 292, 314, 322, 333, 427, 439
Anorexia and Bulimia (Holtzman), 142
anorexia nervosa, x, 43, 56, 64–65, 76, 77, 78, 79–80, 81, 139, 141, 142, 186–187, 199
  overview, 82–89
anxiety, 68, 69, 273
appetite, 170–172, 179
Appetites (Knapp), 288
Appleton, Nancy, 173
  Lick the Sugar Habit, 55
argumentativeness, 421
arrogance, 200, 341
arteries, 168, 169
As a Person, I Have the Right to . . ., 350
ASAM. *See* American Society of Addiction Medicine
aspartame, 21, 23, 177–178
assertiveness, 136
attunement, 131
authenticity, 146, 449–450, 459

authoritarianism, 100
awareness, 454, 455, 460

bargaining, 209–210
beans, 232, 233
Beasley, Joseph D., 155
Beatrice's Eulogy, 446
beef, 229
behaviors, 34, 55, 67–69, 73–74, 315, 434
  manipulation and, 76, 111, 109–114, 132
  mirroring, 97, 101, 104, 131–132, 324–325, 362
  rewards for, 41, 113, 292–293
  See also under children; food addicts
belongingness, 95–101, 136, 315
beverages, 242–243, 254
Bhagavad Gita, 459
Big Book, The (Alcoholics Anonymous).
  See *Alcoholics Anonymous: The Big Book* (Alcoholics Anonymous)
Bill of Rights for Adult Children of Addicts/Dysfunctional Families, 380–381
bingeing, 20, 22–23, 37, 38, 43, 46, 48, 65–66, 67–68, 69, 70, 79, 186, 281, 288
"Biochemistry of Food Addiction" (Sheppard), 42
bipolar disorder, 224
Black, Claudia, 359
  It Will Never Happen to Me, 149
blame, 51, 294, 336, 360
  projection of, 198, 200, 298
blood sugar. *See* glucose
body image, 3, 68, 74–76, 139–141
Bonci, Leslie, 179
boundaries, 76, 98–99, 105, 110, 136, 317–319, 417
Bowlby, John, 97
Bradshaw, John, 105, 121–123, 312–313, 323, 455, 480n121, 480n122
  Healing the Shame That Binds You, 139, 278–279, 315, 317
  "Our Families, Ourselves," 146
  "Shame of Toxic Shame, The," 314

Braggs Liquid Aminos, 242, 249, 250, 255
brain, 40, 46, 154, 158–159, 176, 204,
    237, 291–292, 431
  amygdala, 46
  appetite and, 170, 173
  caffeine and, 183
  cerebral cortex, 46
  changes to, 35, 36, 36, 48, 49, 51, 52,
    55, 60, 65–66, 80, 154–155, 187, 431
  cravings and, 44, 237–238
  executive functioning of, 59
  hippocampus, 46, 165
  hypothalamus, 42, 46, 170, 171
  limbic system, 129, 347
  metabolic adaptation/tolerance and,
    65–66, 431
  nucleus accumbens, 36, 38, 46, 152
  reward circuit, xi, 4, 31, 36, 37, 40–41,
    47–48, 49, 52, 65–66, 150, 152, 221,
    291–292, 388
  rewiring of, 35, 52, 388–389, 396
  thalamus, 46
brain switch analogy, 47–48, 91
bran, 180, 181
BranCrisp Bread, 23
Brand, Russell, 286
bread, 159, 180–181, 254
breakfast, 26, 159, 222, 240, 244, 435,
    477n70
brunch, 239
Buber, Martin
  Way of Man, The, 459
Buddhism, 454
bulimia nervosa, x, 43, 56–57, 64, 66, 76,
    77–79, 81, 109, 141, 142, 292
  overview, 82–89
Butter Buds, 23
Bye, Bye Sugar Blues (JZ), 196

Cabrera, Dena
  Thin to Win, 79
CAC, 24
caffeine, 23, 43, 45, 46, 159, 179,
    183–185, 190, 242, 267, 282, 409
  withdrawal from, 184–185, 237
calcium, 232, 246

calories, 169, 173, 177, 179
Calvelli, Eugene, 8
candy, 46, 243
carbohydrates, x, 23, 65, 157, 163, 175,
    191, 192–193, 233–234
  complex, 163, 192–193
  processed, 193, 234
  refined, 38, 42, 43, 45, 46, 65, 149–150,
    158, 159, 167, 180, 187, 192–193,
    220, 234, 242, 254, 267, 477n70
  simple, 163, 192–193
  unprocessed, 192, 233–234
  unrefined, 192, 233–234
Carpenter, Karen, 64–65
Carter-Scott, Chérie
  "If Life Is a Game, These Are the Rules:
    Ten Rules for Being Human," 461
CASAC, 24
casein, 188
casomorphins, 188
CEA-HOW. See Compulsive Eaters
    Anonymous: Honesty, Open-
    Mindedness, Willingness
celebrations, 292–293
cereals, 23, 159, 187, 242, 254
cerebral cortex, 46
cheese, 188, 267
Cherokee Feast of Days, A (Hifler), 413
chewing, 189, 244
chewing gum. See gum
children
  abandonment of, 1, 104, 112, 127, 147,
    298, 315, 323, 325, 342, 343
  abuse of, 95, 99, 105, 107–109, 113,
    115–117, 130, 136, 140, 289, 294,
    323
  of addicts, 312, 357–360, 370–381
  attachment and, 95, 97–98, 99,
    129–130, 325, 333, 370, 480n123
  behaviors, 132–144, 267–268, 323,
    331
  birth order and, 370, 372, 375
  body image and, 74–75, 139, 141
  boundaries and, 98–99, 105, 110, 136,
    317–319
  as caretakers, 132, 136, 317, 325

characteristics, 92, 97–98, 118–128, 132–139, 337, 338, 465n46

control and, 130, 132, 140, 141–142, 318–319, 366

depression and, 124, 128

development of, 94–139, 291, 311, 323–325, 341–342

dieting and, 139, 141–142

experiences, 48, 49, 109–117, 125–139, 143

families/family systems and, 91–139, 296, 298, 310–332, 432, 444

feelings and needs of, 75–76, 77, 94–103, 105, 110, 111, 114–115, 118–124, 129–130, 132, 133–139, 291, 296, 298, 320–328, 238

hero role, 370–372, 377

holding and touching of, 95, 96, 115, 3 2 5

identification with parents, 100–101, 315

lost child role, 372, 374–375, 377

mascot role, 375–377

nurturing of, 95, 104, 290–291, 295, 328

parental approval and, 316

positive reinforcement of, 102, 316, 323

punishment/discipline of, 95, 100, 108, 112, 295, 323–325, 343

rebellion of, 331, 372

respect for, 105, 314, 319

rights of, 105

roles within families, 296, 319, 324–325, 327, 357, 358–381

routines and, 94, 325

safety/security of, 94–95, 97, 103, 104, 126–127, 327

scapegoat role, 372, 373, 377

separation-individuation of, 101, 328, 414, 442

setting guidelines and limits for, 99, 296–297, 318–319, 323

stress and, 114–115

suicides of, 64

trauma history of, 130–132

trust and, 98, 104, 106, 108, 109, 110,

118, 122, 126, 137, 325, 326, 328, 414

weight and, 335

See also adolescents; families and family systems; self

chips, 187

cholesterol, 166, 172–173

choline, 191

chromium, 223

cigarettes. *See* smoking

cockiness, 421

codependency, 121, 135, 299, 341, 344, 356, 358, 361–369, 378–380, 442

coffee. *See* caffeine

"Coin Principle of Food Addiction," 78–79

cold cuts, 229

Cole, Stephen, 459

Comes the Dawn (Rodriguez), 381–382

communication, 295–296, 304–306, 311, 317–318, 321, 331, 339–340, 345–346, 401, 425, 443

compassion, 387, 456

competition, 327

complacency, 419

compliance, 267–269, 271–281

compulsions, 69, 336, 367, 415, 425

Compulsive Eaters Anonymous: Honesty, Open-Mindedness, Willingness, 407, 411

condiments, 249, 250

control, 8, 66, 67–71, 76–77, 81, 127–128, 130, 140, 205–206, 279, 287, 295, 331, 336

Cooper, Rebecca, 286–287

cooperation, 327

corn, 46, 182–183, 267

cortisol, 161, 164–166, 183

cottage cheese, 188

cravings, x, 23, 33, 36, 42, 43, 44–45, 47–48, 55, 58, 60, 67, 69, 149–150, 175, 177, 182, 185, 191, 192, 220, 221, 223, 237–237, 282, 410, 476n56

Credentialed Alcoholism and Substance Abuse Counselor. *See* CASAC

Index

Credentialed Alcoholism Counselor. *See* CAC

criticism, 200, 345–346, 347

Crumpler, Ann
"Understanding Addictions," 42–43, 50–51, 310

D2 dopamine receptor, 35

Daily Affirmations (Lerner), 347

dairy products, 232

Dayton, Tian
"Denial: Is It Always Pathological?," 326
Emotional Sobriety, 129

Dearest Beloved Sugar (CG), 194

decision-making, 259–264

defense mechanisms, 197–215, 314

defiance, 269–270, 273, 275, 372, 447

De Mello, Anthony
Golden Eagle, The, 355

denial, xi–xii, 1, 34, 60–62, 63, 110, 144, 197–208, 214, 306, 307, 317, 336, 359, 363, 418, 419–420

"Denial: Is It Always Pathological?" (Dayton), 326

depression, 124, 128, 210–211, 282, 423, 437

deprivation, 125, 294, 424

desserts, 159, 180–181, 255

detoxification. *See* withdrawal

diabetes, 158, 168
Type 2, 168, 172

diary keeping. *See* journaling

diet. *See* nutrition

diet industry, xii, 207, 277

diet pills, 206, 478n84

diets, 3, 43, 54, 60, 74–75, 141–142, 206, 209, 278–281, 395, 409
children and, 139–142
restrictive, 46, 68, 69, 70, 163, 186–187
versus food plan, 271–281, 389

dining out, 242, 243

dinner, 240

disappointment, 125, 288

Disease Concept of Food Addiction (C. Starks and P. Starks), 62

diseases, xii, 52, 55, 63
primary, 54–55, 62

dishonesty, 318, 420–421

dissociation, 134, 289, 336

distractions, 286–287

diuretics, 90

diversion, 200

diverticula, 478n90

diverticulitis, 478n90

diverticulosis, 478n90

DMX, 144, 476n64

"Doctor's Opinion, The" (Silkworth), 33

Dodes, Lance
Heart of Addiction, The, 290

dopamine, xi, 31, 35–36, 37, 38, 39, 40, 45, 51, 173, 183, 221

drug addiction, ix, xi, 45, 53, 80, 143, 161, 175–176
relapses, ix, xi
relationship with food addiction, 149–155

dry drunk, 219–220
syndrome, ix, 389

Dufty, William
Sugar Blues, x

DuPont, Robert L., 31–32

dysthymia, 128

"Eat to Kill" (Anderson), 299–300

eating, 1–4, 34, 67–69, 70, 74–75, 103–104, 139–140, 170–172, 201–203, 283–295, 408
normal, 203–204, 212, 433, 452

eating disorders, x, 2–3, 42, 50, 435
versus food addiction, 77–81
See also food addiction

Eating Disorders (American College Health Association), 68

Eating Disorders Anonymous, 408, 410–411

Eckert, Elke, 154–155

EDA. *See* Eating Disorders Anonymous

eggs, 231

ego, 299

emetine, 90

emotional constriction, 133

emotional literacy, 121

Emotional Sobriety (Dayton), 129

emotions. *See* feelings

empathy, 95, 99

emptiness, 291, 294

endorphins, 37–38, 56, 187, 292

endosperm, 180, 181

energy drinks, 46, 190–192, 292

entitlement, 200

environments
chaotic, 312, 320, 325–326, 367
predictable, 325–326

epinephrine, 158

Equal. *See* aspartame

Erik Erikson, 480n122

euphoric recall, 34, 44, 45, 399–400, 423–424

executive functioning, 58, 59

exercise, 3, 141, 186, 221, 245, 401, 419, 452, 477n68

exorphins, 182

FA. *See* Food Addicts in Recovery Anonymous

FAA. *See* Food Addicts Anonymous

"Fabled Truths and Family Lies" (Kaplan), 323

Facing Codependence (Mellody), 314, 344, 347

Facing Love Addiction (Mellody), 343

Facts On: Food Addiction (Fiorentino and Regan), 58, 61–62, 153

Failing at Fairness (Sadker and Sadker), 140

failure to thrive, 96

families and family systems, 91–117, 292, 295, 310–332, 358–360, 431, 444
belongingness and, 95–101, 136, 315
changes to, 416–417
closed/censored/secret versus open, 317–318
competition within, 327
cooperation within, 327
dysfunctional, 105–139, 296, 298, 310–331, 338–339, 357–381, 432
focus within, 327, 328, 358–359, 379

forgiveness within, 322, 323
freedom within, 315
fun within, 315, 320, 368
functional/healthy, 314–328, 332
intergenerational effects, 75, 314, 319, 323, 338
love within, 95–101, 290–291, 315, 316, 317, 338–340
patriarchal, 105
predictability within, 325–326
resolution of issues, 225, 317–319, 322
responsibilities in, 106, 113, 132, 136, 317, 320, 327
roles within, 296, 319, 324–325, 327, 357, 358–381, 444
rules of, 121, 311, 318–319, 322, 329–332, 337, 346
time usage in, 319–320

fantasy, 134, 142, 315

fantasy bond, 315

fat cells, 169, 170–171

fatness, 74–76, 80, 169, 170
fear of, 77, 79–80, 141
See also obesity; weight: gain

fats, 43, 46, 157, 169, 170–171, 172, 187, 233, 234–235, 267
saturated, 234
trans, 234
unsaturated, 234

fault finding, 200, 341

"Fear of Abandonment" (Freundlich), 342–343

fears, 209, 290, 322, 434, 443, 447
of abandonment, 342–343
of fatness, 77, 79–80, 141

Federal Child Abuse Prevention and Treatment Act, 108

feelings, 75–76, 77, 93–103, 105, 110, 111, 114–115, 118–124, 129–130, 132, 133–139, 146–147, 225, 283–308, 320–328, 386, 399, 422, 425, 429, 438–439, 442, 443, 452
changing of, 307, 434
conversion of, 336
identification of, 300–303, 307, 364
language of, 295–308

Index

489

projection of, 198, 200, 294, 336
sharing, 345–346, 386, 398
spectrum of, 299
urges and, 44–45, 238, 400–401, 425,
 429–430
fiber, 192, 478n90
fight or flight response, 183–184
Fiorentino, Nancy
 Facts On: Food Addiction, 58, 61–62,
 153
Firestone, Robert, 315
fish, 230–231, 232
fish oil, 246
flour and flour products, 43, 46, 159,
 180–182, 240, 254, 266
food addiction, x, xi–xii, 1–4, 24, 27,
 43, 50–90, 143–144, 150–153, 186,
 207–215, 411, 412–413, 418, 425,
 431–432, 446–448
 abstinence, 26, 52, 62–63, 126, 131,
 144, 146–147, 154, 219–225, 238,
 262–263, 270, 271–281, 342, 387,
 389, 395, 400, 401, 403, 404, 405,
 408–409, 417, 424, 434–435, 438–
 439, 449–459, 476n56   biochemistry
 and, 25, 42–43, 48–49, 60–61, 77, 78,
 80, 187, 199, 403, 405
 chronicity of, 62–63
 consequences of, 35–36, 56–60, 63–64,
 76–77, 152, 201–203, 204–205, 206,
 261–264, 399–400
 definitions of, 35, 40–41, 53, 55–59,
 79
 development of, 91–117, 124, 125,
 139–140
 disease concept and, 34–48, 54, 60, 62,
 208–214, 387, 395, 401–402, 406,
 407, 411
 eating disorders versus, 77–81
 effect on family and others, 378–380,
 393
 gender and, 4, 141, 152, 477n68
 genetics and, 4, 47, 48, 91, 148
 grief process and, 207–214
 medical issues of, 56–57, 204, 431
 metabolism and, 65–66, 431

progression of, 65–67, 73–74, 79,
 139–144, 207, 453
questionnaire, 465–467
recovery, 3–4, 31, 63, 131, 144,
 146–147, 207–214, 219–225, 259,
 266, 274–275, 342, 385–411, 412,
 414–417, 418, 433–434, 449–452,
 456–459, 463–464
relapse cycle, 426–432
relapses, 36, 63, 144, 152, 214,
 265–266, 307, 394–402, 418–432,
 453
social factors and impacts, 51, 141, 149,
 267–270, 430–432
substance abuse and, 148–155, 205,
 406, 426
symptoms, 54, 58, 60, 411
therapy and treatment programs for, 32,
 54, 146, 161, 298, 401, 433–448, 452
time wasted during, 69, 71, 413
tolerance, 65–67
triggers, 32, 43, 45, 46, 47, 52, 73, 150,
 175–196, 221, 237, 240, 266–267,
 399, 400, 403, 405, 418, 476n56
12 Step programs and, 390–394, 422
withdrawal, 19, 36, 51, 72–73, 80,
 144, 154–155, 184–185, 222–225,
 237–238, 388
 See also anorexia nervosa; bulimia
 nervosa; eating disorders; overeating
"Food Addiction" (Leary and Meyer), 321
Food Addiction (Sheppard), 65–66, 68
Food Addiction 2000, 25
food addicts
 acceptance and, 264, 277–278
 asking for help, 206–207, 388, 391,
 443, 455
 behaviors, 34, 35, 41, 42–43, 55,
 56–59, 66, 67–69, 73–74, 78, 80–81,
 109, 130–131, 139–144, 146, 186–
 187, 197–214, 221, 225, 259–281,
 284–295, 310, 391–392, 399–400,
 414, 430–431, 434
 body image and, 3, 68, 74–76, 139–141
 changes and, 415–417, 423, 426, 430,
 449, 452

compliance and, 267–269, 271–281, 400

compulsion and, 69, 144, 415, 425, 431

control/loss of control and, 66, 67–71, 76–77, 140, 143–144, 205–206, 208, 274, 279, 295, 395, 400, 423

decision-making of, 259–264, 415–416

denial and, xi–xii, 1, 34, 60–62, 63, 110, 144, 197–208, 214, 306, 307, 418, 419–420

economic functioning and, 58

emotional functioning and, 58, 66, 68, 77, 132–139, 146, 422–423

families and family systems of, 91–117, 310–332, 378–380, 416–417, 431, 432, 444

feelings and, 75–76, 77, 94–103, 105, 110, 111, 114–115, 118–124, 129–130, 132, 133–139, 146–147, 225, 283–308, 386, 399, 414–415, 422, 425, 429, 431, 434, 438–439, 442, 452

journaling/diary keeping, 399

personality traits, 118–124, 264, 267–270, 273, 432

psychological functioning and, 31, 57, 76–77, 124, 264–267, 414

relationships and, 205, 225, 286, 288, 414, 453, 456

responsibility for recovery, 426, 451, 459

sabotage and, 414, 415, 417, 419–426

self-esteem and, 340–347, 427–429, 437

social situations and, 425, 430, 447

social skills of, 138, 432

stages of grief and, 207–214

surrender and, 211–214, 264, 265–266, 270, 274, 387, 391–292

Food Addicts Anonymous, 25, 403–404, 411

Food Addicts in Recovery Anonymous, 406–407

Food and Eating (Fox), 2

food funerals, 445–446

food industry, 203–204

food plan. *See* Realization Center food plan

foods, x–xii, 1, 75, 159–163, 175–196, 414

allowed in the plan, 248–249, 250–251

bingeing on, 37, 38, 43, 46, 48, 65–66, 67–68, 69, 70, 79, 142, 186, 281, 288

chewing of, 244

control of intake, 79, 104, 205–206, 287

cravings, x, 23, 33, 36, 42, 43, 44–45, 47–48, 55, 58, 60, 67, 69, 150, 175, 177, 182, 185, 191, 192, 220, 221, 223, 237–238, 282, 411, 476n56

crunchy, 46, 187–188

excluded from the plan, 23, 146, 159, 175–196, 240–242, 254–255, 266–267

memories of, 34, 44, 45, 399–400, 423–424

as metaphors/symbols, 294

obsession with, 51, 58, 60–61, 67–68, 69, 259, 282

portions/volume of, x, 38, 51, 185–186, 202–203, 239, 267, 420

preparation of, 231, 243

processed, 2, 23, 51, 159–160, 171, 186, 187, 189, 478n90

purging of, 38, 43, 46, 48, 56, 64, 66, 142, 206, 287, 292, 294, 322

restriction of, 46, 68, 69, 70, 186–187, 202–203, 267

satiety and, 41, 42, 172, 185

urges for, 44–45, 238, 400–401

use of, 76–77, 104, 109, 197, 284–295, 337–338, 360, 362, 432

weighing and measuring of, 239, 242, 387, 397, 409, 420

See also nutrition; Realization Center food plan; *and see also specific types*

forgiveness, 322, 323, 393

Forgiving Our Parents, Forgiving Ourselves (Stoop and Masteller), 310

formaldehyde, 177–178

Foster, John

I Am Not a Duck, 277–278

Fox, Robin

Food and Eating, 2

Index

Fredericks, Carlton, 24
  Low Blood Sugar and You, 24
Freud, Sigmund, 482n143
Freundlich, Lawrence S.
  "Fear of Abandonment," 342–343
friendships, 111, 113
fructose, 172–174, 177, 179, 191
fruits and fruit juices, 46, 159, 172, 188, 189, 243, 408–409
frustration, 421
  tolerance, 99, 135
fun, 315, 320, 368

GA. *See* Gamblers Anonymous
Gamblers Anonymous, 404
gastric bypass surgery, 152
gender, 4, 140, 141, 152, 477n68
generativity, 333, 480n122
genes, ix, 4, 38, 47, 48, 91, 148
germ (grain), 180, 181
ghrelin, 170–172
ginseng, 190
glucagen, 158, 240
glucose, 23, 24, 43, 58, 150, 163, 166, 168, 175, 182, 184, 191, 233, 476n56
  crash, 158–162, 167, 180, 184, 234, 254, 292
  low, 158–162, 163–166, 191 (*see also* hypoglycemia)
  metabolism, 157–166, 170, 180, 182
  stabilization of, 220, 238, 240
glycogen, 43, 158, 175
goals, 421, 422, 447
Gold, Mark, 35
Golden Eagle, The (De Mello), 355
Gorski, Terence, 418
grain, 43, 46, 159, 171–183, 187, 192, 233, 242
  anatomy of, 180–182
grandiosity, 107, 273, 275, 336, 341
gratification
  delayed, 99, 342–343, 344
  immediate, 343, 344, 414, 416
gratitude, 426
grazing, 70–71

GreySheeters Anonymous, 19, 408–409, 410
grief, 146–147, 293
  giving up carbohydrates and sugar and, 193–196
  stages of, 207–214
GSA. *See* GreySheeters Anonymous
guarana, 190
guilt, 127, 268, 313, 331, 333
gum, 19, 20, 23, 46, 189–190, 243, 409
Gupta, Sanjay, 37

HALT, 221, 399
Healing the Child Within (Whitfield), 298–299
Healing the Shame That Binds You (Bradshaw), 139, 278–279, 315, 317
health, 204–205
heart disease, 168, 169, 172, 232
Heart of Addiction, The (Dodes), 290
Heart Sense for Women (Sinatra), 180
Herman, C. Peter, 75
hero (role), 370–372, 377
HFCS. *See* high-fructose corn syrup
Hifler, Joyce Sequiche
  Cherokee Feast of Days, A, 413
high-fructose corn syrup, x, 172, 179, 183
Hill, Reuben, 100
hippocampus, 46, 165
hitting bottom, 391–392
Hoebel, Bart, 36, 150
Hoffman, Ronald
  Intelligent Medicine, 254
holidays, 292–293
Holtzman, Shaindy
  Anorexia and Bulimia, 142
honesty, 318, 387
honey, 177
hostility, 200
How to Set Effective Limits for Your Child (Markham), 99
Huizinga, Johan, 315
hull (grain), 180, 181
humility, 333
hunger, 60–61, 104, 170
hydrogenation, 234

hyperglycemia, 167
hypertension, 169
hyper-vigilance, 136
hypoglycemia, 65, 160, 163–166, 176
    See also glucose: low
hypothalamus, 42, 46, 170, 171

I Am Not a Duck (Foster), 277–278
I Am Your Disease . . . ., 402–403
I Feel the Feeling (Prather), 307–308
"I" messages, 304–306
idealization, 315
identification, 100–101
identity. *See* self
"If Life Is a Game, These Are the Rules:
    Ten Rules for Being Human" (Carter-
    Scott), 461
imperfections, 454–455
impulsivity, 135, 138, 344
individuality, 328, 459, 463
    defiant, 264, 273
individuation, 101, 328, 414, 442, 463
inflammation, 169
inositol, 190–191
insomnia, 165
insulin, 23, 43, 157–158, 160, 163,
    166–168, 169, 175–176, 177, 184
insulin resistance syndrome. *See* metabolic
    syndrome
insurance companies, 42
intellectualization, 200
Intelligent Medicine (Hoffman), 254
internalization, 334, 335
interpersonal bridge, 334
intuition, 125–126
Ipecac syrup, 90
isolation, 58, 103, 134, 138, 291, 386,
    388, 421–422
It Will Never Happen to Me (Black), 149

Johari's Window, 440–442
joking, 200
journaling, 399, 401
Judith C., 403, 410
Jung, Carl, 211
justification, 199–200

kamut, 182, 255
Kaplan, Debra L.
    "Fabled Truths and Family Lies," 323
Katherine, Anne
    Anatomy of a Food Addiction, 69–70,
    71
Kaufman, Gershen, 139
Kemp, Milton, 10, 12
Kingsley, Emily Perl
    Welcome to Holland, 215
Knapp, Caroline
    Appetites, 288
Kristof, Nicholas D.
    "Poverty Solution That Starts With a
    Hug, A," 114–115
Kübler-Ross, Elisabeth, 207
    On Death and Dying, 211–212
Kurtz, Ernest
    Spirituality of Imperfection, The, 454

Lane, James D., 190
language, 295–306
laxatives, 57, 90, 179, 189
Leary, Amy
    "Food Addiction," 321
leptin, 38, 170–172
Lerner, Rokelle
    Daily Affirmations, 347
Leshner, Alan, 40
"Letter to the Editor" (*Sun*), 59
Lewis, C.S., 459
L-glutamine, 223, 246
Lick the Sugar Habit (Appleton), 55
life span, 63–64, 169
limbic system, 46, 129, 347
liver, 172
loneliness, 287, 291
lost child (role), 327, 374–375, 377
love, 95–101, 136, 290–291, 315, 316,
    317, 333, 338–340, 480n123
Low Blood Sugar and You (Fredericks), 24
lunch, 240
Lustig, Robert, 170, 171, 173

MA. *See* metabolic adjustment
magical thinking, 400, 424–425

Index

Mahler, Margaret, 101
malnutrition, 282, 431
maltodextrin, 23
Margit, 20
marital conflicts, 110, 111
Markham, Laura
  How to Set Effective Limits for Your Child, 99
mascot (role), 375–377
Maslow, Abraham, 93, 102
  Theory of Human Motivation, A, 93
Maslow's Hierarchy of Needs, 93–103
Masteller, James
  Forgiving Our Parents, Forgiving Ourselves, 310
Mate, Gabor, 131
meals, 189, 239, 244, 397, 420
  plans, 242, 243
  skipping of, 239, 267, 282, 397, 420
  timing of, 240, 267, 420
MediResource, 184
meditation, 394, 401, 426
Mellody, Pia, 122, 300, 343
  Facing Codependence, 314, 344, 347
  Facing Love Addiction, 343
memories, 424
  implicit, 34–35, 44
  intrusive, 290
  reprogramming of, 35, 52, 399–400
mental avoidance, 200
mental illness, 42, 49, 224
Mercola, J., 170
metabolic adjustment, 240, 247, 250
metabolic syndrome, 166–168, 172
Meyer, Angie
  "Food Addiction," 321
Mickley, Diane, 435
Milk, Harvey, 65
Miller, Alice, 334, 337
minerals, 235
minimization, 198
mints, 46, 189–190, 243
moods, 53, 78, 157–162, 287, 291–292
moral inventory, 393, 399
morning sickness, 245
mother-child bond, 97–98, 124

muscles, 166–167
My Bill of Rights, 348
My Declaration of Self-Esteem (Satir), 354

NA. *See* Narcotics Anonymous
Narcotics Anonymous, 150
needs-shame bind, 336
negativity, 427–429
negotiating, 209–210
Nelson, Portia
  There's a Hole in My Sidewalk: The Romance of Self-Discovery, 462
neuropeptides, 170, 292
neurotransmitters, 40, 42, 183, 292
nicotine, 23, 150, 176
Noble, Ernest, 35
norepinephrine, 42
nucleus accumbens, 36, 38, 46, 152
numinous, 333, 481n124
nurturing, 95, 104, 290–291, 295, 328, 386
nutrition, x, xi, 154, 156–166, 171, 175–196, 203–204, 219–225, 477n70
nuts, 188, 267

OA. *See* Overeaters Anonymous
obesity, 52, 61–62, 166, 169, 172
  See also fatness; weight: gain
Obesity and Food Addiction Summit (2009), 48
obsessions, 51, 58, 60–61, 67–67, 69, 152, 259, 282
omnipotence, 426
On Death and Dying (Kübler-Ross), 211
openness, 317–318
opioids
  endogenous, 37–38, 187, 292
  receptors, 36, 182
other-esteem, 341–342
"Our Families, Ourselves" (Bradshaw), 146
Overeaters Anonymous, 19–21, 25, 398, 404–406, 410, 411
  Overeaters Anonymous: Tools of Recovery, 398
  "What's the Difference Between Dieting and Abstinence," 276–277

Overeaters Anonymous: Tools of Recovery (Overeaters Anonymous), 398
overeating, 38, 47–48, 69, 70, 171, 185–186, 202–203, 267, 282, 290, 291
   compulsive, 57, 60, 61–62, 65–66, 69, 78, 81, 141, 403, 404, 410, 425
   overview, 82–89
   See also bingeing; bulimia nervosa

Pamela's Eulogy, 445
pancreas, 157, 160, 166–167
parentification, 106, 113
parenting, 94–101, 103, 105–117, 137, 290–291, 296, 310–332
   attunement and, 131
   deficient, 106, 112
   dysfunctional, 105–139, 296, 338–339, 357–358
   inequitable, 109–110, 112
   styles of, 100
parents
   abusive, 107–109
   addicted, 106, 359, 360–361
   controlling, 106–107, 113, 329–331
   perfectionistic, 316, 319, 360
   role of, 324–325
passive-aggressiveness, 137
pasta, 255
Peck, M. Scott
   Road Less Traveled, The, 342
peer groups, 372, 443
peer pressure, 149
people pleasing, 135, 316, 341, 416, 439
perfectionism, 77, 133, 313, 316, 319, 331, 334, 422, 455
permissiveness, 100
phospholipids, 191
physical activity. *See* exercise
Physical Behavior and Obesity Research, 37
pizza, 159
pleasure, 34, 36, 37, 39, 40, 42, 45, 152, 157, 288, 292, 399–400
Podolnick, Dr., 9–10
Polivy, Janet, 75
polypeptides, 182

portions, x, 38, 51, 185–186, 202–203, 239, 420
Positive Affirmations, 350–352
positive regard, 316
post-traumatic stress reaction, 129
poultry, 230
"Poverty Solution That Starts With a Hug, A" (Kristof), 114–115
power, 76, 81, 107, 287, 295, 336, 341
power bars, 46
powerlessness, 48, 107, 108, 150–151, 212, 213, 274, 276, 357–358, 390, 455
Prager, Michael, 35
Prather, Hugh
   I Feel the Feeling, 307–308
prayers, 393–394, 401, 426
prediabetes, 167, 168
pregnancy, 245–246, 372
prime enablers, 361–369
Prin, John Howard
   "Reclaiming Your Destiny," 451
prolactin, 165
protein bars, 46
proteins, 157, 226–233, 240
   complete, 228–229
   incomplete, 228
Psychological Trauma (Van der Kolk), 133
psychotherapy. *See* therapy
punishment, 95, 100, 108, 112, 295, 323–325, 343
purging, 38, 43, 46, 48, 56, 64, 66, 142, 206, 267, 287, 292, 294, 322

Randolph, Theron G., 182
rationalization, 199, 421
Réa, Rashani
   Unbroken, The, 353
Realization Center, 24–25, 26, 433
   Early Recovery group, 443, 445
   Food Addiction Recovery Group, 444
   Food Addiction Treatment Program, 26, 155, 435, 440
   education series, 440, 442
Realization Center food plan, 43, 154, 161–162, 185, 187–188, 219, 220,

222, 225, 265–266, 279–281, 387,
397, 411, 420, 435, 440, 449, 452,
476n56
allowed foods, 248–249, 250–251
men's, 250–252
pregnancy and, 245–246
principles of, 239–246
versus diets, 271–281, 389
women's, 247–249
"Reclaiming Your Destiny" (Prin), 451
recovery, 3–4, 31, 63, 131, 144, 146–147,
207–214, 219–225, 259, 266, 274–
275, 342, 385–411, 412, 414–417,
418, 433–434, 449–452, 456–459,
463–464
reenactment, 311
Regan, Katie
Facts On: Food Addiction, 58, 61–62,
153
rejection, 96, 296
relapses, 45, 154, 161
alcoholism, ix, xi, 161
cycle of, 426–432
drug addiction, ix, xi
food addiction, x, 36, 63, 144, 152,
214, 265–266, 307, 394–402,
418–432, 453
smoking, ix
relationships, 111, 113, 205, 286, 288,
307, 365, 414, 453, 456
intimate, 328, 333, 341, 480n123
religion, 393
repression, 199, 336
respect, 105, 314, 319, 327
responsibility, 426, 451, 459
revenge, 292, 295
reverse tolerance, 67
reward circuit, xi, 4, 31, 36, 37, 40–41,
47–48, 49, 52, 65–66, 151, 152, 221
rice, 181, 232, 233
cakes, 23, 187
ricotta, 188
Risk Taking is Free, 352–353
Road Less Traveled, The (Peck), 342
Rodriguez, Veronica
Comes the Dawn, 381–382

Rogers, Carl, 316
roles (family), 296, 319, 324–325, 327,
357, 358–381
birth order and, 370, 372, 375
Rozanne, 404
rules
healthy, 332
shame-based, 121, 311, 318–319, 322,
329–332, 337–338, 346
Rutledge, Thom, 213

sabotage, 414, 415, 417, 419–426
Sadker, David
Failing at Fairness, 140
Sadker, Myra
Failing at Fairness, 140
sadness, 210–211
safety, 94–95, 97, 103, 104, 126–127,
289–290, 295, 322, 325, 360, 377
salt, 46, 187, 188, 267
satiety, 38, 41, 42, 172, 185
Satir, Virginia, 359
My Declaration of Self-Esteem, 354
scapegoat (role), 372–373, 377
Schatzman, Morton, 115
Soul Murder, 312
Schiavo, Terri, 64
schools, 334
Schwartz, Dianne, 5–27, 456
abstinence, 23, 26, 176, 260
amphetamine addiction, 10–11, 12–13,
14, 15, 17–18, 153
asking for help, 20, 22–23
bingeing of, 20, 22–23
brother (Peter), 5, 6, 13, 16, 21
career, 14, 24–25
CASAC accreditation, 24
codependency, 15
education, 8, 12, 13–15, 16, 24–25
family dynamics, 6–7, 8, 9, 15, 16, 318
father, 5, 7, 12, 13, 18, 22, 368
food addiction of, 8, 10, 18–19, 20,
22–23, 24–26
mother, 5, 12, 13, 15–16, 17
mother's alcoholism and suicide
attempts, 5, 6–7, 11–12, 15, 16–17

psychiatric treatment of, 9–10
recovery, 18–23, 25–26, 260
relapses, 22, 23
relationships, 18, 22
rheumatic fever misdiagnosis, 8–10
smoking, 13, 21, 23, 260
Spain and Spanish, 13–14, 17–18
support systems and, 19–23, 32, 38,
 212
secrecy, 106, 108, 113, 132, 317–318,
 336, 441–443
security. *See* safety
self, 49, 75, 76–77, 101, 104, 108–109,
 115, 124, 127, 130–132, 136,
 146–147, 296, 297–300, 311, 315,
 316, 327, 328, 331, 333, 340–346,
 364–365, 426, 427–429, 434, 436,
 449–451, 455, 480n121, 480n123
 codependency and, 121, 135, 299, 341,
  344, 356, 358, 442
 identification and, 100–101, 315, 335
 internalization and, 335, 427–429
 knowledge of, 440–442
self-actualization, 93, 102–103, 104, 328
self-blame, 294
self-care, 131–132, 331, 342–343, 346,
 414, 419, 423
self-criticism, 345–346, 347
self-doubt, 427–429
self-esteem, 100, 101–102, 128, 131, 135,
 138, 268, 311, 338, 340–347, 437
self-identity. *See* self
self-love, 432
self-pity, 423, 459
self-punishment, 134, 292, 295
seltzers, 185, 243
separation-individuation, 101, 442, 463
serenity, 212, 275, 456
serotonin, 42, 191
Sex and Love Addicts Anonymous, 55
shame, 31, 43, 51, 81, 105, 108, 122, 128,
 139, 268, 279, 290, 310, 312–313,
 323–325, 331, 333–336, 347, 427,
 428–429
 carried, 122
 healthy/natural, 312–313, 333, 455

toxic, 122, 313, 317, 319, 323, 334,
 455, 480n122
shame-bound, 336
"Shame of Toxic Shame, The" (Bradshaw),
 313
shaming, 51, 105, 115–117, 133, 135,
 139, 296, 316, 323–325
share shame, 346
Sheppard, Kay, 224
 "Biochemistry of Food Addiction," 42
 Food Addiction, 65–66, 68
shopping, 242
Silkworth, William D., 409–410
 "Doctor's Opinion, The" 33
Sinatra, Stephen
 Heart Sense for Women, 180
sleep, 47–48, 69, 165, 171–172, 290, 419
Smith, Anna Nicole, 64
Smith, Bob, 33
Smokenders, 21, 260
smoking, ix, 13, 21, 23, 151, 176, 183
snacks, 187–188
sobriety, 219, 410, 447
social pressure, 267
social skills, 138, 432
sodas, 159, 172, 185
 diet, 19, 21, 23, 179, 409
sorbitol, 179, 189
Soul Murder (Schatzman), 312
soy products, 232–233
soy sauce, 242, 249, 250, 255
spelt, 182, 255
Spencer, Frances
 Understanding Children, 327
spirituality and spiritual practices, 205,
 393, 426, 454–456
Spirituality of Imperfection, The (Kurtz),
 454
Splenda. *See* sucralose
sponsors, 220, 243, 387, 395, 396–397,
 400, 422, 452
starches, 159, 172
starchy center (grain), 180, 181
Starks, Charles
 Disease Concept of Food Addiction, 62
Starks, Peggy

Disease Concept of Food Addiction, 62
starvation, 46, 60–61, 79, 142, 163,
  186–187, 267, 282, 288, 292
Statement of Personal Rights—Boundaries,
  348–349
Stice, Eric, 37
stigmatization, 335
Stoop, David
  *Forgiving Our Parents, Forgiving
    Ourselves*, 310
stress, 45, 49, 95, 97, 99, 129–130,
  189–190, 267
  management, 419
  styles, 98
  theory, 97
  toxic, 114–115
strokes, 168
submission, 264
substance abuse. *See* addictions
sucralose, 178
sucrose, 172–174
sugar, x, 19, 23, 24, 36–37, 39, 43, 45,
  46, 63, 151–152, 150–152, 156–157,
  159–160, 163, 171, 172–174, 176,
  177, 183, 188, 191, 194–196, 240,
  241–242, 266, 477n70
  names of, 252–23
Sugar, Sam, 51
Sugar Blues (Dufty), x
Sugar Dearest (BN), 195
sugar substitutes. *See* sweeteners, artificial
suicide, 64
Sun (newspaper)
  "Letter to the Editor," 59
superiority, 200
support systems, 19–23, 305, 388, 415
  See also 12 Step food recovery
    fellowships
surrender, 211–214, 264, 265–266, 270,
  274, 387, 391–392
sweeteners, artificial, 21, 23, 36, 39, 43,
  46, 177–179, 189, 191, 241, 282, 409
  names of, 253
12 Step food recovery fellowships, 32,
  38, 146, 150, 208, 212, 213, 219,
  220–221, 225, 306, 287, 388–390,

392, 394–396, 401, 403–411, 422,
  437, 440, 447, 449, 452
behaviors evidencing defiance to,
  269–270, 422, 447
number of meetings to attend, 395–396,
  422
obligation to/service to, 395, 398
participating in, 398
reading literature of, 398, 422
sponsors and, 220, 243, 387, 395,
  396–397, 400, 422, 452
telephoning others in, 396, 400, 401,
  422, 443
12 Step programs, 274, 298, 385, 387,
  390–394, 410, 436, 440, 453
share shame felt in, 346
sharing within, 345–346, 398
Step 1 (admission), 151, 274, 390–392
Steps 2-3 (discover a higher power),
  392–393
Steps 4-9 (cleaning house), 393, 399,
  422, 440
Steps 10-11 (journey continues),
  393–394
Step 12 (spiritual awakening), 394
syndrome X. *See* metabolic syndrome

tamari, 242, 249, 250, 255
tantrums, 296–297
taurine, 190
tea, 245
teenagers. *See* adolescents
tempeh, 233
temporomandibular joint disorder, 189
terminal uniqueness, 368
thalamus, 46
Theory of Human Motivation, A
  (Maslow), 93
therapy, 32, 54, 146, 161, 298, 401,
  433–448, 452
  goals of, 436–438, 447
  group, 442, 443–445
Thin to Win (Cabrera), 79
thinness, 74–76, 79–80, 141
  See also weight: loss

Tiebout, Harry, 264–265, 266, 273–275, 391

time, 69, 71

TMJ. *See* temporomandibular joint disorder

tofu, 232–233

transference, 444, 482n143

trauma, 129, 130–132, 290, 335

Travis (chimpanzee), 65

Treatment4Addiction, 358

triggers, 32, 43, 45, 46, 47, 52, 73, 149, 175–196, 221, 237, 240, 266–267, 399, 400, 403, 405, 418, 476n56

triglycerides, 158, 166

trust, 98, 104, 106, 108, 109, 110, 118, 122, 126, 137, 325, 326, 328, 360, 414

Turgay, Atilla, 128

Twelve Steps and Twelve Traditions (Alcoholics Anonymous), 390, 398

"twinkie" defense, 65

Unbroken, The (Réa), 353

"Understanding Addictions" (Crumpler), 42–43, 50–51, 310

Understanding Children (Spencer), 327

urges, 44–45, 238, 400–401, 425, 429–430

Van der Kolk, Bessel
Psychological Trauma, 133

vegetables, 228, 232

Vegit, 23

Velveteen Rabbit, The (Williams), 450

victimization, 335

victims and victimhood, 107, 114–115, 129, 136, 294, 298, 423

vitamin B-complex, 246

vitamin C, 246

vitamin D, 246

vitamin E, 246

vitamins, multi-, 235, 245, 246

volume (food). *See* portions

water, 235–236, 242–243

Way of Man, The (Buber), 459

Wegscheider-Cruse, Sharon, 359, 364, 481n134

weight, 52, 61–62, 68, 74–76, 149, 166, 169, 244–245, 276, 395, 405, 410
discrimination and, 335
gain, 54, 60 141, 150, 151, 281–282
loss, x–xi, 43, 56, 90, 207, 239, 241, 271, 279–281, 395
society and, 139–140, 141, 169, 335
tracking of, 221, 244–245, 400

weight cycling, 281–282

Welcome to Holland (Kingsley), 215

"What's the Difference Between Dieting and Abstinence" (Overeaters Anonymous), 276–277

wheat, 46, 175, 182, 240, 267
names of, 255–256

White, Marilyn J., 24, 25, 60, 174, 259, 386

Whitfield, Charles
Healing the Child Within, 298–299

Who Is the Enemy?, 356

Wilbur, Cornelia, 9

Williams, Margery
Velveteen Rabbit, The, 450

willpower, xii, 31, 44, 50–51, 69, 151, 208, 408

Wilson, Bill, 33, 392

Winehouse, Amy, 286

Winnicott, D.W., 131

withdrawal, 19, 36, 51, 72–73, 144, 154–155, 184–185, 222–225, 237–238

Woititz, Janet Geringer
Adult Children of Alcoholics, 377–378

xylitol, 189

"you" messages, 304

Zen Story, A, 460

About Realization Center

Realization Center is a unique, comprehensive, full-service outpatient addictions treatment program located in the Union Square area of Manhattan and in the Brooklyn Heights section of Brooklyn. It is licensed by the New York State Office of Alcoholism and Substance Abuse Services. Realization Center offers specialized treatment for men's, women's, and adolescent's alcoholism, substance abuse issues, food addiction/eating disorders, co-dependency, gambling, and sexual compulsivity, as well as numerous mental health issues such as depression, anxiety, post-traumatic stress, sexual trauma, "family of origin" issues, domestic violence, anger and stress management, school or job difficulties, family conflict, parenting difficulties, and relationship problems as they relate to substance abuse.

From its early founding, Realization Center strove to serve both the under-served (e.g., chronic relapsers, adolescents, LGBTQ community, HIV-positive patients, and those who are dually diagnosed) and the mis-served and under-served addicted population at large. Realization Center became a pioneer in providing the most effective holistic care for people in trouble, with substances, with relationships, with themselves. In a respectful and dignified non-institutional setting, a personal course of treatment is developed jointly by the dedicated clinical staff and the client. The Center offers flexible hours, a 24-hour hotline, crisis intervention, over 90 groups per week, in each location, individual counseling, and programs for family and loved ones. In an intimate and safe environment, with the help of caring professionals, clients with addiction problems are empowered to take charge of their behavior and their lives.

The goal of treatment at Realization Center is freedom from addictions or emotional issues and the discovery of the ability to lead a fulfilling, peaceful life. A multidisciplinary team of professionals, including credentialed alcohol and substance abuse counselors, licensed social workers and mental health counselors, psychiatrists, and food addiction counseling specialists ensure quality care in a safe, supportive environment.

A 12-Step philosophy is an integral part of the clinical program, while group therapy, individual counseling, psycho-education, and family involvement constitute the psychodynamic core of the Center's treatment approach.

The Center is the only outpatient treatment center that treats eating problems as addiction. It features a unique food addiction program where food addiction is treated as a biochemical illness with emotional underpinnings, which help a person regain dignity and freedom. Men, women, and adolescents in the program learn that weight is not the issue, but rather the symptom of their disease. As the disease of food addiction is treated, weight begins to normalize, and energy, mood, and life begin to optimize.

Most clients at the Center, regardless of whether they came into treatment for their alcohol and/or drug problems, are required to attend the series on which this book is based to address the underlying food addiction that plagues most addicts. This focus added the missing piece to our holistic approach to addiction treatment.

About the Author

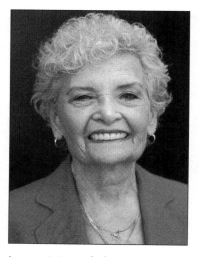

Dianne Schwartz is the co-owner and co-builder of Realization Center, the oldest and largest licensed outpatient addictions treatment program in Manhattan and Brooklyn. She is credentialed as an alcoholism/substance abuse counselor, but because of her recovery from the suffering that comes with food addiction, her interest and passion is food addiction recovery. She developed the Food Addiction Treatment Program at Realization Center in 1993, and as part of the program, she has been offering a 16-week lecture series for all clients on the relationship between their eating behavior and their alcoholism and/or drug addiction, how their eating affects their sobriety and potential for relapse, and how it all began.

Over time, as the reputation of the Food Addiction Treatment Program grew, people with eating problems who did not abuse alcohol or drugs entered the program. Her book *The Big Book of True Recovery from Food Addiction* is an outgrowth of the lecture series. She has lectured at Fordham University's Annual Addiction Institute in a workshop "Broccoli Is Not the Problem: The Real Culprits in Food Addiction." She has presented at master's social work classes at NYU and Fordham University. Her article, "Food Addiction: Chemical Dependency's Twin," was published in *Behavioral Health News* in the Winter 2014 issue.

Made in the USA
Middletown, DE
11 January 2025

68109025R00287